The
Economics
of Mental
Retardation

The Economics of Mental Retardation

Ronald W. Conley

The Johns Hopkins University Press
Baltimore and London

The Johns Hopkins University Press, Baltimore, Maryland 21218
The Johns Hopkins University Press Ltd., London

Library of Congress Catalog Card Number 72-12345
ISBN 0-8018-1410-3

Originally published, 1973
Second printing, 1974

Library of Congress Cataloging in Publication data will be found on the last printed page of this book.

Contents

TABLES

Preface

During the last year prior to publication, several people joked that this manuscript was the most quoted nonpublication in the field of mental retardation. Had I followed my natural inclinations, it might have remained in this status considerably longer than it did. Not that I lacked any desire to see the manuscript in print. Quite the contrary. But during the course of this study, as I thought through issues and evaluated the data, many new research avenues came to light. Some I ventured into, which caused the scope of the manuscript to be considerably larger than originally anticipated and, of course, delayed its completion. For the most part, however, I regretfully, but prudently, refrained from initiating new paths in my work.

Because a member of my family was retarded, early in life I became aware of the problems associated with mental retardation. I admit to a deep-rooted desire to see programs for the retarded greatly expanded, and a conviction that given adequate assistance the great majority of retardates can work and be integrated into society. The fact that many have not done so reflects, I believe, an intolerable and unconscionable indifference and misunderstanding by society. I trust that in the succeeding pages I have separated my personal feelings from my scientific inquiries.

Early in the writing of this manuscript I had to delineate the audience that I was trying to address—economists, professionals associated with mental retardation, the politicians and civil servants who make program decisions, or concerned citizens. The answer was painfully obvious—all four of these groups. After pondering the issue for a while, I decided to write a book that would be intelligible to a college-level audience that had little background in either mental retardation or economics. At the same time, I decided not to hesitate to discuss the most controversial issues in either mental retardation or the economics thereof. In this way I hoped to reach all four of the above-mentioned groups, maintain professional rigor, and strike out into new ground. I doubt that many readers will classify this book as bedtime reading.

The book took longer to write than I or my employers had antici-pated. In part, this was because I covered more topics than I had originally planned. Despite my early involvement in this field, I was astonished to find how incredibly complex and many-faceted is this problem we so simply sweep under the term "mental retardation."

Equally astonishing was the lack of basic data on many important programs that serve the retarded, or of the numbers and characteristics of retardates, or on how well retardates fare in the community. In consequence, the reader will find data spliced together from unlikely sources and in unlikely ways, justified only by the sobering fact that no other data were available.

Even my economics background did not suffice. Neither the eco-nomic theory dealing with health nor with manpower was sufficient for an economic analysis of mental retardation. Instead of trying to eval-uate a specific program (such as vocational rehabilitation), or a specific condition (such as cancer), I was confronted with the task of evaluating a subdivision of the population, within which were people with widely varying abilities and potential, each the utilizer of many services, and with different groups of retardates using quite dissimilar services.

I have resisted occasional efforts to define my work as a narrow comparison of benefits and costs—a task for which economists appear to be noted. I have explored the extent and demographic characteristics of mental retardation, the causes of retardation, the characteristics of programs providing services to the retarded, and the employment and earnings of the retarded. Benefit-cost ratios cannot, after all, be cal-culated without this type of information. Usually, however, I went beyond the narrow needs of benefit-cost analysis. In and of themselves, these areas of exploration are of value and interest.

In the last chapter, I discuss ways to improve services to the retarded, primarily adult retardates. At this point in time, at least one of the programs that is strongly and unequivocally supported—community care for the retarded in group homes or in other forms of community residence—appears to be on the verge of an explosion in the United States. When I began this manuscript, one could count on his fingers the number of such facilities. Now the states are eagerly seeking methods of providing alternatives to institutional care. This movement appears to be gaining momentum concurrently with growing public revulsion at the intolerable standards of care existing in most public institutions.

A word of warning. There is much to learn before we depopulate our institutions. Ill-conceived, hasty efforts to do so may be self-defeating. Problems of continuity of care, fire regulations, transportation, and so on must be solved.

Eventually, we may close down large residential institutions for the retarded. However, recognizing that an institutional population of substantial size will probably be with us for some time to come, concurrently with the development of community facilities, we must improve the quality of care of retardates remaining in institutions.

In the last chapter I also suggest the development of sheltered work in regular employment settings. Unfortunately, a public program to systematically pursue this goal is not yet in sight.

In the development of this manuscript I am greatly indebted to more people than I can name. I initially began work on this manuscript while I was with the President's Committee on Mental Retardation. At that time, David Ray was executive director, and Robert Aldrich was vice chairman of the committee. Allen Menefee was executive secretary. Subsequently, Fred Krause became acting executive director. The manuscript was completed after I moved to the Rehabilitation Services Administration to work for Edward Newman, commissioner, and John Noble, special assistant for research, demonstrations, and evaluation. Without the assistance and patience of each of these persons this manuscript could not have been completed.

Victor Fuchs and Michael Grossman, of the National Bureau of Economic Research, and Paul Imre reviewed and commented on the manuscript. Their suggestions greatly improved the work, but there remain differences of opinion. We wouldn't be researchers if there were not.

Other persons served as research assistants, typists, critics, and in other ways rendered invaluable assistance.

My thanks to all.

The
Economics
of Mental
Retardation

I

Introduction

MENTAL RETARDATION

Mental retardation refers to a condition of inadequately developed intelligence which significantly impairs a person's ability to learn and adapt to the demands of society. Its effects may be devastating. Many retarded persons suffer a greatly diminished capacity to perform effectively as students, workers, or homemakers. Some are reduced to dependency upon others for the provision of the most basic daily needs. Retarded children are frequently a source of anguish and despair to parents who are disappointed in their failure to produce talented offspring and distraught about their children's futures. It must be quickly stressed that the severity of the effects of mental retardation range from the very mild to the very severe and depend not only upon the degree of mental deficit but also upon such factors as physical handicaps, motivation, and the services that are available to assist the retarded.

Two other aspects of mental retardation should be mentioned. The first is its long-term character. Almost all mental subnormality originates during birth or childhood and persists throughout the person's lifetime. The second is its high prevalence. There are about 5½ million mentally retarded Americans.

Mental retardation is clearly a national problem of massive proportions. Moreover, it is a problem that should be of great concern to all Americans for several reasons. To begin with, there is the humanitarian

1

judgment that unnecessary suffering should be eliminated and that all persons should have the opportunity to fully develop their productive and social abilities, no matter how limited. In addition, the effects of mental retardation are, to a greater or lesser extent, borne by all. For example, mental retardation increases the tax burden on the average taxpayer because of the frequent need for publicly provided maintenance and treatment and the reduced tax receipts resulting from lower earnings. Finally, mental retardation may occur in any family, regardless of its social strata, intellectual level, religious affiliation, race, or other distinguishing characteristics. Those fortunate families who have had normal children have no assurance that a future child or grandchild (or other close relative) will not be retarded. There are few families who would not want their retarded child to be given every opportunity to develop his economic and social potential.

It is important to observe that almost all professionals in the field of mental retardation believe that many cases of mental retardation could be prevented and that many of the mentally retarded are capable of achieving far more than they do.

ECONOMICS

Economics is founded on the observations that there are insufficient resources to satisfy everybody's wants and that there must be ways to determine which wants and whose wants will be satisfied. Economics is, therefore, usually, and most correctly, defined as the study of the allocation of scarce resources among competing uses.

It is customary to distinguish between "descriptive" economics and "normative" economics. In "descriptive" economics we ask why resources are allocated as they are and what effect this has on society (e.g., what causes unemployment among the mentally retarded?). In "normative" economics we ask how resources must be allocated in order to achieve specified goals (e.g., how may unemployment among the mentally retarded be reduced?).

"Descriptive" economics and "normative" economics are complementary, not competing (or even distinct) branches of economic inquiry. Before solutions to a problem can be sought, it must first be ascertained that a problem exists, and why. Most of this study is descriptive. It is not until the final chapter that we begin to define goals and suggest ways of achieving them.

The question of allocating resources arises only in the case of *scarce* resources—i.e., those whose use involves a cost. However, examples of nonscarce (free) resources are virtually nonexistent. Many people believe that even the air around us should be cleansed before being inhaled.

Scarce resources are classified as land, labor, and capital. The productivity of a resource depends not only upon its quantity, but also its location, the quantity and quality of other resources that are combined with it, and the many factors which determine its quality. The output of workers, for example, depends upon their health, acquired skills, attitudes, and level of intellectual functioning. The distinction between the quality and quantity of resources is crucial, since most of the goals of society can be achieved only by improving the quality of the available resources.

What are these goals? The wants (goals) which people seek to satisfy must be viewed broadly. From an individual standpoint they include food, shelter, clothing, recreation, physical and mental health, dignity, security, achievement, independence, contentment, and personal liberty; in short, anything that increases enjoyment of life.

Our national goals are, in large part, a reflection of individual wants. Usually we distinguish five goals which are generally accepted by most citizens at any time and of any country. They are: (1) to maximize output which, for reasons to be explained below, should be defined broadly to include the value of homemaking services and other unpaid work and activities that contribute to well-being (this goal requires full employment of the available labor force and the use of the most efficient techniques of production); (2) to maintain reasonably stable prices; (3) to achieve an equitable distribution of income and wealth consistent with ethical judgments as to individual need and merit; (4) to increase per capita output each year at some desired rate; and (5) to preserve individual freedoms of thought, expression, and action, insofar as these are consistent with the rights and welfare of others. These five goals may be summarized by observing that society seeks a high and increasing level of well-being for its citizens.

The role of the economist in the health and rehabilitation field has often been questioned by other professionals, who stress the fact that many of the qualities that make life worthwhile cannot be valued in monetary terms. These apprehensions are based on a misunderstanding of the nature of economics. Economists are, or at least should be, as fully cognizant and appreciative of esthetic, intangible, and humanitarian values as are other professionals. It is the contribution to human welfare, not measured output, that is relevant when deciding how resources should be allocated.

Most economists agree that the ultimate goal of economic inquiry is to ascertain the most efficient allocation of resources. Nevertheless, economists rarely report unambiguous conclusions and often disagree vigorously among themselves as to the most appropriate use of available resources.

In part, these disagreements arise because economists are usually uncertain of the magnitude of the effects of a policy decision. Also, since economists must frequently work with fragmentary and sometimes misleading data, it is not at all surprising that they often differ in their interpretations of these data and that their conclusions are usually tentative.

Another source of disagreement stems from the fact that the goals of society often conflict with one another. High levels of employment may not be consistent with stable prices. Progressive taxation and income maintenance may be inconsistent with high levels of work effort. In short, in a normally functioning economy the increased attainment of any one social goal usually requires some partial sacrifice of other worthwhile goals. Economists disagree among themselves as to the relative importance of various goals as often and as vehemently as any other group of citizens. Finally, there are many unresolved conceptual issues in evaluating the use of resources, especially when these resources are invested in people.

It follows that decisionmaking as to the proper use of resources ultimately becomes a philosophical issue that is further obscured by many uncertainties as to the effects of a given use of resources. Since economists are no more qualified than others to make philosophical judgments, what is their role in decisionmaking?

Economic analyses aid decisionmaking by reducing uncertainty as to the effects of alternative uses of resources. These analyses develop a framework for evaluating the benefits and costs of various programs and then fit available information within this framework. The identification and manipulation of benefit and cost variables is a task for which economists are uniquely qualified. These analyses not only aid decisionmakers in selecting among alternative ways of achieving given goals, but may, in fact, influence the selection of goals. Economic analyses should not be disparaged because they do not always yield clear cut answers. *If* their limitations are understood, they can be of major value to decisionmakers.

How does mental retardation fit into this economic framework? For one thing, the mentally retarded are a significant part of our labor resources. Most can be trained to produce the goods and services that satisfy many of society's wants. In some cases mental retardation may be prevented, thus maintaining the quality of our labor resources. Moreover, the retarded are people to whom a reasonable share of our national output should be allocated. Their roles as producers and consumers are related, since their earnings provide the means to supply most of their consumption needs. In the last chapter we will conclude that the productive capabilities of many retardates are not being fully utilized and that a considerable number have an unacceptable and sometimes miserably low standard of living.

II

The Epidemiology of Mental Retardation

DEFINITION

Several difficult and controversial issues must be considered before defining mental retardation. Perhaps the least important of these is terminology. Many terms have been used as synonyms for "mental retardation." Such an abundance of terminology would be of little consequence if there were general agreement as to the precise meanings of the different terms. Unfortunately, there is not.

To illustrate, the terms "mental retardation" and "mental deficiency" are frequently used interchangeably by modern authors. But the term "mental deficiency" has also been used to describe the inadequate *social* functioning resulting from "mental retardation."[1] More often, the two terms are distinguished by using the term "mental retardation" to "refer only to those whose educational and social performance is markedly lower than would be expected from what is known of their intellectual abilities,"[2] and by reserving the term "mental deficiency" for those conditions "of mental arrest resulting in a social inadequacy which is not amenable to fundamental improvement through education and experience and any known treatment."[3] Others

[1] T. L. McCulloch, "Reformulation of the Problem of Mental Deficiency," *American Journal of Mental Deficiency* (October 1949): 130–36.

[2] World Health Organization, *The Mentally Subnormal Child*, Technical Report Series, 1954, pp. 6–7.

[3] Thorlief G. Hegge, "Psychological Aspects of Mental Retardation," in *Vocational Rehabilitation of the Mentally Retarded*, Salvatore G. Dimichael, ed. (Washington: USGPO, 1950), p. 21.

have further restricted the term "mental deficiency" to include only those cases "with demonstrable neurological damage or pathology."[4] When a distinction is made between "mental retardation" and "mental deficiency," the term "mental subnormality" is sometimes used as a general term to cover both cases.[5]

For purposes of this study, the terms "mental retardation," "mental deficiency," and "mental subnormality" will be used synonymously. These are the most important terms in modern use. Other terms will be utilized only when citing from the work of others. Our equating of these terms is motivated by the facts that: (1) it is a practice followed by many professionals in the field; and (2) the leading citizen's organization concerned with mental retardation is the National Association for Retarded Children and the leading professional organization is the American Association on Mental Deficiency. It hardly seems appropriate to use a definition of terms that would erroneously imply that these organizations are concerned with different problems.

The most generally accepted definition of mental retardation was prepared by Rick Heber for the American Association on Mental Deficiency.[6] The three crucial elements of this definition are: (1) subaverage intellectual functioning (2) which originates before adulthood and (3) which causes social incompetence.

No authority would dispute the necessity for the criterion of subaverage intellectual functioning. The purpose of the second stipulation is to distinguish mental retardation from mental deterioration caused by mental illness. Although one may question whether adults who become intellectually impaired after extensive brain damage shouldn't also be considered retarded, the issue is of minor significance.

The criterion of social competence is more controversial. Many authorities believe that a deficit in intelligence must be associated with impairment in adaptive behavior before a diagnosis of mental retardation can be made. Among school-age children adaptive behavior is measured by ability to learn, and among adults it is measured by social adjustment, i.e., "the degree to which the individual is able to maintain himself independently in the community and in gainful employment as

[4] William I. Gardner and Herschel W. Nisonger, *A Manual on Program Development in Mental Retardation, Supplement: American Journal of Mental Deficiency* (January 1962): 16.

[5] Seymour B. Sarason, "Mental Subnormality," in *The Theory and Practice of Psychiatry*, Frederick C. Redlich and Daniel X. Freedman, eds. (New York: Basic Books, Inc., 1966), p. 654. Also, World Health Organization, *Mentally Subnormal Child*, p. 7.

[6] Rick Heber, "A Manual on Terminology and Classification in Mental Retardation," *American Journal of Mental Deficiency*, Monograph Supplement, 64 (1954), no. 2, p. 3.

well as by his ability to meet and conform to other personal and social responsibilities and standards set by the community."[7]

At least three reasons have been advanced in defense of the criterion of social competence:

1) The criterion of social competence reduces the importance of determining how mentally subnormal a person must be before he is diagnosed as mentally retarded. The problem, as noted long ago by Terman, is that "Since the frequency of the various grades of intelligence decreases gradually and at no point abruptly on each side of the median, it is evident that there is no definite dividing line between normality and feeble-mindedness. . . . The number of mentally defective individuals in the population will depend upon the standard arbitrarily set up as to what constitutes mental deficiency."[8] The importance of choice of a standard becomes manifest when we observe that there are twice as many people with IQs below 75 as there are people with IQs below 70. Although the criterion of social competence does not eliminate the necessity for selecting a cut-off point, it ensures that only those persons whose deficient mental functioning actually results in social incompetence will be labeled as retarded.

2) Many authorities distrust the results of IQ tests. These tests are subject to substantial errors of measurement, depending on the person doing the testing, the physical conditions surrounding the test, and the attitudes and physical alertness of the person being tested. In addition, it is believed that the best-known IQ tests misrepresent the abilities of nonwhites, the poor, and persons with physical and mental handicaps. Finally, intelligence tests are imperfect measures of "intelligence"—an abstraction that lacks a generally agreed upon definition, and all of whose components are not equally accessible to testing. The criterion of social competence serves to, in effect, validate a measure of intellectual subnormality.

3) Many authorities believe that, regardless of degree of intellectual subnormality, a person should not be labeled as mentally retarded if he is able to conduct himself satisfactorily in the community. The label causes derogatory connotations and may become a self-fulfilling prophecy as the retarded and their instructors, relatives, and other associates gauge their expectations to the level expected of a retarded person.

Although these arguments appear compelling, there are, in my opinion, even stronger arguments against the use of the criterion of social competence. The basic criticism of this criterion is that it confuses

[7] Ibid., p. 4.

[8] Lewis M. Terman, *The Measurement of Intelligence* (Cambridge: The Riverside Press, 1916), p. 67.

cause and effect. Social incompetence may result from mental subnormality, but cannot be considered as diagnostic of this condition, unless a one-to-one relationship between the degree of social competence and the degree of mental subnormality can be demonstrated. No such one-to-one relationship exists. Social competence depends not only upon the extent of intellectual subnormality but also upon the myriad of social, personal, economic, political, and cultural factors which influence success or failure.

The use of the criterion of social competence makes a diagnosis of mental retardation dependent on all of these factors. In consequence, persons facing job discrimination—nonwhites, the middle-aged, the physically handicapped, and others—are more likely to be labeled retarded than their counterparts who are no more intelligent but are younger, white, or healthier. Subnormal women who marry may avoid the label of retardation *until* separated from their spouses. And during periods of rising unemployment the prevalence of mental retardation would rise substantially. Many other such absurd situations exist.

A definition of mental retardation based solely on IQ has the following advantages:

1) By defining mental retardation in terms of the *one* variable that almost all professionals agree is its primary characteristic, the ambiguity surrounding the term would be reduced. All persons within a given level of intellectual functioning would be considered as either retarded or not retarded—a diagnosis that would be unaffected by occupational pursuit, age, the economic climate, etc.

2) Viewing mental retardation as one among many factors affecting social competence emphasizes the necessity for a meaningful appraisal of the importance and interrelationships among these factors. This will provide needed guides to appropriate social policy. In the past, there has been an unfortunate tendency to place great stress on compensating for the intellectual deficits of the retarded while neglecting the other factors that lead to social incompetence.

3) A definition based solely on IQ would be more definitive of the population that is likely to require special assistance. Although many of these persons will be satisfactorily maintaining themselves at a given point in time, they represent a high-risk group, many of whom will need services if conditions change, e.g., a death in the family, job loss, etc. It is not necessary to know which persons among all those of a given level of mental subnormality will require services, but it is necessary to be prepared to provide services when needed.

For purposes of this study, an IQ of 70 or below will be considered the cut-off point that distinguishes retardation from nonretardation. This choice is based on the considerations that: (1) it has been the most frequently used dividing point; (2) available empirical studies are usually concerned with persons whose IQ falls below this level; and (3) above an IQ of 70, social incompetence is usually caused by factors other than intellectual deficit.

Two points must be stressed:

1) A definition of mental retardation based on IQ alone should be used *only* for purposes of program planning and evaluation. At a clinical level it is altogether unnecessary and potentially hazardous to label a socially competent person as retarded, even if his IQ falls into the range arbitrarily designated as subnormal.

2) The use of a cut-off point of 70 is solely for the purpose of delimiting the scope of the study. Certainly no one would wish needed services denied to persons whose IQs fall slightly over this or any other arbitrarily designated threshold.

Several other points with respect to the definition of mental retardation should be clarified:

1) Mental retardation is not synonymous with illiteracy or mental illness. Although some persons who are illiterate or mentally ill are retarded, many function at normal and even superior levels.

2) Many persons, because of adverse environmental conditions, function at IQ levels below their potential. In some cases, this is sufficient to push them below the threshold of retardation. However, those persons who function below their potential but above the threshold of retardation are not defined as mentally retarded, although a literal interpretation of the term would suggest otherwise. In a similar vein, it has been suggested that brain damage, to a greater or lesser extent, may occur throughout the intellectual spectrum, even among those in the above-average and near-genius ranges.

3) Cases of retardation caused by environmental deprivation are potentially "curable." It has been often questioned whether these cases of "pseudo" mental retardation should, in fact, be considered retarded. In this study they will be so considered for the practical reasons that a distinction between the "curable" and "incurable" retarded is usually not possible at the time of initial diagnosis, and in any event, the "curable" cases may not be cured if appropriate services are not provided, and the intellectual defect may become permanent and incurable.

4) Mental retardation has been defined in many different ways. Some authorities have preferred to exclude retardation caused by environmental deprivation. Others have not only included this group, but expanded the term to include all mental defects, including mental illness. Many different IQ cut-off points have been used.

For the most part, these differences in definition do *not* reflect substantive disagreement among the various authorities, since they all agree on the basic nature of the problems presented. The question as to which of these groups should be included under the overall term of "mental retardation" ultimately resolves into a matter of choice.

CAUSATION AND CLASSIFICATION

The retarded vary enormously with respect to the cause of retardation, the degree of intellectual impairment, and the existence of other handicapping conditions. This results in an equally large variation in the services needed by different groups of retardates and their potential for social adjustment. Classification systems are therefore necessary.

There are over 200 known causes of mental retardation. For purposes of this study, however, it is sufficient to group them under three major headings under which almost all of the known and unknown causes could be subsumed. They are:

1) Mental retardation due to a significantly below-average genetic endowment of intelligence. This simply reflects the fact that the genetic variation in human intelligence is unavoidably broad.

2) Mental retardation that results from physical damage to or maldevelopment of the brain. Among the many ways that this can occur are: infections in the mother during pregnancy or in the infant after birth, ingestion of toxic agents by the mother during pregnancy or by the infant after birth, birth injuries, accidents among children, disorders of metabolism, chromosomal malformations, etc.

3) Mental retardation due to environmental deprivation. The effect of environmental deprivation among the children of poor and nonwhite Americans is well known. Since environmental deprivation is not a necessary consequence of low income, but rather a result of modes of thinking and perceiving, attitudes toward achievement, and emotionally traumatizing experiences, it must be emphasized that not all poor or nonwhite children are predestined to be culturally deprived (hopefully, only a minority are), nor are all children from affluent white families insulated from mind-retarding environmental deprivation.

Loss of sight or hearing and mental illness may also retard mental development by interfering with mind-developing experiences.

Mental retardation often has more than one cause. This is due in part to the semirandom manner in which genetic endowments of intelligence, brain injuries, and physical and emotional handicaps are distributed in the population. Necessarily, a small percentage of brain-injured persons will have begun life with a poor genotype for intelligence. A similar statement is true for the blind, the deaf, and the mentally ill. More importantly, persons who suffer from one cause of retardation have an above-average chance of suffering from another cause. The injury that causes blindness or deafness may also destroy part of the brain. In addition, retardation may create its own form of environmental retardation due to the difficulty retardates have in maintaining normal peer relationships and the unfortunate tendency of many people to shun contact with the mentally subnormal.

In recent years it has become increasingly common to distinguish four levels of intellectual deficit among the mentally retarded: (1) profound retardation (IQ 0 to 19); (2) severe retardation (IQ 20 to 34); (3) moderate retardation (IQ 35 to 49); and (4) mild retardation (IQ 50 to 69).

Retarded children are often classified as educable, trainable, or totally dependent. The educable child is unable to profit to any great degree from regular school programs, but is able to learn basic reading, writing, spelling, and arithmetic skills and provide for most of his personal needs. The trainable child is unable to learn these basic skills, but can be taught to provide for most of his personal needs. The totally dependent child has little developmental potential.

Retarded adults are often classified as marginally dependent, semidependent, and dependent. The marginally dependent adult is capable of self-support and independent living, but needs special assistance when under unusual stress. He will often need assistance in budgeting funds, locating work, etc. The semidependent adult is capable of some work, usually under sheltered conditions, and needs guidance in meeting the day-to-day stresses of normal life. The dependent adult requires constant care and supervision.

Usually mildly retarded children are educable as children and marginally independent as adults, and moderately retarded children are trainable as children and semi-independent as adults. However, there is not perfect equivalence between these categories. Physical or mental impairment, as well as many other factors, can sharply reduce the educability and capacity for independence among the various levels of intellectual deficit.

In the succeeding pages, these terms will be frequently used. Because of data limitations, however, it was not possible to use the four categories of intellectual deficit as defined above. Often only a two-way division is used—IQ below 50 and IQ between 50 and 70. In these cases I usually refer to the former group as severely retarded, although it encompasses the profoundly, severely, and moderately retarded. Other atypical uses of terms will be noted as needed.

EPIDEMIOLOGICAL SURVEYS

Epidemiology in the field of mental retardation would be a simple matter if intelligence test scores were distributed according to the normal curve. Unfortunately, they are not. The prevalence of mental retardation must, therefore, be measured by epidemiological surveys.

Table 1 summarizes the results of the more important epidemiological studies of mental retardation within the United States. With one exception, each study is identified by the last name of the author reporting the study or, in the case of multiple authors, by the last name of the first author listed on the publication. The one exception is the Onondaga study, which refers to the area where the investigation was undertaken.

The rates of mental retardation ascertained by these various studies vary broadly; the highest rate is 46 times the lowest. Nor is there any tendency for these rates to cluster around a modal value. The following factors explain most of the variation in these studies:

1. Method of conducting study. Epidemiological studies are of two types: agency surveys and household surveys. In agency surveys, schools, clinics, institutions, and other agencies that are likely to be in contact with cases of mental retardation are asked to report the number of such cases (or the clients of such agencies are tested for mental retardation). Agency surveys invariably report lower prevalence rates of mental retardation than household surveys. One reason is that not all retardates are known to agencies. This is because the retarded are not usually brought to these agencies until they present problem behavior. The mildly retarded are especially apt to be underreported. When young they may be considered lazy or immature and their deficits may not be recognized until several years after entering school. After leaving school their intellectual limitations are usually less handicapping. Even when the retarded present problem behavior, their parents or guardians may be unaware of available assistance, or may be unwilling to avail themselves of outside aid. Another problem with agency surveys is that it is difficult to reach all the facilities that come in contact with the retarded. Multiply-handicapped retardates may be taken to one of the many agencies that specialize in serving persons with these additional handicaps.

Even when there is fairly comprehensive coverage of agencies, not all multiply-handicapped retarded children are identified as retarded. In the Wishik study, two-thirds of the cases identified as mentally retarded were initially referred for clinical evaluation on the basis of some other handicapping condition. Moreover, not all agencies may be cooperative in surveys of this type, especially those concerned with the confidentiality of their relationship with their clients.

These limitations of agency surveys were clearly shown by the Richardson study. Both agencies and households were surveyed. Rates based on the household survey were twice as high as those based on the agency survey (not given in Table 1).

2. **Criteria of mental retardation.** Epidemiological surveys have utilized widely different IQ cut-off points with obvious effects on prevalence rates. The most extreme case is the Onondaga study, which apparently had no IQ limit. Over 60% of the persons reported as having "suspected" mental retardation had IQs above 75, and almost 25% had IQs of 90 or more. Apparently, any child with a known learning difficulty was reported as possibly retarded (e.g., emotional or cultural factors, physical handicaps, etc.).[9]

Several studies employed the criterion of social competence. The use of this criterion is implicit in most agency studies where identification of retardation is contingent on problem behavior.

Apparently, the Wishik study did not consider as retarded those persons whose intellectual limitations were not causing adjustment problems.[10] This probably explains why the Wishik study reported a prevalence of mental retardation that was less than half of two other household surveys (Richardson and Imre) in spite of the fact that the IQ cut-off in the Wishik study was a relatively high 79.

The Jastak study made the most rigorous use of the criterion of social competence, counting a person as retarded only if his intellectual deficiency was matched by a correspondingly severe occupational and educational deficiency. In consequence, less than one in five persons in the lowest 2% of the population intellectually was counted as retarded; about one in four at the 9% level, and one in three at the 25% level. The more restrictive the criterion of intellectual deficiency the smaller was the probability of a correspondingly severe social inadequacy.

3. **Method of identifying the retarded.** Rates of mental retardation are usually higher in surveys that are based on IQ tests than in surveys that rely on respondents' replies. In household surveys parents may be reluctant to admit, or perhaps do not know, that their child is retarded. In the Richardson (Alamance County) survey, rates of retardation based on an IQ test administered to a sample of children identified as retarded, physically handicapped, or normal found a rate of retardation

[9] Samuel A. Kirk and Bluma B. Weiner, "The Onondaga Census—Fact or Artifact," *Exceptional Children* (January 1959): 228.

[10] Elizabeth J. Levinson, *Retarded Children in Maine* (Orono, Maine: University of Maine Press, 1962), p. 43.

Table 1. Rates of mental retardation reported by various epidemiological studies

Name of study	Year of study	Place of study	Number of persons in population	Upper IQ limit	Confirmed by IQ test by investigator	Rate[j]	Age range covered
Agency studies							
1. Lemkau[a]	1936	Eastern Health District of Baltimore					
2. Onondaga[b]	1953	Onandaga County New York	55,000	70	No	1.2%	all
3. Levinson[c]	1957	Maine	108,000	90+	No	3.5	1–17
4. Kennedy[d]	1960–61	Five south-eastern states	148,000	75	No	3.2	5–20
5. Taylor[e]	1962	Oregon	1,800	69	Yes	18.4	6–14
			215,000	75	No	1.9	0–20

[a]Paul Lemkau, Christopher Tietze, and Marcia Cooper, "Mental Hygiene Problems in an Urban District," *Mental Hygiene* (1942): 275–88. In the case of adults, social incompetence rather than an IQ score was usually the means of diagnosing mental retardation, primarily because test scores were not available.

[b]New York State Department of Mental Hygiene, Mental Health Research Unit, "A Special Census of Suspected Referred Mental Retardation, Onondaga County, New York," *Technical Report of the Mental Health Research Unit* (Syracuse: University Press, 1965). No clear criteria of mental retardation were employed. Agencies were asked to report all persons "... identified as definitely mentally retarded, or suspected of mental retardation on the basis of developmental history, poor academic performance, IQ score, or social adaptation when contrasted with their age peers."

[c]Elizabeth J. Levinson, *Retarded Children in Maine* (Orono, Maine: University of Maine Press, 1962). Test scores were not avail-

able for all children, and those that were available were often of poor quality. The rate is adjusted to allow for the fact that not all 5-year-olds were in kindergarten at the time of the survey. The population survey included all schools and all child-serving residential facilities.

[d]Wallace A. Kennedy, Vernon Van Do Riet, James C. White, Jr., *A Normative Sample of Intelligence and Achievement of Negro Elementary School Children in the Southeastern United States*, Monographs of the Society for Research in Child Development (Yellow Springs, Ohio: The Antioch Press, 1963). The subjects were all Negro school children.

[e]Joseph L. Taylor et al., *Mental Retardation Prevalence in Oregon, A Survey by the Oregon State Board of Health* (Portland, Oregon: Oregon State Board of Health, 1965). This survey was probably the most thorough of all agency studies. The survey population encompassed about one-third of the State's population and

Table 1. (Continued)

Name of study	Year of study	Place of study	Number of persons in population	Upper IQ limit	Confirmed by IQ test by investigator	Rate[j]	Age range covered
Household surveys							
6. Jastak[f]	1953–54	Delaware	2,002		Yes		10–64
2% level				f		.4	
9% level				f		2.0	
25% level				f		8.3	
7. Wishik[g]	1954	Clark and Oconee Counties, Georgia	1,373	79	Yes	3.7	0–20
8. Richardson[h]	1961–62	North Carolina					
Alamance County Household study			3,100	h	No	7.9	0–20
Clinical study				70	Yes	9.0	0–20
Halifax County Household study			2,600	h	No	7.7	0–20
9. Imre[i]	1965	Unidentified Maryland county	14,500	69	Yes	8.2	1–59

was believed to be reasonably representative of its demographic composition. Most of the retardates were identified by individual intelligence tests.

fJoseph F. Jastak, Halsey M. MacPhee, and Martin Whiteman, *Mental Retardation—Its Nature and Incidence* (Newark, Delaware: University of Delaware Press, 1963). The criteria of mental retardation used in this study were unique. Four indices were constructed, when possible, for each individual: (1) the average of 15 separate standard standard intelligence scores; (2) The highest subtest standard score (altitude); (3) A scholastic achievement index which, for each individual, was the number of completed grades divided by the average for his age group; (4) An occupational achievement index based on skill level, salary, increase in salary from previous

note i. The study sought to measure the prevalence of a wide range of handicapping conditions among children. It was conducted in two parts. The first was an intensive three-week campaign to solicit voluntary referrals from schools, physicians and nurses, families, and other agencies. The second stage was a sample survey of 8.5% of the children in the two counties. All reports of handicapped children, both from the voluntary campaign and the canvass, were examined by pediatricians, and children tentatively diagnosed as handicapped were asked to attend clinics set up to clinically confirm the diagnoses. Apparently children were diagnosed as retarded only after a clinical judgment that the retardation actually constituted a handicap (criterion of social competence).

hWilliam P. Richardson and A. C. Higgins, *The Handicapped*

job, supervisory status, mobility from father's occupation, and mobility from his own first job. An occupation achievement index could be constructed for only about half the sample. Three alternative definitions of mental retardation were used. In one, persons were considered as retarded if they fell in the lowest 25% of the population on *all* indices. Corresponding definitions were used for the 9% and the 2% levels. "The cutoff points were determined separately for American-born whites, foreign-born whites, and Negroes to avoid biases due to foreign language background and lack of educational opportunities."

The use of the four indices to diagnose mental retardation was an attempt to combine rigorous indices of social competence (scholastic and occupational achievement) with an index of intelligence. The use of the highest score achieved on a subtest of the intelligence test was an attempt to reduce the effect of errors of measurement and reflected the philosophy that people might frequently perform below their intellectual potential, but rarely above it.

[g]Samuel M. Wishik, "Handicapped Children in Georgia: A Study of Prevalence, Disability, Needs, and Resources," *American Journal of Public Health* (1956): 195–203. Additional statistical data concerning this survey was obtained from Levinson, *Retarded Children in Maine*; Lemkau, "Mental Hygiene Problems"; and Imre, see footnote *Children of Alamance County, North Carolina* (Wilmington, Delaware: Nemours Foundation, 1965). The study sought to determine the prevalence of a number of handicapping conditions. Five percent of the households in Alamance County and 4% of the house-

holds in Halifax County were surveyed. A diagnosis of mental retardation was based on household responses to such question as "Is . . . mentally retarded or slow-witted, or does he have serious difficulty in learning or remembering things?"

In Alamance County 456 children were clinically examined and retardation was apparently diagnosed on the basis of IQ tests.

[i]The data reported in this study were obtained from Paul Imre, the director of the study. Preliminary results were published by Paul V. Lemkau and Paul Imre in "Preliminary Results of a Field Epidemiologic Study," a paper presented at the Scientific Symposium for the dedication of Joseph P. Kennedy, Jr., Memorial Laboratories, March 15, 1966. This is one of the best available epidemiological studies in mental retardation. Every family in the county was interviewed. Every child over the age of one, including those not in school, every adult under 35 who had not completed high school, and every adult over 35 who had not completed the eighth grade were screened for possible mental retardation on the basis of some form of IQ test or child-behavior check list (for preschool children). Persons scoring below 80 were given more extensive tests.

Henceforth this unidentified county will be referred to as "Rose County."

[j]In calculating the prevalence of mental retardation, all studies, whether of the agency or household type, took account of the number of institutionalized retardates that originated from the area being surveyed.

14% higher than in the household survey, although in the latter case interviewers aided parents in making a diagnosis through the use of leading questions. The Wishik study also supports this observation, since most retarded children were not originally reported as such. The influences are conflicting however, since the Wishik study also found that one-fifth of the cases voluntarily reported as retarded were not so diagnosed when tested for IQ. One can assume that agency responses are more reliable than parents' responses, but less so than IQ tests.

4. Demographic differences. In the next section we will show that the prevalence of mental retardation varies strikingly by race, social class, and other demographic variables. Much of the variation in results of epidemiological studies can be explained by differences in their demographic composition. The high rate of the Imre study, for example, is due to the fact that it was conducted in a rural, relatively poor county with a high proportion of nonwhites.

DEMOGRAPHIC CHARACTERISTICS OF THE MENTALLY RETARDED

Not all of the epidemiological studies provided information on the demographic variables that we shall evaluate. In addition, the studies often employed different demographic groupings, especially in the cases of age and IQ. The awkwardness of Tables 2 and 7, and the complexity of the ensuing analysis is a direct result of these problems.

Age. In almost every study, the reported prevalence of mental retardation increased steadily with age until the middle teens (Table 2), after which it began to decline. In addition, the low prevalence of mental retardation among adults and very young as compared to teenage children is considerably more pronounced in agency studies than in household studies. It is noteworthy that the Imre study, which diagnosed mental retardation on the basis of IQ tests, reported a considerably higher prevalence rate among preschoolers than did the Richardson study, which based a diagnosis on parental responses. The Wishik study found a low prevalence of mental retardation among preschool children, apparently because this study employed the criterion of social competence. Each of these three studies was a household survey.

Sex. Agency studies reported higher rates of mental retardation among males than females (Table 3), generally by a ratio of about 2 to 1. Among the household surveys, the percentage of retarded males still exceeded that of retarded females, but was much smaller. In the Imre study, the difference in rates was not significant; in fact, under the age of 20, females were slightly more likely to be retarded.

Table 2. Rates of mental retardation among various age groups (per 100 persons)

Age range	Lemkau	Onondaga	Levinson	Taylor	Jastak 2% level	Jastak 9% level	Jastak 25% level	Wishik	Richardson Alamance Co.	Richardson Halifax Co.	Imre
0– 4	0.07	0.46						0.87	4.8	4.3	
1– 4											7.24
0– 2				0.45							
3– 5				1.02							
5– 6		3.00	0.9								
7– 9		4.70	2.3								
6– 8				1.83							
5– 9	1.18							5.71	8.1	9.2	7.49
10–14	4.36	7.74	3.9	2.77				6.08	9.7	8.7	8.47
15		7.75									
10–16					0.49	1.95	9.31				
15–17			2.7								
16–17		2.81		2.76							
15–19	3.02								8.9	8.7	10.39
15–20								1.94			
18–20			1.1	2.10							
17–35					0.38	1.33	6.28				
20–34	0.76										8.00
35–59											8.12
36–64					0.33	2.28	9.51				
35–44	0.83										
45–54	0.64										
55–64	0.26										
65+	0.19										

Table 3. Rates of mental retardation by sex (per 100 persons)

Name of study	Male	Female
Lemkau[a]	5.05	3.68
Onondaga	4.47	2.53
Jastak		
2% level	0.34	0.30
9% level	2.35	1.48
25% level	8.96	7.20
Richardson[b]		
Alamance County	10.0	5.9
Halifax County	8.5	6.7
Imre	8.45	7.94

[a] Based upon 10- to 14-year-old subjects.
[b] Not clinically adjusted.

Both the Onondaga and Imre studies reported on the sex composition of retardates with IQs below 50. In both cases, the prevalence was about one-third again as high among women as among men.

Race. The prevalence of mental retardation among Negroes is strikingly higher than among whites.

The Imre study, which combined a household survey with clinical evaluation, indicated that Negroes were almost nine times more likely to be retarded than whites. In contrast, the Richardson studies, which depended upon parental responses for a diagnosis of mental retardation, found a higher rate of retardation among whites and a much lower rate among Negroes than did the Imre study (possibly because of different expectations); however, the rate was still considerably higher for Negroes than whites.

Agency studies also reported a less pronounced difference in the rates of mental retardation between Negroes and whites than the Imre study (which probably indicates that retarded Negroes are less likely to be served by social agencies).

Even the Jastak study, which utilized different cut-off points for Negroes and whites, reported higher rates of mental retardation among Negroes, especially at the 9% and 25% levels. Because the criteria of mental retardation differed between the two racial groups, it is difficult to draw firm inferences.

The Imre study indicated that the rate of mental retardation among Negroes tended to increase with age, while whites showed the opposite trend.

The Kennedy study reported one of the highest rates of retardation among Negroes and understates the actual rate for this population, since it included only school children. Most of the children in this study were from the lowest socioeconomic levels.

Table 4.   Rates of mental retardation by race (per 100 persons)

Name of study	White	Non-white
Lemkau[a]	2.61	9.82
Onondaga[b]		
Both sexes	3.05	10.31
Male	3.87	13.74
Female	2.18	7.12
Kennedy		18.4
Jastak		
2% level	.30	.43
9% level	1.37	5.58
25% level	5.85	23.61
Richardson		
Alamance County	6.5	14.1
Halifax County	6.2	8.5
Imre		
All ages	1.78	15.76
Ages 1–4	2.45	10.95
Ages 5–9	2.33	12.03
Ages 10–14	1.60	14.55
Ages 15–19	1.55	19.46
Ages 20–34	1.85	16.17
Ages 35–59	1.45	20.90

[a] Based on 10- to 14-year-old subjects.
[b] Race was reported for about 85% of the cases of suspected retardation.

Social class. Two studies reported on the prevalence of mental retardation among social classes.

In the Richardson studies the "lower" social class in Alamance County had a rate of retardation over five times that of the "upper" and "middle" classes. In Halifax County the differential was much less pronounced. As compared with Alamance County, the rate of retardation was higher for the "upper" and "middle" classes and lower for the "lower" class.

Imre distinguished five social classes on the basis of the education, occupation, and source of income of the household head. The three highest social classes were combined because of a paucity of cases.

Table 5 shows the prevalence of mental retardation among 5- to 19-year-old children by social class. This analysis is restricted to children, since adult retardates will almost inevitably gravitate to one of the two lower social classes.

Children born into the lowest social class were almost 13 times as likely to be retarded as children born into one of the upper three social classes. Part of the reason for this remarkable difference is the high percentage of nonwhites in the lowest social class. Lower-class white children were about 7 times as likely to be retarded as white children

Table 5.   Prevalence of mental retardation among persons 5 to 19 years
old in Rose County,[a] Maryland, by social class and race (per
100 persons)

Socioeconomic status	IQ 0–69	IQ 0–49
SES 1, 2, 3	1.19	0.26
White	0.64	0.18
Nonwhite	8.53	1.22
SES 4	6.09	0.48
White	1.89	0.15
Nonwhite	11.14	0.88
SES 5	15.43	1.78
White	4.93	0.87
Nonwhite	17.45	1.89

[a]A fictious name for the real county studied.

born to the upper three social classes, and among nonwhites the corresponding ratio was about 2. Within each social class, the prevalence of retardation among children was much higher for nonwhites than for whites, by a factor of about 3 in the lowest social class and 13 in the highest three social classes.

A somewhat less expected observation is that the prevalence of children with severe retardation (IQ below 50) also showed strong race and social status variations. The prevalence of severe retardation was 7 times as large in the lowest socioeconomic class as in the highest three classes. Moreover, within each social class, nonwhites were far more likely than whites to suffer severe retardation, by a factor of 2 in the lowest class and 7 in the upper three classes.

Rural versus urban. Several studies have reported that the average IQ score of rural residents is below that of urban residents. In addition, it appears that the discrepancy widens as older age groups are considered. McNemar reported that the average IQ of urban and suburban children remains relatively constant at about 106 between the ages of 2 and 18, while the average IQ of rural children falls from about 100 to 96.[11]

Wheeler studied the intelligence of East Tennessee mountain children in 1930 and again in 1940. In 1930 he found a mean IQ of 95 among 6-year-olds and 74 among 16-year-olds. In 1940 the corresponding figures were 103 and 80.[12] Other studies appear to contradict these observations.

[11] Q. McNemar, *The Revision of the Stanford-Binet Scale* (Boston: Houghton-Mifflin Co., 1942), p. 37.

[12] Lester Wheeler, "A Comparative Study of the Intelligence of East Tennessee Mountain Children," *Journal of Educational Psychology* (May 1942): 3, 22.

During 1963–65 the Health Examination Survey reported that the estimated IQs for 6- to 11-year-old children from rural and urban areas were almost identical, nor were there any significant variations by age.[13]

The Jastak study, the only epidemiological study which explicitly distinguished between rural and urban areas, found that at all three cut-off levels, rates of retardation were slightly lower in rural than in urban areas.

In the Richardson study, Alamance County was described as highly industrialized and rapidly growing, while Halifax County was described as typically rural. Alamance County had a lower proportion of Negroes (17% to 55%) and a higher per capita income ($1,800 to $1,491 in 1959). Despite these differences, the overall rate of mental retardation, as measured by household survey, was slightly lower in Halifax County. Since mental retardation was diagnosed on the basis of household responses, this could be interpreted to mean that rural populations have a lower awareness of the milder handicapping conditions, or, perhaps, different standards for a satisfactory social adjustment.

The Imre study was carried out on a clearly rural population. However, the high rate of mental retardation reported is largely explainable by the racial and social class composition of "Rose County." In fact, rurality appears to be of value as an explanatory factor of the prevalence of mental retardation only insofar as it serves as a proxy variable for racial and social class differences between rural and urban populations. Perhaps this is too strong a statement. Some isolated rural populations may find themselves hemmed in by lack of cultural, educational, and occupational opportunity, which not only relegates them to a low social class but also restricts their knowledge of how to move to areas with greater opportunity and limits their motivation and financial ability to do so. The more isolated the area the more restrictive would be the effects of rurality. High rates of retardation become self perpetuating as people have limited opportunity to break out of the cycle. This would explain the high rate of retardation found by Wheeler among Tennessee mountain children and the relatively low rate found by Jastak among rural residents in Delaware.

Urban ghettos. Despite the attention that has been focused on urban ghettos, only one of the epidemiological studies (the Onondaga study) provides any information on rates of retardation in these areas

[13]U.S. Department of Health, Education, and Welfare, Health Services and Mental Health Administration, *Intellectual Development of Children*, Series 11, Number 110, December, 1971, p. 41.

(Table 6). Given the social class and racial composition of these areas, the rates are about as expected. As in the case of isolated rural areas, lack of educational and occupational opportunity may perpetuate a cycle of retardation that would be broken in some cases if the inhabitants were able to move to more favored areas.

Table 6. Prevalence of suspected mental retardation in Onondaga
County by race and region (per 100 persons)

	White	Non-white
Nonwhite area	6.43	13.22
Rest of city	2.81	9.95
Rest of county	3.00	8.89

Further analysis of age and sex variations in retardation. The distressingly high prevalence of mental retardation observed among nonwhites and the lower social classes is by far the most important demographic characteristic of mental retardation. Discussion of the reasons for these differences will be deferred until the next chapter. The possible causal relationship of mental retardation and life in rural areas and urban ghettos has already been described. This leaves age and sex variations in the prevalence of retardation for further discussion here.

Agency studies consistently report a higher prevalence of mental retardation among males than females and among teenagers than among younger children or adults. This reflects the fact that retarded males and retarded teenagers are more likely to behave in ways that will make them known to public agencies.

Lemkau has suggested that the visibility of mental retardation among males is caused by "two characteristics of the male that are well recognized; first, his retardation in comparison with the female as regards communication skills and second, his greater aggressiveness that tends to lead to lower grades in deportment, reflecting his greater capacity to 'make trouble' and thus have his defect discovered in the course of a fundamentally unrelated investigation."[14] Levinson has additionally suggested that cultural expectations are more lenient for girls than for boys.[15] The Imre study (based on a census of households) supports these critical observations by reporting a much less pronounced sex

[14] Paul V. Lemkau, "Epidemiological Aspects," in *The Evaluation and Treatment of the Mentally Retarded Child in Clinics* (New York: National Association for Retarded Children, 1956).

[15] Levinson, *Retarded Children in Maine*, p. 99.

ratio. In fact, among persons with IQs of less than 50, females predominated, perhaps because of higher mortality among severely retarded males.

Differences in rates of mild mental retardation (IQ 50 to 69) between men and women in the Imre study were minor. The small differences that occurred may reflect nothing more than a slightly less cooperative attitude on the part of males taking intelligence tests than females. We can conclude that mild retardation is as prevalent among men as women.

A similar appraisal may be made of age variations in the prevalence of retardation. Mildly retarded children find the academic requirements of early school years less exacting than those encountered later, and mildly retarded adults find work less demanding than school, so that failure to maintain the normal expected role is most likely for the mildly retarded during their teenage years.

One would expect, therefore, that a household survey such as the Imre study would find roughly comparable rates of mental retardation among all age groups. However, even in this study the prevalence of mental retardation among teenagers was significantly higher than for other age groups. This led Lemkau and Imre to hypothesize that the excess frequency consisted of persons who are "made" mentally retarded. This hypothesis entitles one to ask if the decline in the prevalence of mental retardation among adults represents cases that are "unmade."

When the Imre study data are broken down by severity and race (Table 7) it becomes apparent that the peaking of the prevalence of mental retardation among 15- to 19-year-olds is entirely due to the influence of nonwhites. If mental retardation can be "made" and "unmade" the "making" appears to be concentrated in the nonwhite population and the "unmaking" in the white population.

When looked at in this way, the Imre data does not support a teenage peaking hypothesis, except possibly among nonwhites. If such peaking does occur, however, it is noteworthy that it occurs in those ages where academic and social pressures are greatest. It would be no surprise if some borderline cases, unable to cope with school or find jobs, sensing failure and social disapproval, should be indifferent and perhaps even hostile to an intelligence test. Adult status and responsibility usually change attitudes and may result in somewhat improved performance.

For subsequent purposes, we will assume that age variation in the prevalence of mental retardation results only from the above-average rates of mortality among the retarded. This is not, strictly speaking, true. Environmental circumstances may systematically vary the intelligence levels of particular groups, especially among the culturally deprived where IQ test performance decreases as children grow older.

The implications of this assumption for our estimates of the prevalence of mental retardation are: (1) in younger age groups we will be measuring the number of children who score below 70 on an IQ test, or who *will* do so in the near future; and (2) we may omit some teenagers who will test in the retarded range for only a few years.

PREVALENCE OF SEVERE MENTAL RETARDATION

Table 7 shows the estimated prevalence of various degrees of mental retardation reported by different epidemiological studies. To simplify the complicated task of synthesizing these studies, we will first estimate the prevalence of severe retardation (IQ less than 50).

School-age children. The first step will be to estimate the prevalence of severe retardation among 5- to 19-year-old children, since most of the epidemiological studies focus on this group.

Despite the incomparabilities among these epidemiological studies, they should be reasonably comparable with respect to estimates of the prevalence of severe retardation among school-age children. The great majority of such children are almost certain to be brought to the attention of one or more agencies at a relatively early age. Household surveys should not, therefore, uncover significantly more cases of severe retardation than agency studies.

If we confine our attention to the 10- to 14-year age group, three of the epidemiological studies appear to support this hypothesis. The Lemkau, Imre, and Levinson studies reported that 0.33%, 0.37%, and 0.39% of the persons in this age group had IQs below 50 (the upper limit of the IQ of "imbeciles" in the Lemkau study can be assumed to be about 50).

When we look at other age groups, however, this consistency is lost. In the Levinson study, 0.26% of those age 5 to 9 had IQs below 50 compared to 0.57% in the Imre study. Moreover, the Imre study reported a remarkable increase (to 1.93%) in the prevalence of severe mental retardation in the age group 15 to 19, while the Levinson study found no change. The Imre estimate for the late teens is probably a consequence of unusual chance variation. On the other hand, Imre's estimate for 10- to 14-year-olds is the lowest of all of the age groups he considers and is probably an underestimate.

If we consider all age groups together, agency studies consistently yield lower rates of severe retardation than household studies. In the Onondaga, Levinson, Taylor, and Richardson studies, the rates were

0.32%, 0.33%, 0.33%, and 0.2%. In the Wishik and Imre studies, on the other hand, the rates were 0.59% and 0.97%.

The unusually high rate of severe mental retardation in the Imre study is not representative of the United States. To begin with, the high rate of severe retardation among children one to 4 years old is undoubtedly due to a bias in the testing instrument. Despite high death rates among severely handicapped children, it is unlikely that three-fourths of these children die before the age of 10. In addition, nonwhites constituted a much larger proportion of the population of Rose County than of the United States, and rates of severe retardation were much higher among nonwhites than among whites. Finally, children from lower-class families were more likely to be severely mentally retarded than those from higher-class families. Lower-class families predominated in Rose County.

If we weight the rates of severe mental retardation for whites and nonwhites in the Imre study by the percentage of whites and nonwhites in the United States (about 86% and 14%) and restrict our analysis to persons age 5 to 19, then we obtain an adjusted rate of severe mental retardation of 0.43%. Corresponding adjustments of the Wishik data would undoubtedly yield a similar rate. An adjustment for social class would lower the Imre rate still further.

The adjusted rate of the prevalence of severe mental retardation derived from the Imre data is not inconsistent with the results of the Levinson study when roughly comparable ages are considered. Levinson reported that 0.39% of 10- to 20-year-old children had an IQ below 50. On balance, an estimate of 0.40% as the percentage of school-age children (5–19) with IQs below 50 is as reasonable as existing data will allow.

Three studies have estimated the prevalence of persons with IQs under 25. The prevalence rate reported by the Onondaga study was 0.08% (school-age children); 0.11% by the Levinson study (children between 5 and 20); and 0.07% by the Lemkau study (children 10 to 14 years old and assuming the "idiot" category to have an IQ cut-off point of 25). The Onondaga rate was based on children with known IQs and is therefore low. We might also expect that the Levinson rate is low because of underreporting in the youngest age group. A reasonable estimate for the percentage of school-age children (5–19) with IQs below 25 is 0.12%, which, combined with our estimate of the number of persons with IQs below 50, would indicate that about 0.28% of this age group has an IQ between 25 and 50. These estimates are consistent with those of the Taylor study, which reported that 0.15% of children below age 20 had IQs of 30 or less.

Table 7. Rates of mental retardation by severity (per 100 persons)

Name of study, IQ and other characteristics	Ages								
	All Ages	1–4	5–9	10–14	15–19	15–20	20–34	35–59	20+
Lemkau									
Idiots				0.07					0.028
Imbeciles				0.26					0.189
Morons				3.96					0.243
Feebleminded				0.07					0.209
Levinson[a]									
IQ 0–24			0.08	0.14		0.14			
25–49			0.18	0.25		0.25			
50–59			0.28	0.47		0.27			
60–69			0.58	1.33		0.63			
70–75			0.70	1.57		0.66			
76+			0.97	0.16		0.05			
Imre									
IQ 0–49	0.97	1.92	0.57	0.37	1.93		0.95	0.74	
White	0.38	1.29	0.56	0.10	0.12		0.45	0.19	
Nonwhite	1.68	2.41	0.57	0.62	3.79		1.61	1.79	
Male	0.82	1.27	0.51	0.18	1.63		0.95	0.69	
Female	1.14	2.68	0.62	0.57	2.26		0.94	0.78	
IQ 50–69	7.22	5.31	6.92	8.10	8.45		7.05	7.38	
White	1.40	1.16	1.77	1.50	1.43		1.40	1.27	
Nonwhite	14.08	8.54	11.46	13.93	15.67		14.56	19.11	
Male	7.63	5.91	6.82	8.17	8.59		7.20	8.49	
Female	6.80	4.62	7.03	8.02	8.30		6.92	6.27	
Onondaga[b]									
Males									
IQ 0–24	0.06								
25–49	0.21								
50–74	1.32								
75–89	1.64								
90+	1.23								

28

Females		
IQ	0–24	0.10
	25–49	0.26
	50–74	0.81
	75–89	0.87
	90+	0.48
Both sexes		
IQ	0–24	0.08
	25–49	0.24
	50–74	1.07
	75–89	1.26
	90+	0.84
Wishik		
IQ	0–49	0.59
	50–69	1.37
	70–79	1.74
Taylor		
IQ	0–30	0.15
	31–40	0.07
	41–50	0.11
	51–60	0.24
	61–70	0.65
	71–75	0.62
	Unknown	0.09
Richardson		
Alamance Co.		
(clinically adj.)		
	Presumptive	0.8
	Educable	7.0
	Trainable	0.9
	Custodial	0.2

[a] Estimated from Table 8, Levinson, *Retarded Children in Maine*, p. 39.
[b] Based on data contained in Table 28a, New York State Department of Mental Hygiene, "A Special Census," p. 115. The rates are based on school-age children with known IQs.

Preschool children. To estimate the number of severely retarded persons under 5, it is necessary to consider the unusually high mortality among this group. Penrose has stated that "if intelligence could be measured at birth in every child, the incidence of mental defect would be found to be much higher than that observed at school age. About 1 percent would be idiots."[16] By "idiots," Penrose is referring to persons with IQs below 25. The proportion of newborn infants with potential IQs between 25 and 50 is probably no greater and may be less than the proportion with IQs below 25, since severe retardation is almost always caused by malformation of the brain, which has devastating effects on intellectual capacity. The percentage of children who are severely retarded when born is therefore apparently between 1.3% and 2%. The lower figure adds together Penrose's estimate of the percentage of new births with IQs below 25 and the percentage of school-age children with IQs between 25 and 50. The unknown factor is the percentage of children in the 25 to 50 IQ range who die before age 5. Mortality in the higher-IQ range is considerably less than in the lower-IQ range so the actual prevalence of severe retardation at birth is probably of the order of 1.5% to 1.7%.

Several observations are of interest:

1) Most severely retarded persons—apparently almost 9 out of 10 of those with IQs below 25, and perhaps 1 in 2 of those with IQs between 25 and 50—die within the first five years of life.

2) Most of the deaths occur in the first year of life. Data from the Pacific State Hospital in California indicates that after the first year, 3 out of 4 of even the most severely retarded (IQ below 20) survived an additional five years.[17]

3) In 1966, 2.3% of all children born alive died during the first year of life. Evidently about half of these infants would have been severely retarded had they survived.

4) These high death rates are not a consequence of low intellect, but of the serious physical ailments that frequently accompany severe retardation.[18]

5) If we extended the analysis backward to take account of fetal deaths, the figures would be even more dramatic. Bierman reported that there were 311 fetal casualties for every 1,000 live births on the island

[16] L. S. Penrose, *The Biology of Mental Defect* (New York: Grune and Stratton, Inc., 1963), p. 197.

[17] George Sabagh et al., *Differential Mortality in a Hospital for the Mentally Retarded*, International Population Conference (Vienna, 1959).

[18] Ibid.

of Kauai (Hawaii) during 1962, and this included only fetuses with a gestation period of four weeks or more.[19] Fetal defect is an important cause of spontaneous abortion.

Adults. Mortality rates among severely retarded adults have declined drastically during the last fifty years as former major causes of death have been brought under control. During the early 1900s, tuberculosis, pneumonia, and influenza were responsible for 50% to 60% of all deaths among the severely retarded. These causes of death occurred 3 to 13 times more frequently among the retarded than among the general population.[20]

Nevertheless, mortality rates among the severely retarded are still considerably above average. One study reported that the mortality of adults, 18 to 34 years, admitted to Pacific State Hospital (of whom three-fourths had IQs below 50) was approximately eight times that of the general population during the first five years after admission. The authors of the study cautioned: "it may be that patients are admitted to the hospital because they are in such poor condition that death is imminent."[21]

No study of the mortality of both institutionalized and noninstitutionalized retardates is available. In a Massachusetts study of the mortality of all persons who "were admitted to, were in residence within, or were discharged or died while in residence or on the books" of the three state schools during the years 1917 through 1930, it was reported that mortality among idiots (IQ below 25) between the ages of 20 and 60 was approximately three times the mortality of the general population. Among imbeciles (IQ 25 to 49) of the same age, mortality was about twice that of the general population.[22] Unfortunately, there may still be adverse selection in this study (causing mortality among the retarded to be overstated). In addition, mortality rates forty to fifty years ago were far higher than at present.

Given this limited information, the most reasonable approach is to assume that the *relative* mortality between the severely retarded and

[19] Jessie M. Bierman et al., "Analysis of the Outcome of all Pregnancies in a Community," *American Journal of Obstetrics and Gynecology* (January 1, 1965): 37–45.

[20] Eugene W. Martz, "Mortality among the Mentally Deficient during a Twenty-Five Year Period," *Training School Bulletin* (February 1934): 189, 191, 193. Neil A. Dayton et al., "Mortality and Expectation of Life in Mental Deficiency in Massachusetts: Analysis of the Fourteen Year Period 1917–1930," *New England Journal of Medicine* (March 1932): 616.

[21] Sabagh et al., *Differential Mortality*, p. 4.

[22] Dayton et al., "Mortality and Expectation of Life," pp. 559, 560.

the general population has remained roughly constant over time—i.e., that it is three times the average among persons with IQs below 25 and twice the average for persons with IQs between 25 and 50.

If this assumption is correct, age-specific rates of mental retardation should be about the same among younger age groups because of relatively low mortality rates. Higher rates of mortality among older age groups, however, should affect prevalence rates, and, in fact, Imre reports a 22% decrease in the prevalence of severe retardation among persons age 35 to 59 as compared to those age 20 to 34. If Imre's prevalence rates are adjusted to reflect the relative proportion of whites and nonwhites in the adult population, the decrease would be of the order of 36%. This is greater than would be expected on the basis of our assumption of constant differential mortality, but is readily explainable in terms of the much higher mortality rates prevailing prior to 1940.[23]

Table 8 shows what the prevalence by age of severe retardation would be if death rates were those prevailing in 1966[24] and given our assumption of constant relative mortality rates. It represents the rates of severe retardation that *may* prevail in the future. High mortality rates in the past, however, would cause these rates to overstate the

Table 8.   Estimated prevalence of severe retardation in population with unchanging mortality

Age	IQ 0–24	IQ 25–49
20–24	0.12%	0.28%
25–29	0.12	0.28
30–34	0.12	0.28
35–44	0.11	0.27
45–54	0.10	0.26
55–64	0.08	0.23
65–69	0.05	0.19
20–64	0.11	0.26

[23] Prior to World War II, various studies placed the life expectancies of persons with IQs below 25 at about 20 years and of persons with IQs between 25 and 50 at about 30 years. Dayton et al., "Mortality and Expectation of Life," p. 652; Martz, "Mortality among the Mentally Deficient," p. 193; Oscar Kaplan, "Life Expectancy of Low Grade Mental Defectives," *Psychological Record* (March 1940): 300.

[24] Average mortality rates for each age group were used in these calculations. The data are not sufficiently refined to adjust for age and sex variations in mortality.

prevalence of severe retardation that currently exists among older age groups.[25]

Unfortunately, I have little information with which to adjust for this factor. It is, however, consistent with (but not necessarily indicated by) the Imre study to reduce the age-specific prevalence rates of both levels of retardation that are predicted by the static model as follows:

Age	Reduction in prevalence (%)
20–24	0
25–29	5
30–34	10
35–44	15
45–54	20
55–64	25
65–69	30

This gives rise to adjusted and, as far as we are concerned, final estimates of the age-specific prevalence of severe mental retardation (Table 9). The rate for the 20- to 64-year age group was calculated by

Table 9.   Estimated prevalence of severe retardation, by age (per 100 persons)

Age	IQ 0–24	IQ 25–49
5–19	0.12	0.28
20–24	0.12	0.28
25–29	0.11	0.26
30–34	0.10	0.25
35–44	0.10	0.23
45–54	0.08	0.21
55–64	0.06	0.17
65–69	0.04	0.13
20–64	0.09	0.23

[25] A very simple example will suffice to demonstrate the effect of changing mortality rates on the prevalence of mental retardation. Suppose we assume that the annual death rate among normal people is 2%, and the corresponding rate among the retarded is 6%, and that the prevalence of profound retardation is, in a specific age group, 0.12%. After ten years the prevalence of profound retardation in this age group will decline to 0.08%. On the other hand, if the relevant mortality rates were 1% and 3%, after ten years the prevalence rate would be 0.10%.

weighing each age-specific rate by the proportion of the adult population in that age group.

Despite the uncertainty surrounding the assumptions that have been employed to develop these estimates, the final results are consistent with the fragmentary evidence provided by epidemiological studies. On the basis of the discussion in this section, the total number of severely retarded persons in the United States is estimated to be of the order of 675,000, of whom almost 200,000 had IQs below 25 in 1968. By contrast, ten years earlier, Dingman and Tarjan estimated that the prevalence of severe retardation was around 437,000,[26] of whom 87,000 had IQs below 20. Adjusting this earlier estimate to allow for population growth would increase it to about 500,000. A 35% discrepancy does not seem unreasonable in view of the fact that Dingman and Tarjan believed that their estimates were conservative. The most important difference between these estimates is that I have estimated that almost 200,000 persons had IQs below 25, while even adjusting for population growth would raise the Dingman-Tarjan estimate of the number with IQs below 20 to only about 100,000. A part of the discrepancy is accounted for by the difference in IQ cut-off points. Another part is due to the effect of decreasing mortality rates that become increasingly important as the impact of high mortality rates prior to 1940 recedes.

PREVALENCE OF MILD MENTAL RETARDATION

Despite the limitations of agency studies, they should fairly accurately measure the prevalence of mild mental retardation among persons in their early teens. Compulsory school attendance and the intellectual competence required to perform satisfactorily in school make it unlikely that more than a handful of retarded teenagers could avoid detection.

We will therefore begin our assessment of the prevalence of mild mental retardation by restricting our attention to the 10- to 14-year age group. Only three of the epidemiological studies provided age-specific rates for persons with IQs between 50 and 70. Lemkau reported that 3.96% of the 10- to 14-year-olds in his study were in this IQ range; Levinson reported a figure of 1.80% and Imre 8.10%. If Imre's rates for

[26] H. F. Dingman and G. Tarjan, "Mental Retardation and the Normal Distribution Curve," *American Journal of Mental Deficiency* (May 1960): 991. The number of persons with IQs below 20 was estimated by assuming that the institutional population represented only half the total number, and the number of persons with IQs between 20 and 50 was estimated by assuming that the institutionalized population represented about one-fifth of the total.

whites and nonwhites are weighted by the relative proportion of whites and nonwhites in the United States, the rate falls to 3.24%. A similar adjustment to the Lemkau estimate yielded an almost identical rate of 3.21%.

The lower rate reported by Levinson is attributable to the fact that this is predominantly a Caucasian rate (nonwhites constituted only 0.6% of Maine's population in 1960). Race is clearly a crucial variable. Our estimate of the prevalence of mild mental retardation will therefore proceed by considering whites and nonwhites separately.

Prevalence among whites. Imre reported that 1.5% of whites age 10 to 14 in Rose County, Maryland, had IQs between 50 and 70. Levinson reported 1.8% for this age group. Both studies were conducted in areas that were predominantly rural and that had per capita incomes below the U.S. average. It can be assumed, therefore, that the prevalence of mild mental retardation among whites will be no greater than the 1.8% found in Maine.

Several possible sources of bias in the Levinson study may have caused this estimate to slightly overstate the prevalence of mild retardation among whites. About one-fifth of the reported IQ scores were estimates, and almost all of the remainder were based on group rather than individual tests. Also, Levinson's estimate for 10- to 14-year-olds may be affected by the broad distribution of intelligence scores usually recorded among this age group. This causes a greater percentage of scores to fall below 70 than will occur in other age groups where the distribution narrows. The Lemkau study may have presented a similar problem. Imre, however, corrected his test score results for differences in standard deviations among different age groups.[27]

On balance I am inclined to accept the Imre study rate as the more representative of the prevalence of mild mental retardation among 10- to 14-year-old whites. This is much lower than the overall rate (all ages) among whites reported in the Richardson studies. In these household surveys mental retardation was diagnosed by the use of leading questions which may have resulted in a significant number of children with IQs above 70 being counted as mentally retarded. Other problems with the Richardson studies are that there were relatively few subjects (only 34 cases of mental retardation were discovered or confirmed in the

---

[27] The age-specific standard deviations of scores on the Stanford-Binet IQ Test range from 13 among 6-year-olds to 20 among 12-year-olds. Thus a person who maintains his rank in the intellectual distribution will nevertheless have varying test scores at different ages. The test scores in different age groups are standardized by basing them on a person's percentile rank within an age group. See Q. McNemar, *The Revision of the Stanford-Binet Scale* (Boston: Houghton-Mifflin, 1948).

clinical examination) and the method of diagnosing mental retardation during the clinical examination was not made explicit.

Even the low Rose County rate probably overstates the national rate of mild retardation among 10- to 14-year-old whites. A large proportion of the white population in that county, over half, fell into the two lowest socioeconomic classes, where the rates of mental retardation were far above average. Any adjustment for social class differences between Rose County and the United States would, however, be highly speculative and likely to be small, probably of the order of one-tenth of one percent. In view of these considerations, we will accept a rate of mild mental retardation of 1.4% among 10- to 14-year-old whites as being as accurate as can be inferred from existing data.

Prevalence among nonwhites. Imre reported that 13.9% of 10- to 14-year-old nonwhite children in Rose County were mildly retarded; Kennedy reported a rate of 16.8% among Negro children in elementary school; and Lemkau estimated that 9.8% of 10- to 14-year-old non-white children were either mildly or severely retarded.

It is probable that the Imre rate overstates the prevalence of mild mental retardation among Negroes. In Rose County, over *90%* of all nonwhites fell into the two lowest socioeconomic classes; over half fell into the lowest. A similar situation prevailed among the children in the Kennedy study.

If we assume that the rates of mental retardation for nonwhites within each social class in Rose County are accurate for these social classes among all nonwhites, and if we further assume that we can estimate the number in the lowest social class in the United States by the proportion of nonwhite families with annual incomes of less than $3,000, the number in the next lowest social class by the proportion of nonwhite families with incomes between $3,000 and $5,000, and the number in the highest three social classes by the proportion of non-white families with incomes over $5,000, then Imre's estimates can be adjusted to yield a rate more reflective of the national rate of mild mental retardation among nonwhites. After weighting each rate by the estimated percentage of nonwhite families in each social class, an adjusted estimate of 11.8% is derived. (Income figures are for 1968.)

This procedure assumes that social class directly affects the prevalence of mental retardation, and that social class in Rose County is in part determined by the limited opportunities available in a southern rural county. In effect, it assumes that if the population in Rose County had been situated in more favorable circumstances, more people would have entered into the higher social classes, and the prevalence of mental retardation among these persons would have declined. Of course, this process may take a generation to work itself out. It should be noted that it is possible for the first part of this assumption to be valid, i.e., that part of the population would move into higher social classes, and the second part invalid, i.e., that there would, in fact, be no reduction in the prevalence of mental retardation.

A number of studies have shown that, on the average, the mean intelligence score of Negroes is about 85 with a standard deviation of about 12 points. On this basis we would expect to find that 10.3% of Negroes were mildly retarded. The agreement between this rate and the adjusted Imre rate is, considering the roughness of the data, quite close.

The adjusted Imre rate of 11.8% will be accepted as the most reasonable estimate of mild mental retardation among nonwhites that can be derived at the present time. This conclusion is based on the considerations that we would expect the distribution of IQ scores to be slightly skewed toward the lower scores and that the prevalence of mild retardation among 5- to 9-year-old nonwhites in Rose County was just slightly less than 11.8%. The effect of cultural impoverishment would be expected to be less pronounced among this group than among 10- to 14-year-olds. Among older age groups the prevalence of mild retardation among nonwhites increases, as would be expected.

This rate is very tentative. It should be noted that had Imre found one more or one less case of mental retardation among Negroes in the upper three socioeconomic classes in Rose County, it would have changed the estimated rate for the United States by 1.3 percentage points. A rate of 11.8% is, however, consistent with the results of other epidemiological studies and is probably within 2 percentage points of being correct.[28]

Age-specific prevalence rates. In the Massachusetts study cited in the preceding section, age-specific death rates among the mildly retarded ranged between 1.2 and 4.0 times those of the general population, and averaged 1.9 times normal mortality rates if each age group is given equal weight. This certainly overstates excess mortality among the mildly retarded. Only 7% of the mildly retarded in the state were included in the study (assuming a low prevalence rate of 1.4%) and all either had been or were institutionalized. Mildly retarded individuals

---

[28] In these calculations we have sometimes used information about Negroes and sometimes about all nonwhites. Nonwhites include American Indians and persons of Oriental extraction. Indians may not, and Orientals certainly do not have as high a rate of mental retardation as Negroes. However, since Negroes comprise the great majority of nonwhites, this will not cause an important bias in these estimates.

with medical conditions have a much greater chance of being institutionalized than those without medical problems. Mortality among the latter group is probably no greater than for the population generally.

If it were assumed that all of the mildly retarded not encompassed by the survey had no more than an average risk of death, then excess mortality among the mildly retarded would be only 1.06 times normal. This is undoubtedly too low. However, it is probable that mortality among the mildly retarded is nearer to 1.06 times average than 1.9 times average, because of the strong element of adverse selection in the higher figure and because about 75% of the mildly retarded are apparently free of major physical handicaps (as will be discussed later in this chapter). We will assume an excess mortality rate of 25% among the mildly retarded, which is the approximate figure that would be derived if we assume that 75% of these persons have normal death rates and 25% have death rates that are 1.9 times normal.

Table 10 shows our estimates of the age-race-specific rates of mild mental retardation. The effect of excess mortality on the prevalence of mild mental retardation was calculated on the basis of age-specific mortality rates for the total population. Had age-race-specific mortality rates been used, higher mortality among nonwhites would have caused a slightly greater decrease with age in the prevalence of mild retardation. Age-race-specific mortality rates were not used because the bulk of mild retardation among nonwhites is probably culturally based, which should lower the rate of excess mortality. In addition, mild retardation

Table 10.   Estimated prevalence of mild mental retardation (IQ 50–69) by age and race (per 100 persons)

Age	White	Nonwhite	Combined white and nonwhite[a]
Under 5	1.4	11.8	3.2
5–9	1.4	11.8	3.0
10–14	1.4	11.8	2.9
15–19	1.4	11.8	2.8
20–24	1.4	11.7	2.6
25–29	1.4	11.7	2.6
30–34	1.4	11.7	2.6
35–44	1.4	11.6	2.5
45–54	1.4	11.5	2.4
55–64	1.3	11.0	2.2
65–69	1.2	10.4	2.0

[a]The white and nonwhite rates are weighted by the relative percentages of each racial group in each age group. The decreasing proportion of nonwhites as older age groups are considered is part of the reason for the decrease in the combined rate with age.

among nonwhites rose slightly with age in the Imre study. No adjustment was made in these estimates for the effect of higher mortality in past years. Because of the relatively small excess mortality among the mildly retarded, such an adjustment would be slight.

NUMBER OF MENTALLY RETARDED

Table 11 shows estimates of the number of mentally retarded, by selected age and IQ groupings, based on the rates developed in the previous two sections and the 1968 and 1970 populations. Prevalence rates for children under 5 with IQs below 50 were increased by 5% to allow for those who die between the ages of 1 to 5. No adjustment was made for the large number who die during the first year of life. The prevalence rates for persons 65 to 69 were imputed to all persons 65 and over, although this figure does not appear too useful in view of the increasing numbers of senile aged whose needs and problems are often indistinguishable from those of retardates.

Table 11. Estimated number of persons in specified IQ ranges by age, United States, 1968 and 1970 (in 000's)

IQ	Age				
	0 to 4	5 to 19	20 to 64	65 and over	0 to 64
			1968		
0–24	24	71	94	7	189
25–49	57	166	232	25	455
50–69	605	1,699	2,529	369	4,833
Total	686	1,936	2,855	401	5,477
			1970		
0–24	25	72	96	7	193
25–49	58	169	237	26	464
50–69	618	1,734	2,582	376	4,934
Total	701	1,975	2,915	409	5,591

Although there were an estimated 5.6 million retarded persons under age 65 in the United States in 1970 who had IQs under 70—almost exactly 3% of the population—most were mildly retarded; 88.2% had IQs between 50 and 70, 8.3% had IQs between 25 and 50, and 3.5% had IQs below 25. The overall estimate of the prevalence of mental retardation is almost identical to what would be predicted if intelligence were normally distributed with a mean of 100 and a standard deviation of

16. A closer scrutiny of the demographic composition of mental retardation, however, destroys any resemblance to the normal distribution curve.

Among children, the prevalence of mental retardation is slightly greater, and among adults slightly less than predicted by the normal distribution curve. The normal curve would indicate that there should be 167,000 persons under age 65 with IQs between 25 and 49 in 1970 and only about 600 with IQs below 25. Our estimates are 464,000 and 193,000 respectively.

Among whites the prevalence of mental retardation is just slightly over half of what would be predicted by the normal distribution curve; among nonwhites the prevalence is about four times the predicted rate. It is a fortuitous balancing of these unpredicted rates that made the estimate of the total prevalence of mental retardation almost identical to what would be predicted by the normal distribution curve.

PHYSICAL AND BEHAVIORAL HANDICAPS

Many retardates suffer physical or emotional handicaps which greatly complicate their vocational, social, and academic adjustment. In this section, we will estimate the prevalence of selected handicaps among the retarded and assess the extent to which retardation exists among groups defined by selected handicaps other than retardation.

One difficulty in such an evaluation is that most physical and emotional handicaps are as difficult to define operationally as mental retardation. Handicaps usually range from the barely noticeable to the totally incapacitating. Any survey of the prevalence of potentially handicapping conditions will find a very large proportion of the population suffering from such conditions, although in most cases they will not impose any significant restriction on the individual. For example, National Health Survey figures indicate that one-half of the population suffers from one or more chronic conditions, but that only one of every twelve persons reports any limitation in their major activity. We must not overstate the problem of multiple handicaps by dramatizing a large number of minor and relatively unrestricting conditions. Another difficulty is the usual one of fragmented, inadequate data and ill-defined studies.

The following discussion will be primarily concerned with multiple handicaps among retarded children, largely because there is an almost complete lack of such information about noninstitutionalized retarded adults. The prevalence of multiple handicaps will be considerably higher among retarded adults than among retarded children because of the greater prevalence of almost all types of handicaps among adults.

Hearing loss. Kodman reviewed studies of the prevalence of hearing loss among the retarded and concluded that hearing loss among retarded children was three to four times that of public school children.[29] Health Examination Survey tests conducted by the National Center for Health Statistics found that 2.9% of the population would have difficulty with normal speech because of a hearing impairment, and over one-third of these persons would have difficulty with loud speech.[30] Much of the hearing loss in the population is concentrated among persons over 45. Significant hearing loss occurs less than 1% of the time among children, so that if Kodman is correct, serious hearing loss among mentally retarded children would occur in about 3% of the cases. Total deafness occurs only about 0.1% of the time among school-age children.[31]

Levinson reported a hearing problem among 1.6% of the school-age retarded children in her survey and a serious hearing problem among 0.34%. The latter figure is in accordance with the Kodman prediction and is probably reasonably accurate, since serious hearing loss can usually be detected among the mildly and moderately retarded. The former figure probably understates the true prevalence of hearing problems. Imperfect hearing often goes unrecognized, especially among persons unable to effectively describe their problems or to respond to standard testing techniques for hearing. In one study, an auditory problem was mentioned in the patient's file in only one-third of the cases of persons with suspected hearing loss.[32]

The prevalence of mental retardation among persons with *severe* hearing defects (the other way of looking at the problem) appears to be considerably above average. A 1968 survey in California found that about 15% of the deaf children of school age in the state were retarded.[33] In a national survey of facilities for the deaf in 1960, it was reported that 4.9% of the students in public day classes or schools for

[29] Frank Kodman, Jr., "Sensory Processes and Mental Deficiency," in *Handbook of Mental Deficiency*, Norman R. Ellis, ed. (New York: McGraw-Hill, 1963), p. 467.

[30] *Health, Education and Welfare Trends*, 1966–67 edition, Part 1, *National Trends*, pp. 5–25.

[31] Paul A. Harper, *Preventive Pediatrics* (New York: Appleton-Century-Crofts, 1962), p. 447.

[32] Clarence Webb et al., *Procedures for Evaluating the Hearing of the Mentally Retarded*, Cooperative Research Project No. 1731 of the Cooperative Research Program, Office of Education, U.S. Department of Health, Education, and Welfare, p. 115.

[33] Myron Leenhouts, "The Mentally Retarded Deaf Child," *Proceedings of the Thirty-ninth Meeting of the Convention of American Instructors of the Deaf*, U.S. Senate Document No. 62, 86th Congress, 2nd Session (Washington, D.C.: USGPO, 1960), p. 56.

the deaf and 5.0% of the students in public residential schools for the deaf were retarded.[34] This survey evidently understated the actual number of retarded. A study by Frisina reported that 10% to 12% of the students in residential schools for the deaf were retarded.[35] The percentage of retarded children in facilities for the deaf would understate the true prevalence of retardation among the deaf, since many deaf retardates are cared for in facilities for the retarded.

All things considered, the California estimate that 15% of deaf children are retarded appears reasonable, although it must be emphasized that it applies only to children with *serious* hearing loss. In terms of the overall problem of retardation, the number of deaf child retardates does not loom large. Using Levinson's estimate that 0.34% of the retarded have serious hearing problems would yield an estimate of about 6,700 for the 5 to 19 age group in 1970 (all subsequent estimates of the number of retarded with handicapping conditions will be based on the 1970 estimates).

An alternative estimate can be derived on the basis that 0.1% of 5- to 19-year-olds are profoundly deaf and that the rate of retardation among them is 15%. This would lead to an estimate of 9,000 deaf child retardates. The two estimates are reasonably close, and we can conclude that there are between 6,000 and 9,000 retardates of school age in the United States with serious hearing problems. There are, of course, many more retarded children with lesser hearing problems.

Loss of sight. Levinson reported that 0.77% of the retarded had severe visual problems. If less serious visual defects are included, the figure rises to 2.31%. The latter figure is presumably low, since it is based on respondent replies, in most cases without the benefit of clinical examination.

Several studies of the blind have reported high rates of retardation. A comprehensive 1956 study of blind children in New York State reported that 21% had known IQs below 75.[36] IQ was unknown in one-fourth of the cases. Of these retarded blind children with known IQs, almost one-third had IQs below 25 and almost as many had IQs between 25 and 50.

In a study encompassing almost three-fourths of the pupils in residential schools for the blind, it was reported that 25% of the children

[34] *American Annals of the Deaf* (January 1961): 129, 151, 152, 157.

[35] Dominic Robert Frisina, *A Psychological Study of the Mentally Retarded* cited in *Dissertation Abstracts*, 1955, p. 2288.

[36] William M. Cruickshank and Matthew J. Trippe, *Services to Blind Children in New York State* (Syracuse: Syracuse University Press, 1959), p. 73.

were retarded.[37] In view of the large number of cases of unknown intellectual status in the New York study, this is probably a closer indication of the prevalence of mental retardation among the blind.

Levinson's rate for severe visual problems among the retarded would indicate that about 15,000 retardates between the ages of 5 and 19 are blind. If we estimate the total number of blind children in this age group by extrapolating the New York State experience to the nation and assume that one in four of these children will be retarded, then this would indicate that about 7,700 blind children will be retarded. This estimate is considerably lower than the one based on the Levinson study.

At least one other study supports the lower figure. In a study of about 9,000 *multiply*-impaired blind children between the ages of 6 and 21 in 1966, 4,700 were retarded (IQ 0–75).[38] The author believed that his sample constituted about two-thirds of the total population of multiply-impaired blind children. If so, then, allowing for population growth, there should be about 7,400 blind retarded children between the ages of 6 and 21. We can only conclude that there are between 7,000 and 15,000 retardates of school age who are blind. There will, of course, be many more thousands of retarded children with less severe visual problems.

Cerebral palsy. Levinson reported that 1% of retarded children in Maine had cerebral palsy. A study of 406 retarded children, 7 to 14 years of age, in Edinburgh in 1964, found that 16% had cerebral palsy.[39] The former rate seems unduly low and the latter rate exceptionally high. Definitional differences may account for part of this variation. In addition, reliance on nonmedical assessments may have depressed the rate in Levinson's study. The high rate in Edinburgh is at least partly attributable to the fact that many mildly retarded persons were not identified, probably over half. Most of these unidentified cases would not have had cerebral palsy.

Cardwell summarized the results of thirteen studies which evaluated the intelligence of cerebral palsied children.[40] In nine studies the per-

[37] James M. Wolf, *The Blind Child with Concomitant Disabilities* (New York: American Foundation for the Blind, 1967), p. 30.

[38] Milton D. Graham, *Multiply-Impaired Blind Children: A National Problem* (American Foundation for the Blind, 1967), p. 49.

[39] C. M. Drillien, S. Jameson, and E. M. Wilkinson, "Studies in Mental Handicap, Part I: Prevalence and Distribution by Clinical Type and Severity of Defect," *Archives of Diseases of Childhood* (October 1966): 531.

[40] Viola Cardwell, *Cerebral Palsy* (New York: Association for the Aid of Crippled Children, 1956), p. 341.

centage of children with IQs below 70 ranged between 40% and 50%. The lowest reported rate was 30% and the highest was 59%. Many of these children are severely retarded. In an assessment of 354 cerebral palsied children in Birmingham and the neighboring counties, 22% had IQs below 50.[41] Another study of 141 cerebral palsied children in Leeds reported that 12% had IQs below 50.[42]

Estimates of the prevalence of cerebral palsy range from 0.1% to 0.2%[43] (depending, in part, on how it is defined). If 0.15% of 5- to 19-year-old children suffer from cerebral palsy, then there would be about 91,000 cerebral palsied children in this age range in the United States. If 45% of these are retarded, then about 41,000 would have IQs below 70. This would indicate that about 2% of the retarded suffer from this additional handicap, which is the best estimate that can be derived from existing data.

Epilepsy. Epilepsy was reported in 7.2% of the cases in the Lemkau study, 1.5% of the cases in the Levinson study, and 9.6% of the cases in the Edinburgh study. Most of this variation is undoubtedly due to differences in the way epilepsy was defined. Almost all of the cases of epilepsy reported in the Levinson study were severe. The Lemkau and Edinburgh studies, on the other hand, apparently included all persons with a history of convulsions, even though isolated occurrences of convulsions are not uncommon among young children and do not necessarily indicate epilepsy.[44] In addition, Lemkau felt that his rate may be high because epileptics are more likely to be psychologically tested than nonepileptics.

The percentage of epileptics who are retarded is considerably above average. In a study of children treated for epilepsy in Contra Costa and San Bernadino counties, California, 37% were diagnosed as mentally retarded.[45] In another study of epileptic children admitted to a Los Angeles hospital, it was reported that 21% had IQs below 70.[46]

[41] Patricia Asher and F. Eleanor Schonell, "A Survey of 400 Cases of Cerebral Palsy in Childhood," *Archives of Diseases of Childhood* (January 1950): 375.

[42] Irene M. Holoran, "The Incidence and Prognosis of Cerebral Palsy," *British Medical Journal* (January 26, 1952): 215.

[43] Paul A. Harper, *Preventive Pediatrics* (New York: Appleton-Century-Crofts, 1962), p. 447; Asher and Schonell, "A Survey of 400 Cases of Cerebral Palsy," p. 361; Holoran, "Incidence and Prognosis of Cerebral Palsy," p. 216.

[44] Given a sufficiently high temperature or sufficient tension anyone may be subject to a convulsion.

[45] *Children with Epilepsy and the California Crippled Children Services Program, A Report to the State Legislature*, January 1963, p. 35.

[46] Ellen B. Sullivan and Lawrence Gahagan, "On Intelligence of Epileptic Children," *Genetic Psychology Monographs* (October 1935): 333.

The subjects of these studies represent the more serious cases and therefore overstate the prevalence of retardation among all epileptics. Estimates of the prevalence of epilepsy range from 0.5 to 2%. The higher figure represents the more recent estimates and encompasses mild cases that are sometimes overlooked. If we take the mean value of this range of estimates and assume that 10% of these have IQs below 70, it can be estimated that about 4% of the retarded have epilepsy, about 75,000 in the case of 5- to 19-year-old children. This estimate probably errs on the low side.

Psychiatric disorders. Lemkau explicitly explored the relationship between psychiatric disorders and mental retardation. Of almost 700 mental deficients located by the study, 9.7% were psychotic or had psychotic traits, 6.6% were classified as adult neurotics, and 24.8% had other forms of personality disorder. In total, over 40% of the mentally retarded had a psychiatric problem.

Looked at from the other point of view: "of the 393 psychotics and persons with psychotic traits included in the survey, 17.0 percent were mentally defective; of the 425 'adult neurotics,' 10.8 percent were mentally defective; and of the group with other forms of personality disorder, 16.0 percent showed mental deficiency." Lemkau hesitated to infer a close association between mental deficiency and mental illness. It seemed "more likely that the large number of mentally deficient cases among those with personality disorders is an expression of the forces active in bringing individuals to attention for social case work, psychiatric examination, and psychometric testing."

Despite this disclaimer, it is generally agreed that mental retardates are more prone to behavioral disturbances than most other people.[47] Indeed, in view of the frustrations of the retarded, their frequent exclusion from normal activity, and the indifferent and occasionally cruel way in which many are treated, one wonders how they can escape some form of personality disorder. Wortis reported that "about 80% of the retarded children seen at our clinic present some associated psychiatric problems, and at least 5% could be diagnosed as primarily schizophrenic." Excessive fearfulness, found in 24% of the cases, was a major problem.[48]

It is one thing to say that most of the mentally retarded enjoy something less than perfect mental health and another to categorize

[47] Delton C. Beier, "Behavioral Disturbances in the Mentally Retarded," in *Mental Retardation, A Review of Research*, Harvey A. Stevens and Rick Heber, eds. (Chicago: The University of Chicago Press, 1964), p. 454.

[48] Joseph Wortis, "Schizophrenic Symptomatology in Mentally Retarded Children," *American Journal of Psychiatry* (November 1958): 430.

mild personality disturbances as mental illness. The criteria employed by various investigators will, therefore, greatly affect estimates of the prevalence of psychiatric disorders among the retarded. Lemkau, for example, undoubtedly employed more stringent criteria for mental illness than Wortis. For the present, the Lemkau study provides the best base by which to estimate the association of mental retardation and mental illness—or at least the extent to which psychiatric problems among the retarded are sufficiently severe to attract attention.

Multiple handicaps. A mentally retarded person suffering from an additional psychiatric and physical disorder is, by definition, multiply-handicapped. Frequently, the mentally retarded suffer from *two or more* additional handicaps. Over half of 62 epileptic and retarded children found in one California study had at least one other associated handicap: 19 had cerebral palsy, 12 had severe emotional problems, and one had cerebral palsy *and* severe emotional problems.[49]

In a recent study of 240 deaf-blind children in California, it was reported that over two-thirds were mentally retarded. The average number of handicaps for these retarded deaf-blind children was in excess of four.[50] Three out of four of 220 blind and retarded children in public institutions in New York in 1956 (most in institutions for the retarded) had one or more additional physical disabilities, the most common being cerebral palsy (34%) and epilepsy (23%).[51]

In the previously mentioned study by Wolf it was reported that two out of three of 453 children attending special classes for the mentally retarded in residential schools for the blind had three or more disabilities. Personality and speech defects were the most common (30% and 29%). Cerebral palsy occurred in 6% of the cases and epilepsy in 9%—much lower percentages than those found among the blind mentally retarded in public mental institutions in the New York study mentioned in the preceding paragraph. It is obviously speculative to generalize from such fragmented data. On the other hand, even this limited data points out clearly that a significant number of the mentally retarded have two or more disabilities in addition to mental retardation.

Physical handicaps by severity of retardation. Only one epidemiological study, the Edinburgh study, has assessed the relationship between physical handicaps and severity of retardation.[52] The results are

---

[49] *Children with Epilepsy and the California Crippled Children Services Program*, p. 36.

[50] Berthold Lowenfeld, *Multihandicapped Blind and Deaf-Blind Children in California*, a report submitted to the California State Department of Education, Division of Special Schools and Services, May 1968, pp. 78, 80.

[51] Cruickshank and Trippe, *Services to Blind Children*, p. 201.

[52] Drillien et al., "Studies in Mental Handicap," p. 531.

striking. Almost 95% of those with IQs below 30 and almost 78% of those with IQs between 30 and 55 suffered from at least one major physically handicapping condition. Among the mildly retarded, this percentage declined markedly to 37%.

Table 12. Physical handicaps by IQ level for Edinburgh children aged 7–14

Clinical type	IQ and percentage of cases		
	0–29	30–54	55–69
No other abnormality	5.6%	22.4%	62.8%
Epilepsy[a]	11.3	7.5	10.6
Cerebral palsy[b]	46.5	11.6	6.9
Down's syndrome	14.1	40.9	1.6
Other major recognizable conditions[c]	22.5	17.6	18.1
Total	100.0	100.0	100.0
	(71 cases)	(147 cases)	(188 cases)

[a] Cases without other defects or with other defects causing little additional handicap.

[b] Includes cerebral palsied with epilepsy or other defects.

[c] Many children in this group had multiple congenital abnormalities. Some had a single defect such as blindness or deafness. Also included were children with phenylketonuria, the cerebral lipoidoses, hydrocephalus, etc.

There is little reason to doubt the accuracy of the Edinburgh figures for the severely retarded. However, they probably overstate the prevalence of physical handicaps among the mildly retarded. The study directors believed that they failed to locate about one-sixth of the mildly retarded. Even if these additional cases are added to the survey results the estimated prevalence of mild retardation among children age 7 to 14 would be only 0.63%—about half the comparable rate for white children in the United States. It is unlikely that the prevalence of mental retardation in Edinburgh is that much lower than in the United States, so that the number of missed cases may be substantially greater than estimated by the study directors. It is probable that the missed individuals suffer from fewer physical ailments than those cases which were located.

Another consideration in the United States is that a disproportionate number of nonwhites are mildly retarded. If part of the reason for this disparity is lack of adequate learning stimuli, then it is unlikely that these culturally deprived retardates suffer the same proportionate number of physical handicaps as the genetically inadequate.

Observations. Slightly over 30% of retarded children suffer additional physical handicaps, and perhaps 40% suffer psychiatric problems. These percentages cannot be summed because they overlap, but it is probable that at least one in two retarded children are multiply-handicapped. It is necessary to note that this ratio will be considerably higher among retarded adults (because of the natural increase of physical infirmities with age) and among the more severely retarded. Among persons with IQs below 25, the prevalence of multiply-handicapping conditions is almost universal. Among mildly retarded children, the prevalence of multiply-handicapping conditions is probably about 25%.

SUMMARY

This has been a long and laborious explanation of existing epidemiological data relevant to mental retardation. Although many crucial issues were posed, few definite answers emerged. Some important questions could not be answered at all. And many conclusions depended upon weakly supported assumptions that will be modified as future research generates improved information.

Yet such an effort was necessary. A meaningful evaluation of the effects of mental retardation and of programs for the retarded could not be undertaken without an understanding of the size and the many dimensions of this extremely complex problem that arises from a wide number of genetic, neurological, and environmental causes, has strikingly different levels of severity, and is often complicated by physical and psychiatric handicaps which interfere with social adjustment.

The major points of this chapter are:

1. Although there are over 200 known causes of mental retardation, they can, in general, be summarized under three headings: brain damage, poor genetic endowment, and deprivation resulting from environmental conditions and the sensory limitations imposed by physical and mental handicaps.

2. Epidemiological studies of the prevalence of mental retardation have produced widely varying results, most of which are explainable by differences in the definition of mental retardation, differences in methods of identifying the retarded, and differences in the demographic characteristics of the population being sampled.

3. Overall, an estimated 5.6 million persons in the United States under the age of 65 have IQs below 70—slightly over 3% of the population. About one in eight has an IQ below 50.

4. Nonwhites are six to seven times more likely to have IQs below 70 than whites, and the children of the poor are about thirteen times

more likely to be retarded than the children of the middle and upper classes.

5. The high prevalence of mental retardation in urban ghettos and in isolated rural areas is largely explainable in terms of the racial and socioeconomic composition of these areas. The limited opportunities for environmental stimulation probably contribute to a perpetuation of poor socioeconomic conditions.

6. Physical and psychiatric handicaps occur frequently among the retarded, especially the more severely intellectually limited.

III

The Etiology of Mental Retardation

In the previous chapter the major causes of mental retardation were classified as poor genetic endowment, brain damage, and environmental or sensory deprivation. The relative importance of these causative factors, however, cannot be assessed precisely. In fact, a precise cause of mental retardation can be clearly diagnosed in only about one-fourth of the cases.

It was also concluded that the prevalence of mental retardation is considerably above average among nonwhites, the physically and psychiatrically handicapped, and the lowest socioeconomic classes. In the latter case we are referring to the prevalence among children born to lower social class parents. One would expect that most adult retardates would be in the lower social classes. Explanations of the significance of these demographic variations have ranged from denials that such variations have validity to assertions that particular demographic groups are genetically inferior.

In this chapter we will examine the major issues concerning the relative importance of the causes of retardation and the explanation of demographic differences, topics which are highly interrelated.

Findings of excessive rates of retardation among particular demographic groups are often criticized on the grounds that intelligence tests that are standardized on white, middle-class populations cannot be used to gauge the intelligence of groups with different cultural backgrounds and perspectives on life, and, in the case of the handicapped, different sensory perceptions. If intelligence tests are rigidly interpreted as a measure of innate intelligence, such criticisms have considerable validity. But if intelligence tests are interpreted as a measure of the qualities needed for success in modern society, then such criticisms are of questionable value. A low intelligence test score, for whatever cause, is a clear indication of the need for some type of remedial action.[1]

Part of the explanation for the uneven distribution of the prevalence of mental retardation is probably due to the increased hazard of brain injury among certain demographic groups. This is obviously an important reason for the high rates of mental retardation among the physically disabled.

Although brain damage or malformation is indisputably an important cause of mental retardation, estimates of the prevalence of brain injury among the retarded vary widely. On one point, however, there is general agreement. Severe retardation (IQ less than 50) usually results from brain injury or malformation. This is suggested by the enormous prevalence of physically disabling conditions among the severely retarded and has been fairly conclusively verified on the basis of autopsy reports.

In reviewing the results of 1,410 successive autopsies performed in 3 hospitals in California over a 14-year period, Malamud found neurologic damage in 97.5% of the cases.[2] About 90% of these autopsies were performed on persons classified as "idiots" or "imbeciles."

In the Imre study, severe retardation was highest among Negroes and the lower socioeconomic groups and was most common among the lowest socioeconomic class of Negroes, where almost 2% of school-age children had IQs below 50. If severe retardation primarily results from brain damage, then brain damage must be more extensive among these demographic groups.

The extent of brain damage among the mildly retarded cannot be assessed. Malamud reported that brain pathology was 2½ times more prevalent among the severely retarded than among the mildly retarded, and also that the former suffered more severe lesions. Thus, although Malamud did not supply this information, it would appear that the incidence of brain injury or malformation among the mildly retarded in his sample was of the order of 35 to 40%. Since the Malamud survey

[1] In a 1965 follow-up study of 312 Negro children who had been tested for IQ in 1960, Kennedy found that the Stanford-Binet IQ was an excellent predictor of academic achievement. Wallace A. Kennedy, *A Follow-up Normative Study of Negro Intelligence and Achievement*, Monographs of the Society for Research in Child Development, vol. 34, no. 2 (Chicago: University of Chicago Press, 1968), p. 30.

[2] N. Malamud, "Neuropathology," in *Mental Retardation, A Review of Research*, Harvey A. Stevens and Rick Heber, eds. (Chicago: University of Chicago Press, 1964), pp. 431, 449.

was conducted on an institutional population, this estimate is probably high.

It is clear, however, that brain damage is a significant cause of mild retardation. And if brain damage causing severe retardation is greater among nonwhites and the lower socioeconomc classes, then it is almost certain that less extensive damage causing mild retardation also occurs more frequently among these groups.

Explanations for the greater prevalence of brain injuries among the poor and the nonwhite are not difficult to find. Hurley has summarized much of the evidence on this point.[3] One problem is the lack of adequate prenatal care. Hurley writes (references omitted):

. . . in 1964 in New York City 40.9 percent of all mothers living in four poor housing areas had late or no prenatal care, as compared with 12.3 percent of all mothers living in four good housing areas. At the charity hospital serving the poor of Atlanta, Georgia, some seventy percent of all mothers in 1962 had late or no prenatal care, while at Newark City Hospital in the same year one-third of all maternity patients had received no prenatal care at all.

More than ten percent of all non-white mothers in this country in 1964 gave birth without a physician in attendance, the rate of such births being above twenty percent in several Southern States.

In addition, poor women, as compared to their middle-class counterparts, are likely to be younger when they have their first child and older when they have their last child, are more apt to suffer nutritional and dietary deficiencies, and are more prone to suffer diseases that may damage an unborn child. These factors result in an increased incidence of prematurity and maternal complications associated with childbirth.

In 1966 the rate of fetal deaths among nonwhites was twice as high as among whites; the rate of infant deaths was also twice as high, and maternal deaths were almost three times as high.[4] One can only speculate that differences in infant morbidity roughly parallel these differences in infant mortality.

Infants in poor families who survive unscathed the hazards of birth continue to face above-average hazards. The association of poverty and lead poisoning is well known. Inadequate pediatric care for many poor children leaves them especially susceptible to the ravages of diseases such as meningitis, encephalitis, diphtheria, whooping cough, scarlet fever, nephritis, influenza, and pneumonia.

[3] Rodger L. Hurley, *Poverty and Mental Retardation: A Causal Relationship* (Trenton, New Jersey: State of New Jersey, Department of Institutions and Agencies, Division of Mental Retardation, April 1968), pp. 41–53.

[4] *Statistical Abstract of the United States*, 1968, p. 55.

Differential rates of brain damage, alone, however, cannot explain all of the differences in rates of mental retardation among demographic groups. This leads us into the environment-heredity debate: to what extent are differential rates of retardation among demographic groups due to a combination of environmental deprivation *and* above-average rates of brain damage, and to what extent, if any, are they due to genetic differences?

The importance of this question cannot be overemphasized. If the entire population had the same rate of mental retardation as white children in the three highest social classes (about 1 in every 150 according to the Imre study), the number of retarded persons under the age of 65 would have been only 1,180,000 in 1970. In short, if one assumes that there are no differences in genetic intellectual potential between whites and nonwhites and among the social classes, it could be concluded that almost 80% of mental retardation in the United States is caused by environmental conditions which lead to brain injury or in some other way impede intellectual development. This would be only a small part of the total problem. There would also be millions of Americans functioning intellectually at levels far below their genetic capacity, even though above the threshold of retardation.

This conclusion, however, requires a critical and controversial assumption, i.e., that there are *no* significant differences in the genetic endowment of intelligence among persons of different races or in different social classes. A number of scholars believe that there are, in fact, genetic differences in intelligence between whites and nonwhites and among the various social classes, and they have presented plausible arguments in support of their contentions. Three hypotheses are required to support a genetic explanation of differences in intelligence among demographic groups. The first hypothesis is that there is biological variation in the genes that determine intelligence, just as there is in the genes that determine height, weight, hair color, etc. Since measured intelligence depends upon both environmental and hereditary factors, the obvious problem in demonstrating a genetic basis for differences in intelligence is to separate these two factors. As Burt points out, "the obvious procedure would be to keep first one and then the other as constant as possible, and observe the results in either case."[5]

Burt approached this difficult task in two ways. First, as psychological consultant to the London County Council, he was given free access to orphanages and other residential institutions and was able to study

---

[5] Cyril Burt, "The Inheritance of Mental Ability," *American Psychologist* (January 1958): 6.

the case records of large numbers of children who had been brought up in an environment that was much the same for all since the earliest weeks of infancy. He found "that individual differences in intelligence, so far from being diminished, varied over an unusually wide range."

Second, to secure cases of identical genetic endowment, Burt and his coworkers collected information on over thirty cases of identical twins raised in different homes almost from birth. He reports: "As regards intelligence the outstanding feature is the high correlation between the final assessments for the monozygotic twins, even when reared apart: it is almost as high as the correlation between two successive testings for the same individual."

Other studies confirm Burt's findings. Jensen, reporting on four surveys of identical twins reared apart, found a median correlation of IQ of 0.75 as compared to 0.87 (fourteen studies) for identical twins reared together.[6] If genetic endowment was unimportant, the expected correlation of the IQ of identical twins reared apart would be 0.00.

Advocates of both a genetic and an environmental explanation of the varying rates of mental retardation among demographic groups can accept, and most do, the hypothesis that the contribution of heredity to intelligence varies sharply among individuals. In general, both groups also accept the assertion that intelligence tests do not measure intellectual capacity, but the interaction of genetic endowment and environment. A favorable environment may enable persons to perform at the limit of their genetic potential, but an unfavorable environment may depress intelligence to a greater or lesser extent.

If innate intelligence at birth is conceived of as a series of empty bottles of varying sizes, then environment can be conceived of as one of the forces determining the extent to which each bottle is filled. Intelligence tests measure the contents of each bottle.

Necessarily the resulting distribution of intelligence will be shifted to the left as illustrated by the diagram on the opposite page. The divergence between the two curves measures the effect on IQ of environment plus the effects of brain damage which can, analogously, be described as the accidental breaking or cracking of bottles.

Two points to be made are: (1) half-filled or cracked bottles may fall to the left of smaller, but more completely filled bottles in the distribution of phenotypes; (2) since we do not know the genotypic distribution of intelligence, we cannot be certain as to the extent of divergence between the two curves. In these observations lie the points of conten-

---

[6] Arthur R. Jensen, "How Much Can We Boost IQ and Scholastic Achievement?" *Harvard Educational Review* (Winter 1969): 49.

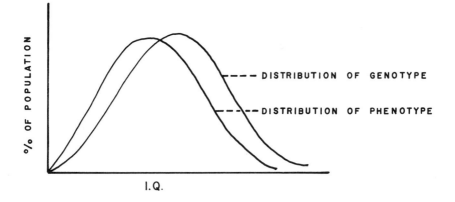

tion between advocates of an environmental and a genetic explanation of the causes of mental retardation.

A second hypothesis needed for a genetic explanation of differences in rates of retardation among various demographic groups is that intellectually subnormal parents will tend to have intellectually subnormal children. This matter is not as straightforward as it appears. A genetic endowment of intelligence is not the result of a single pair of genes, but of multiple genes. At least ten pairs must be involved and perhaps many more.[7]

The polygenic theory of intelligence states that intellectual capacity at conception is determined by a chance combination of genes, half of which are contributed by the father and half by the mother. Now, if each gene specific for intelligence had a small but cumulative effect, then the genetic endowment of a child would, on the average, be midway between the genetic endowments of the parents.

In fact, such a one-to-one relationship between the intelligence of parents and children does not take place. The children of both very bright and very dull parents tend to regress toward the mean.

In genetic theory, there are two mechanisms to explain regression. One is that some genes are recessive and their effects are not manifested unless they are paired with another recessive gene at the same locus in the chromosome. The other explanation, technically termed "epistasis," is that genes are not always independent of each other so the combined effect of two or more genes may be less than, or more than, the sum of their individual effects.

[7] Irving I. Gottesman, "Genetic Aspects of Intelligent Behavior," in *Handbook of Mental Deficiency*, Norman R. Ellis, ed. (New York: McGraw-Hill, 1963), p. 289.

Given the factors of epistasis and recessive genes, it becomes possible to construct plausible *genetic* theories of intelligence which range from predicting no relationship between the intelligence of parents and children to predicting almost complete resemblance between the intelligence of parents and children. Until we understand better the actual mechanics of the way in which genes determine intelligence, the degree to which a child's innate intelligence resembles that of its parents must be inferred through empirical data.

It should be observed that the high correlation of intelligence between identical twins raised apart, although indicating a strong genetic component to intelligence, does *not* demonstrate that the intelligence of children is closely correlated with that of the parents. Yet, it is the latter that must be shown if a genetic explanation for demographic differences in the prevalence of mental retardation is to be supported.

There have been a number of attempts to demonstrate such a correlation. One of the most sophisticated efforts was made by Burt, who studied 954 pairs of sibs between the ages of 8 and 13. He assessed the intelligence of at least one of the parents and divided both children and parents into three groups—bright, average, and dull—in the proportions 1:2:1.[8] The correlation between the intelligence of child and parent was 0.481. This corresponded closely with a theoretical value estimated by Burt on the assumptions of complete dominance, assortive mating, and Mendelian segregation. Moreover, Burt noted that differences in intellect are themselves a function of genetic variability and concluded that "at least 75 percent of the entire variance must be due to genetic influences, probably far more." In a later article, Burt stated that as much as 88 percent of the variance may be due to genetic variables.[9]

Additional evidence for the transmittibility of intelligence is derived from kinship studies. Jensen has recently summarized almost all such correlations reported in the literature. In general, he found a close relationship between the theoretical value of the correlation of IQs of relatives and the actual correlation.[10]

Perhaps the most alarming evidence on the transmittibility of mental retardation is derived from studies of the relatives of retardates. Such studies have a long history beginning in 1877 with Robert L. Dugdale's study of "The Jukes." The frightening results of most of these early studies have been largely discounted because of a lack of objectivity in assessing mental retardation.

[8] Cyril Burt, "The Evidence for the Concept of Intelligence," *British Journal of Educational Psychology* (November 1955): 172–73.

[9] Burt, "Inheritance of Mental Ability," p. 9.

[10] Jensen, "How Much Can We Boost IQ?" p. 49.

The Reeds have summarized the results of recent studies of this nature as an introduction to their own massive study.[11] They began with 289 patients with IQ scores below 70 who had been institutionalized between 1911 and 1918 in Minnesota. An investigation was made of as many of the descendants of the patients' grandparents as could be found. The sample finally consisted of over 80,000 persons of whom 2.7% were retarded.

Of the original 289 patients, 28% of their first-degree relatives (parents, sibs, and children) were retarded, compared to 7.1% of second-degree relatives (grandparents, uncles, aunts, half-sibs, nephews, nieces, and grandchildren), and 3.1% of third-degree relatives. The Reeds noted that "these must be underestimates because all persons of unknown intelligence were counted as normal."

Fourteen hundred and fifty retardates were located other than the original patients, their parents, or grandparents. Of this group, 48.3% had at least one retarded parent. This corresponded closely with a figure of 49.8% for the original group of patients.

The Reeds concluded that mental retardation was highly transmittible. Two startling conclusions were that "1 to 2 percent of the population, composed of fertile retardates, produced 36.1 percent of the retardates of the next generation . . ." and that approximately five-sixths of the retarded "would have at least one parent, or an aunt or uncle, who is or was, retarded."

The Reeds also surmised that very little retardation was due to social deprivation. They argued that about 1% of the population would be retarded as a result of Down's syndrome, rare recessive genes, and obvious calamaties, such as syphilis, and that "on any polygenic theory of intelligence we are forced to assume an appreciable fraction of the retarded to be the result of the unfavorable multiple gene combinations." Thus, "we have surprisingly little residue of our 2 to 3 percent of the population which is retarded and which could be ascribed as primarily the result of social deprivation."

This is an unwarranted conclusion. The normal curve of the distribution of intelligence is derived by assessing phenotypes, not genotypes as the Reeds' conclusion requires. Although most retarded undoubtedly have below-average intellectual potential, it may well require a combination of an adverse environment and poor heredity to push many below the threshold of retardation. In the *absence* of social deprivation, the prevalence of mental retardation may be substantially less than 2% to 3%.

---

[11] Elizabeth W. Reed and Sheldon C. Reed, *Mental Retardation: A Family Study* (Philadelphia: W. B. Saunders Co., 1965), p. 206.

That there is a significant relationship between the IQ of parents and children can hardly be questioned. But this does not prove that the relationship is genetically determined, since it could be caused by a similar environment as well as common genes.

There is one bit of evidence, however, that is difficult to explain on other than genetic grounds. Skodak and Skeels found that the correlation between the IQs of foster children and their *true* mothers was 0.44 when the former were 13 years of age, while there was *no* correlation between the IQs of foster children and their *foster* mother's educational level.[12] Other studies have reported slightly higher correlations between foster children and their true mothers and verified the lack of correlation of IQ between foster children and their foster mothers.

A correlation between the IQ of the true parent and a foster child, however, is not sufficient to prove the genetic inferiority of a particular subgroup in society, even if the average IQ of that group is considerably below average. If foster children are placed in an environment superior to that of their true mothers, the net effect may be to move the IQ distribution of the children to a higher level without disturbing the correlation of IQ between the true parent and foster child. Of course, such a shift in the intellectual distribution could hardly occur quite this smoothly, so we would expect the correlation to be lower than between children and parents generally.

A *third* hypothesis needed to support a genetic explanation of demographic differences in rates of retardation is that environment has only a small effect on intelligence test performance. If environment causes a small part of the variance of intelligence, it necessarily follows that the bulk of social class and race differences in intelligence are due to genetic factors. Jensen has recently suggested that this may, in fact, be the case.[13]

A genetic explanation of these differences is straightforward. As Jensen observes: " . . . genetic differences are manifested in virtually every anatomical, physiological, and biochemical comparison one can make between representative samples of identifiable racial groups. There is no reason to suppose that the brain should be exempt from this generalization." In the case of social class, the dullards of society tend to fall into the lowest class, to marry within it, and, if the genetic hypothesis is correct, to transmit their intellectual inadequacies to future generations.

[12] Marie Skodak and H. M. Skeels, "A Final Follow-Up Study of One Hundred Adopted Children," *Journal of Genetic Psychology* (1949): 110.

[13] Jensen, "How Much Can We Boost IQ?"

Jensen did not deny the importance of environment to intellectual development. In his words: "There can be no doubt that moving children from an extremely deprived environment to good average environmental circumstances can boost the IQ some 20 to 30 points and in certain extremely rare cases as much as 60 to 70 points." He emphasizes, however, that "it is doubtful that psychologists have found consistent evidence for any social environmental influences short of extreme environmental isolation which have a marked systematic effect on intelligence."

To sum up the discussion thus far, three hypotheses are needed for a genetic explanation of the demographic differences in the prevalence of mental retardation: (1) genetic variability of intellectual potential; (2) transmission of below-average intellectual potential to future generations; and (3) minimal effect of environment on intellectual performance. Logically and empirically, the first hypothesis appears indisputable. The second hypothesis is supported by foster child studies. The third hypothesis, however, is more suspect, largely on the basis of evidence from foster child studies.

It cannot be denied that the IQs of foster children correlate more closely with their biological parents than with their adoptive parents. Most foster child studies have also found, however, that the average IQ of foster children is above the national average,[14] well above the average IQ of the biological mothers, and close to what would be expected for the natural children of the adoptive parents. Moreover, the average IQs of adopted children are considerably higher the earlier they are removed from the home of their natural parents. Although these observations support the hypothesis of genetic variability of intelligence and the transmission of intelligence from parent to child, they also indicate that there is a *substantial* environmental influence on intelligence that begins at birth and persists throughout most of childhood.

Consider these findings. Skodak and Skeels followed the lives of 100 children who were placed in adoptive homes between 1933 and 1937.[15] The great majority were under 6 months of age at the time of adoption. Some thirteen years later, the average IQ of these children was 117. The IQs of 63 of the true mothers were known and averaged some 20 points below those of their children (although the correlation between the IQs of the true mothers and their children was 0.44). Skeels and Skodak considered two groups of children: one whose mothers were known

---

[14] Boyd R. McCandless, "Environment and Intellectual Functioning," *Mental Retardation, A Review of Research*, Harvey A. Stevens and Rick Heber, eds. (Chicago: The University of Chicago Press, 1964), p. 186.

[15] Skodak and Skeels, "Follow-up Study," pp. 112–14.

to have IQs below 70 and the other whose mothers had IQs above 105. The average IQs of these two groups at the time of final test were 106 and 130, which would indicate substantial genetic transmission of intelligence, although, as Skeels and Skodak point out, selective placement could also be a factor. The children in the high-IQ group had been placed in far superior homes.

A study by Speer of 59 adopted children found an average increase in IQ of 5.1 points after a short period in the adoptive home.[16] Speer reported that most of these children had come from unsuitable natural parents and homes of a low economic level. Those placed before the age of 2 had a median IQ of 103, while those who were not adopted until after the age of 12 had an IQ of 79, with intermediate ages having intermediate IQs. Adoption into superior homes reversed the downward trend in intelligence, but could not completely undo the damage that had been done to older children.

One of the most striking studies of foster children has recently been summarized by Skeels.[17] In the early 1930s, 13 children under 3 years of age were transferred from an Iowa orphanage to an institution for the mentally retarded as "house guests." At the time of transfer, their mean IQ was 65, and they were generally believed unsuited for adoption. The children were placed with older mentally retarded girls who became very fond of them and provided extensive individual care. The children remained in the institution for an average of one and one half years. Substantial increases in IQ were reported for all 13 children. At the end of the experimental period their average IQ was 92. Eleven of the children were adopted. One remained in the institution until adulthood, and another was returned to the institution after a time at the orphanage. Individual intelligence tests were given to all of the children approximately 2½ years after the close of the experimental period. Their average IQ had risen further to 96, and only two tested below 90.

A contrast group of 12 children of approximately the same age remained in the orphanage, which was described as an extremely bleak and unstimulating environment. Although the average IQ of this group was originally 87 they were not, for various reasons including possible mental retardation, considered immediately suitable for adoption. The average IQ of the contrast group declined to 66 and at one point fell to 60 during approximately the same period as the experimental group.

[16] George S. Speer, "The Intelligence of Foster Children," *Journal of Genetic Psychology* (September 1940): 49–55.

[17] Harold M. Skeels, *Adult Status of Children with Contrasting Early Life Experiences* (Chicago: Society for Research in Child Development, 1966).

On the basis of occupation and educational history, Skeels concluded that the true parents of both the environmental and contrast group represented the lower levels in society. IQs were known for five of the mothers in the experimental group and nine of the mothers in the contrast group. The mean IQ for the former was 70 and for the latter 63.

In view of the results of adoptive studies, on what grounds can the effect of environment be challenged? One problem is that there is a selective factor which tends to exclude low-IQ orphans from the study results. Obviously retarded children are usually screened out as unsuitable for adoption.[18] In addition, adoptive parents frequently have the option of returning a mentally retarded child.[19] The importance of these factors cannot be assessed, but they are probably minor among adopted infants (those under the age of 1), and it is precisely in this group that the highest IQs are eventually found.[20]

Jensen relied heavily on studies of adopted children by Leahy and by Burks, both of which found a relatively small correlation between the intelligence of foster children and an environmental rating of their foster homes.[21] However, in both of these studies the adopted children being investigated went into above-average and often superior homes. Burks estimated that the average mental age of the foster parents was between two and three years above the population average. Leahy observed that: "The distribution of homes of the children in this investigation are probably somewhat skewed towards a superior level. Adoptive homes of even the lowest occupational and economic levels are undoubtedly superior in respect to other traits since society's control and imposition of standards on this type of home is much greater than on the ordinary home." Jensen's belief that above "a certain threshold of environmental adequacy . . . environmental variations cause relatively small differences in intelligence" appears to be borne out by these studies. But because of the superior nature of the adoptive homes, it would be difficult to infer from these studies that this hypothetical

[18] McCandless, "Intellectual Functioning," p. 186.

[19] Rick Heber, Richard Dever, and Julianne Conry, "The Influence of Environmental and Genetic Variables on Intellectual Development," in *Behavioral Research in Mental Retardation*, J. J. Prehm, L. A. Hamerlynck, and J. E. Crosson, eds. (Eugene, Oregon: University of Oregon Press, 1968), p. 16.

[20] Skodak and Skeels, "Follow-up Study," p. 91.

[21] Barbara S. Burks, "The Relative Influence of Nature and Nurture upon Mental Development: A Comparative Study of Parent-Foster Child Resemblance and True Parent-True Child Resemblance," in *Yearbook of the National Society for the Study of Education, 1928*, pp. 219–316. Alice M. Leahy, "Nature-Nurture and Intelligence," *Genetic Psychology Monographs* (June 1935): 241–305.

threshold is much, if at all, below average environmental conditions for the population as a whole. It is noteworthy that the foster children in these studies had IQs that were above average and similar to the IQs of the natural children of their adoptive parents, which ought to say something for the importance of environment.

Jensen attempted to explain away the remarkable results of the Skeels study by distinguishing between the culturally disadvantaged and the severely deprived. The orphanage children were, of course, severely deprived, and lower-class children were culturally disadvantaged. He observed that the culturally disadvantaged do not suffer from the extreme sensory and motor deprivation that characterized the children in the Skeel's study, and he noted that while the IQs of the severely deprived rise rapidly, markedly, and permanently when exposed to normal environmental stimulation, the culturally disadvantaged are only slightly affected by the "environmental enrichment afforded by school attendance." Jensen does not explicitly derive any conclusions from these observations, but he seems to imply that the orphanage children are below the threshold of environment that depresses intellect, while the culturally disadvantaged are above this threshold.

There is an alternative interpretation. Judging from the family histories of the orphans in the Skeel's study, it is likely that, had they remained with their true mothers, they would have been among the culturally disadvantaged. And although their IQs would have been higher than ascertained in the orphanage, they would have been considerably below the IQs they finally achieved. Perhaps the major difference between the orphans in the Skeel's study and the culturally disadvantaged is that for the former the environmental change was total and early in life, while for the latter the environmental change was too little and too late. There is no reason to believe that the culturally disadvantaged could not do at least as well as the orphanage children in comparable environmental situations.

Jensen also emphasized that the culturally disadvantaged show no early deficit and are sometimes even precocious, inferring that the decline in IQ among older culturally disadvantaged children depends upon the increasingly abstract nature of IQ tests and not the inherent disadvantages of the environment. In this regard, one can only note that the decline in IQ observed as the culturally disadvantaged grow older has not been observed in foster child studies when adoption took place at an early age.

The question of innate intellectual differences among children in different social classes cannot be definitely answered on the basis of existing evidence. The relatively high mean IQs of foster children, many of whom originate from the disadvantaged strata of society, do suggest, however, that environment significantly depresses intellectual performance among the lower social classes.

The most that can be inferred from the foster child studies cited by Jensen is that environment may be a minor but not altogether insignificant factor explaining intellectual variability among children in *above-average* homes. The threshold above which environment does not have a marked and systematic effect on intelligence appears to be considerably higher than inferred by Jensen and generally above the environmental levels existing among deprived populations.

This conclusion does not deny the possibility of social class differences in innate intelligence. If such differences exist, however, they are much narrower than observed through conventional IQ measures. In fact, given the positive correlation between parent-child intelligence and the inherent tendency for the less intelligent to gravitate to the lower social classes, it would be surprising if some small innate intellectual differences did not exist among children in different social classes.

It is reasonable to suppose that the lower social classes can be subdivided into two groups: one which has gravitated to the lower class because of limited intellect, and another which was never able to escape the environmental bonds holding it there—bonds that would be especially strong in areas where educational and occupational opportunities are limited. Although environmental conditions would have a depressing effect on the intelligence of the children of both groups, one would expect on both genetic and environmental grounds to find a substantially higher rate of mental retardation among the former group. Heber et al. in a study of the families of 88 low economic class mothers in Milwaukee, found that children over the age of 6 were five times as likely to have an IQ below 80 if their mother's IQ was below 80 than if their mother's IQ was above 80.[22]

The children observed in foster child studies were generally white and of North European extraction. If, however, environmental conditions exert a depressing influence on the intelligence of lower-class whites, no other inference can be drawn but that environment exerts an influence that is at least as important among lower-class nonwhites. Since more nonwhites than whites are concentrated in the lower social classes, the next step is to compare white and nonwhite children of the same social class.

We observed in the Imre study that rates of retardation among Negro children in each socioeconomic class were substantially above those of

[22] Heber et al., "Influence of Environmental and Genetic Variables," pp. 7–8.

whites in the same class. Shuey has noted that when the comparison is restricted to persons in the same class, the average IQ of Negroes is about 11 points lower than that of whites.[23]

These differences are striking, and not all observers believe they can be explained on purely environmental grounds. Shuey, for example, notes that upper-status Negro children have slightly lower IQs than lower-class white children and doubts that the latter have more cultural opportunities than the former.[24] Jensen observes that this is consistent with the hypothesis of a lower average IQ among Negroes and therefore a greater regression to the mean.

Although the unquestioned fact of hundreds of years of servitude, cultural impoverishment, and discrimination is fully sufficient to explain the lower-class status of many Negroes, the question remains, why do Negroes in all social classes have intellectual deficits substantially greater than their white counterparts?

One obvious answer to this question is that gross socioeconomic differences alone cannot take into account all of the environmental influences that affect intelligence—influences that are numerous, complex, and not well known.[25]

Jensen, however, doubted that environmental differences could explain the intellectual discrepancy between whites and Negroes. Perhaps his most impressive argument was based on the nationwide 1966 Coleman study.[26]

In that study the many environmental variables and socioeconomic indices that are believed to contribute to differences in scholastic performance were assessed. Jensen notes that:

These factors are all correlated—in the expected direction—with scholastic performance within each of the racial or ethnic groups studied by Coleman. Yet, interestingly enough, they are not systematically correlated with differences between groups. For example, by far the most environmentally disadvantaged groups in the Coleman Study are the American Indians. On every environmental index they average lower then the Negro samples, and overall their environmental rating is about as far below the Negro average as the Negro rating is below the white average . . . (American Indians are much more disadvantaged than Negroes, or any other minority groups in the United States, on a host of other factors not assessed

[23] A. M. Shuey, *The Testing of Negro Intelligence* (New York: Social Science Press, 1966), p. 519.

[24] Ibid., p. 520.

[25] Benjamin Pasamanick, "Some Socio-biologic Aspects of Science, Race, and Racism," *American Journal of Orthopsychiatry* (January 1969): 8, 11.

[26] J. S. Coleman et al., *Equality of Educational Opportunity*, U.S. Department of Health, Education, and Welfare, 1966.

by Coleman, such as income, unemployment, standards of health care, life expectancy, and infant mortality.) Yet the American Indian's ability and achievement test scores average about half a standard deviation higher than the scores of Negroes. . . . If the environmental factors assessed by Coleman are the major determinants of Negro-white differences that many social scientists have claimed they are, it is hard to see why such factors would act in reverse fashion in determining differences between Negroes and Indians, especially in view of the fact that *within* each group the factors are significantly correlated in the expected direction with achievement.

Contrary to Jensen's assertions, American Indians do have some environmental advantages over Negroes, notably in the schools they attend. Their teachers are probably superior. According to the Coleman report, the teachers in the schools Indians went to scored higher on a vocabulary test and were far more likely to have attended colleges which had white students and conferred advanced degrees. The school facilities used by Indians also appeared more favorable, especially at the secondary level. Indians were more likely to have access to biology, chemistry, physics, and language laboratories. In addition, they had considerably more library books available per pupil and had somewhat smaller classes than Negroes.

Perhaps the most striking difference between Indians and Negroes in the Coleman report was that while only 10% of Negroes had mostly white classmates at the secondary level, 72% of Indians were so situated. This explains, of course, the superiority of their schools.

Even in terms of home environment, Indians had a few advantages over Negroes. Fewer had five or more brothers and sisters, and their mothers were more likely to be high school graduates. In view of these differences, it hardly requires a genetic hypothesis to explain the superior scholastic achievements of Indians over Negroes.

Perhaps a better comparison than the one made by Jensen would be to compare the test scores of Indians with those of Negroes who have attended integrated schools. The Coleman study reported that twelfth grade Negro students who attended schools which were more than half white and who attended integrated schools at some time during the first three grades had reading comprehension and math achievement scores midway between Indians and whites. This is about what would be expected, given the other environmental disadvantages of American Indians.

Social class is, at most, a proxy variable designed to measure differences in life styles among various segments of society. There is, necessarily, great diversity within each social class. Being born into a low social class does not predestine an infant to be culturally deprived, nor is birth into a high social class a guarantee against deprivation. It requires more than a lack of access to middle-class comforts to depress intelligence, and more than an occasional visit to a cultural event to stimulate intellectual growth. About the only positive statement that can be made is that lower-class attitudes and responses to the external environment will, on the average, be less conducive to intellectual development than middle- and upper-class attitudes and responses.

Although a Negro child may be born into the same socioeconomic class as a white child, this by no means guarantees equality of learning stimuli or the development of comparable attitudes. Negro children are, in fact, almost certain to be more disadvantaged than whites, regardless of social class. There is the ubiquitous element of neighborhood and school segregation. In addition, there is the pervasive nature of white culture which glorifies the white man's achievements but rarely gives the nonwhite child any basis for pride in his own heritage. The nonwhite child is, in fact, surrounded by hints of his own inferiority.

The attitudes surrounding even middle- and upper-class Negroes are unlikely to be the same as for their white counterparts. Most Negroes moving into these classes are new arrivals. Merely moving into a higher social class does not mean that previous attitudes and ways of thinking are automatically discarded. Nor are the children of middle- and upper-class Negroes insulated from the spectre of failure. Many, through daily contact with lower-class Negroes, absorb attitudes that are not always conducive to intellectual achievement. Middle- and upper-class white children, on the other hand, are more likely to fall heir to attitudes emphasizing intellectual growth and achievement that have developed over several generations and are by now firmly entrenched.

Lower-class Negro children are likely to be swamped in a culture of poverty and failure. Few, if any, have successful relatives to emulate. Lower-class white children, on the other hand, often have successful relatives who are spoken of approvingly within the family. They are more likely to be taught, and to believe, that scholastic attainment will be rewarding.

Rather than compare the intellectual attainments of lower-class Negroes and whites, perhaps a fairer comparison would be between lower-class Negroes and isolated groups of whites, such as Wheeler's Tennessee mountain children, where one might expect an equivalent pervasiveness of poverty, lack of achievement, and dubious attitudes toward scholastic attainment. Compared to the white children in Wheeler's study, Negroes do rather well. Although the mean IQ of 6-year-olds in Wheeler's study was 103, among 16-year-olds the mean IQ declined to 80.

Although the possibility of genetic differences between Negroes and whites and among social classes cannot be disproved, the existing data, meager as it is, suggest that environmental differences explain much, probably most, of the observed intellectual inequalities.

If there are genetic differences in intelligence among social classes, not only do they appear slight but they are probably more pronounced among whites than Negroes for the simple reason that Negroes have had less opportunity to develop and take advantage of their innate capacities.

If one accepts the importance of the role of environment in determining IQ, then two conclusions must be drawn. First, it is futile to talk of genetic differences among different demographic groups until environmental opportunities for all groups are raised at least to the threshold where environment ceases to be a major factor in determining intellectual performance. Second, many of the mildly retarded did not need to become retarded. Perhaps it would be too optimistic to argue that 80% of the retarded have an innate genetic capacity that would enable them to score above 70 on an IQ test (as would be the case if the rate of mental retardation among all demographic groups was the same as it is among the white middle and upper classes), but it may not be unrealistic to visualize reducing the percentage of persons with IQs below 70 by one-half if appropriate policies are pursued.

The emphasis must be on prevention. Although unusual cases of "cures" in retardation are occasionally reported, it is doubtful if the consequences of prolonged deprivation can be eradicated when this is the cause of retardation.

SUMMARY

Environmental deprivation and an excessive prevalence of brain injury appear to explain most of the variation in rates of retardation among the various social classes and between whites and nonwhites. Although genetic endowment is unquestionably an important factor in determining intelligence, foster child studies show that when children of the poor are adopted at an early age by middle-class parents, their mean IQs tend to be approximately the same as would be expected from the natural children of their foster parents. Most adoptive studies have been restricted to children of North European extraction, but it is reasonable to believe that environmental disadvantages among poor Negroes are at least as great as among poor whites, and that even when gross socioeconomic class is held constant, Negroes face more disadvantages than whites.

IV

Programs for the Mentally Retarded

GENERAL OBSERVATIONS ON SERVICES TO THE RETARDED

Services provided to the mentally retarded are generally of the same type and have the same general goals as those provided to the nonretarded. These services seek to develop the intellectual, physical, social, and vocational skills of the retarded, to help them adjust to the problems they encounter in the day-to-day process of living and working, and to protect them from situations with which they would be unable to cope. The difference is one of degree. The retarded sometimes require additional services and sometimes require them in modified form. Frequently, however, the retarded utilize the same services as the nonretarded. Their skills develop slower and less completely than those of the nonretarded, and as adults they are more likely to need supportive aid, sometimes of a lifelong nature.

The types of services needed by the retarded will vary according to their particular intellectual and physical limitations and their stage in the developmental process. Retarded children have very different needs from retarded adults. The severely retarded have needs different from the mildly retarded. The environmentally deprived require different services from the brain injured.

In this chapter we will identify and describe those programs which provide services specifically as a consequence of the effects of mental retardation. Several limitations of this analysis should be borne in mind.

First, it will not encompass all of the services needed or utilized by the retarded, in part because statistical information was not always available and in part because many *essential* services are not motivated primarily by the fact of retardation (e.g., adequate medical care, recreation).

Second, this chapter will not discuss programs designed to prevent mental retardation. There are few activities whose *sole* concern is with the prevention of mental retardation,[1] and it is fair to say that relatively few cases of mental retardation are prevented by these activities.

One should not infer, however, that prevention is quantitatively unimportant. In Chapter VI we will argue quite the opposite. There are many mechanisms by which mental retardation is prevented; in fact, they encompass almost all aspects of our daily lives—prevention of accidents, proper medical care, etc. For the most part, each of the various mechanisms would be carried on even if mental retardation were not a possible outcome of an accident or disease.

To identify and describe all of these activities would not only be a monumental task, but would give a misleading impression of the quantity of resources being devoted to the field of mental retardation. To illustrate, prevention would encompass *all* obstetrical care and, indeed, almost all pediatric care, but one can hardly imagine that parents and prospective parents would forgo such care even if they could be assured that their child would not be retarded.

We should distinguish between a particular type of service (e.g., vocational training) and the facility which provides the service (e.g., public institutions for the mentally retarded). Statistical information is usually available only by facilities, most of which provide a range of services and many of which serve several types of clients, not just the retarded. Our analysis of services to the retarded, therefore, will be primarily based on a classification of facilities.

Before embarking on this subject, we will briefly discuss the terminology used to describe various types of expenditures on people. A basic distinction must be drawn between expenditures on people that increase present consumption and those that increase future consumption. The latter expenditures are called investments in people and increase a person's earning capacity, health, ability to cope with life's problems, etc. Present consumption refers to expenditures on items such as food, shelter, clothing, recreation, relief from pain, etc., which may be provided through income transfers (e.g., social security, public

---

[1] The most common examples are the providing of shunts to hydrochephalic children, the detection and treatment of phenylketonuria and galactosemia, and abortion after the interuterine detection of chromosomal abnormalities.

assistance) or direct services (as in residential care). These items provide for immediate necessities, but their benefits are quickly exhausted. The dichotomy is not precise, since any of these consumption items may themselves be a factor contributing to future consumption—e.g., the amount and type of food consumed will affect a person's health status, which in turn will influence his productivity.

Investments in people take many forms. Specific types of investments that may be identified are:

1) *Education*, which is broadly defined as any activity that stimulates learning. It includes all formally organized education at elementary, secondary, and higher levels, including special education and vocational training; on the job training, home study programs, armed forces training programs, church programs, and all the learning that goes on as people cope with the day-to-day problems of living.

2) *Health and medical care*, which following Schultz, will be "broadly conceived to include all expenditures that affect the life expectancy, strength, and stamina, and the vigor and vitality of a people."[2] We should also include all services designed to improve the mental health of the population and many of the services designed to improve their physical appearance (e.g., plastic surgery).

3) *Child care*, which includes the forgone earnings and the value of other forgone activities of parents who care for their children.

4) *Migration* of individuals and families when such migration stems from a desire to improve job opportunities, or to improve educational opportunities, or to live in a more healthful environment.

5) *Counseling*, which includes diagnostic services and case finding, to assist people in finding employment or a suitable field of study.

6) *Elimination of discrimination* when this interferes with the optimal allocation of resources or in any way adversely affects a person's enjoyment of life.

7) *Modification of the work or social environment*, when this is necessary to enable a person with unusual physical or mental limitations to increase his productive capacity or his ability to make a satisfactory social adjustment. These modifications may take many forms. Staircases can be replaced by ramps for people in wheelchairs. Special work tools for the physically disabled and stools for people unable to stand for long periods can be provided. Living arrangements can be modified.

[2] Theodore W. Schultz, "Investment in Human Capital," *American Economic Review* (March 1961): 9.

8) *Other services provided in support of the above mentioned activities*, e.g., transportation to and from educational or medical facilities, occupational tools, and licenses.

Another way of classifying services provided to people (both for the present and the future) is the following:

1) *Developmental services* are designed to increase a person's intellectual, vocational, personal, or social capabilities. Obviously, these services are usually provided during childhood. Most education and child care and much counseling and health care falls into this category.

2) *Supportive services* are needed by people to help them to make effective use of their intellectual capabilities or to enable them to cope with the rigors of an impersonal and competitive society. Supportive services include the provision of normal maintenance, occupational tools and licenses, transportation, job placement, periodic counseling, etc.

3) *Protective services* protect individuals from situations they are unable to cope with. In the case of the retarded, three important protective services can be distinguished—sheltered living, sheltered work, and advocacy programs.

4) *Rehabilitative services* are designed to restore a person's productive capacity or his ability to manage his own affairs in part or entirely as he had previous to his incapacity, usually through training and medical programs.

5) Services that modify the work or social environment (previously described).

All protective services and many supportive services would be classified as present consumption in the first classification of expenditures on people.

We should also draw the distinction between direct (or internal) and indirect (or external) investments in human beings. Direct investments are those embodied in particular persons that would be lost if that person should die or not utilize the benefits of the investments—i.e., education, health, child care, assistance in obtaining employment, etc. Indirect investments are those that benefit a class of people—i.e., reduction of discrimination, reducing the prevalence of infectious diseases, altering the work milieu, etc.

At least one other distinction among the various types of investments in human beings should be drawn. Some investments have a "general" purpose in that they increase the ability of the person to perform in a wide range of areas. Others are highly "specific" in that they improve a person's capability to perform in a particular activity. Vocational training and on-the-job training are the major types falling into this category.

Investments in people and investments in physical capital have many similarities. Like physical capital, human capital represents a sacrifice of present consumption in order that future consumption may be increased. Moreover, like physical capital, human capital may become obsolete (especially when it is "specific" in nature), it may require maintenance (physical check-ups, reviews of past learning), it may deteriorate if not used, and it probably should be depreciated over the lifetime of the individual as a legitimate expense of productive activity (although this is only feasible when it is "direct" in nature). Perhaps the most important distinction between physical and human capital is that the great bulk of the latter is embodied in living persons and can be sold in the marketplace only through the sale of the labor of the individual.

We have distinguished four different dimensions in which investments in humans might be delineated. The first described the different ways in which such investments might be made; the second (which included services for consumption needs) sought to classify each of these investments according to whether they are developmental, supportive, protective, rehabilitative, or whether they changed the milieu within which people function; the third—our direct-indirect dichotomy—questioned whether these investments were embodied in particular individuals or whether they benefited a group of individuals; and the final categorization grouped these investments according to whether they enabled a person to perform more satisfactorily in many possible areas of activity or in a specific one.

It may be questioned whether some of the investments described above should be encompassed under the rubric of investments in people. Usually, investments in people are defined as intangible and embodied in the person for whom the expenditure is made (as opposed to physical capital which is tangible and independent of the persons who work with it). Some of the investments in people that we have identified, although intangible, are not embodied in people (such as eliminating discrimination) and some are not embodied in people and, in addition, have a tangible existence (violating both of the customary criteria), such as many of the ways of altering the work milieu to enable the physically and mentally disabled to work.

The identification of efforts to reduce discrimination as a way of investing in people will probably not be seriously challenged by many economists, since these efforts are clearly designed to aid a defined group of people and do not result in a tangible asset. Economists are more likely to challenge the identification of *tangible* changes in the work milieu as investments in people. Their inclusion appears justified when their purpose is to enable the disabled to work and live within their limitations and are of benefit only to a specific group of disabled persons. In each case, these changes increase the productive potential of only a small group of persons. It is the orientation of these expenditures toward increasing the productivity of a small group of people rather than establishing new or improved productive facilities that leads me to classify them as investments in people.

Looked at in this way, the distinction between physical capital and investment in people is not always clear cut. Suppose all forms of investment were ranged along a continuum according to the number of persons whose productivity could conceivably be increased by each investment. At one extreme, only a single person is benefited, as in the case of mobility training. At the other extreme, almost everyone's productivity is increased, as when a truck is purchased which could be used by anyone who could drive (note that it is the number of persons who conceivably could benefit, not the number that actually benefit that is relevant). Near the first extreme are prosthetics which may, with modification, be used by more than one person, but the possibilities of their being so used are restricted. Crutches and ramps occupy intermediate positions.

Basically, tangible investments can be identified as increasingly of a "human" nature as the number of persons who could conceivably be benefited by these investments decreases. This generalization is not valid in the case of intangible investments, all of which are considered to be human capital.

Clearly, mobility training is an example of human capital, and elevators are an example of physical capital. Most economists would consider prostheses as human capital; crutches or ramps (and perhaps elevators installed in homes for the use of the physically disabled) are debatable items, which we include as human capital.

It is important to emphasize that the concept of human capital that has been developed in this discussion is broader than the usual concept, which includes only investments that are intangible and embodied in people. The last criterion means that they benefit primarily those persons in whom they are embodied, and therefore last only as long as those individuals live.

Our concept of human capital includes all intangible investments, whether embodied or disembodied. Disembodied intangible investments (e.g., efforts to reduce discrimination) are long-lasting and serve many people. In addition, we have defined as human capital, tangible investments that are embodied in a single person (such as specific types of prostheses) and tangible investments that are designed to offset the physical or mental limitations of a limited number of workers (such as ramps for persons in wheelchairs).

There is not a neat dichotomy between investments labeled "physical" and those labeled "human." Some investments could fall into either category (tangible investments that benefit few people) and some could be defined as falling in neither category (disembodied intangible investments). Agreement as to labeling is not crucial as long as it is made clear how specific types of investments are handled and there is recognition of the various types of investments (whether called "physical" or "human") that are essential for the social and vocational adjustment of the physically and mentally disabled.

A lack of statistical data has imposed major limitations on this study. Often, the number of retardates served by existing programs could not be estimated. In other cases the estimates had to be based on questionable assumptions. These statistical limitations do not reflect a lack of resources being devoted to the collection of data. Indeed, the amount of data available from state, federal, and private sources is bewildering. The fault lies in the total absence of any meaningful coordination among the various data-collection agencies and sometimes in the failure to ask appropriate and meaningful questions.

Most agencies collect data to serve their own needs. This leads to large gaps in the data, large overlaps in the populations covered by different statistical series, and frequent duplication of effort. The problem of overlap is compounded because some agencies collect data on particular types of services, others on particular types of facilities, and still others on particular demographic groups.

Many of these problems could be resolved if the data-collection efforts of different agencies were better coordinated and if data were collected simultaneously on facilities, services, and demographic groups. This could then be accumulated into a master register of all health and educational resources. Admittedly, some difficult definitional problems would have to be resolved, but the end result would be well worth the effort. For example, we would be able to ascertain the various services offered to nursing home residents, and the number of residents in nursing homes, with a breakdown as to the number of residents who are blind, deaf, retarded, aged, orthopedically handicapped, etc. Because of integrated survey design and data bases among agencies, more complete and accurate information would be achieved with fewer survey instruments being mailed to harried facility managers than at present.

In empirical studies, one always faces the problem that there may be a considerable time lag between the initiation of a study and when the pages are ready to go to press. This study was primarily based on the data available for 1968. However, as it is about to make the last trip to the publisher, it becomes possible to update many of the figures. Whenever it is possible, therefore, two sets of data are presented, one for 1968 and one for the latest year for which data was available at the time of this final editing. In most cases, the latest available year was 1970. In some cases, however, especially when dealing with the demographic characteristics of the retarded receiving different types of services, the data could not be updated beyond 1968. In a few cases, even earlier years had to be used. The updated information that is available, however, indicates that the characteristics of the retarded receiving various kinds of services have not changed significantly in the last few years.

Another small problem is that data were sometimes available on a calendar year basis and sometimes on a fiscal year or school year basis. Fiscal year or school year data were treated as if they belonged wholly to the calendar year in which they terminated for purposes of aggregating data from different sources. Sometimes, in order to simplify the exposition, these data are identified only by their year of termination in the text. Thus, the 1967–68 school year is usually referred to as the 1968 school year.

RESIDENTIAL CARE

Residential care is provided on a 24-hour basis and usually encompasses a wide range of services. However, the quality of care provided by different institutions varies widely. In some institutions, often described as human warehouses, the retarded are provided little more than subsistence. Other institutions devote a large share of their resources to developing the physical and mental capabilities of the retarded, enabling many to return to the community.

Sources of data. Estimates of the number of mentally retarded persons in residential care are presented in Table 13. All data *except* that for schools for the blind, schools for the deaf, other chronic disease hospitals, private institutions and other private facilities for the mentally retarded (hereafter private institutions), and federal and state prisons were obtained from the Office of Biometry of the National Institute of Mental Health (NIMH) of the United States Department of Health, Education, and Welfare (USDHEW) or from the Division of Developmental Disabilities of the Rehabilitation Services Administration (RSA), USDHEW. These data represent a reasonably complete census of these facilities, although in some cases the data were adjusted upward to allow for nonreporting.

Three data sources were used to estimate the number of mentally retarded persons in private institutions for 1967. In 1968 the American Association on Mental Deficiency (AAMD) published a directory of public and private residential facilities for the mentally retarded and estimated the resident population for the previous year.[3] Another survey was made by the National Center for Health Statistics (NCHS) of the U.S. Public Health Service, USDHEW, of all public and private facilities for the retarded as of July 1, 1967. A final source of data was derived from an inventory of resources for the mentally retarded submitted to the Division of Mental Retardation, Social and Rehabilitation Service (SRS), USDHEW, by each state sometime between 1965 and 1967 for the purpose of developing a state plan for the retarded. NCHS provided a computer printout of all facilities providing residential care, and the Division of Mental Retardation prepared a listing (unpublished) of all of the facilities reported by each state.

In all three surveys the listings were acknowledged to be incomplete. In addition, the AAMD survey limited its listings to facilities serving twenty-five or more patients. (The other two surveys listed facilities serving as few as one person.) The state plans survey reported on the total number served, including those in day care and diagnostic and evaluation services, rather than on the number of full-time residents in a given facility. The NCHS survey systematically (and for unknown reasons) understated the number of resident patients in facilities by substantial amounts—usually around 50%, but occasionally much more.

An estimate of the number of retarded persons receiving private residential care in 1967 was calculated as follows. Whenever possible, AAMD estimates of the resident population of private facilities were used. Of those facilities reported by one or both of the other two surveys, but not by AAMD, the following were eliminated: those with fewer than 5 residents and those with more than 5 residents if they appeared to be foster homes, general or pediatric hospitals, or institutions for the deaf, blind, and crippled. Of the remainder, if the patient population was reported by *both* of these surveys, the invariably higher state plans estimate was used if the facility provided only residential care, and the NCHS estimate was utilized if the facility also provided day care and/or diagnostic and evaluation services. The estimates of the

---

[3] *Directory of Residential Facilities for the Mentally Retarded* (Albany, New York: The American Association on Mental Deficiency, 1968).

two surveys had to be used as given if a facility was reported by only one of these surveys, except when a residential facility reported only by the state plans survey also provided day care or diagnostic and evaluation services. In such a case it was assumed that one-third of the mentally retarded persons being cared for by that facility were residents. This was the approximate ratio of the number of persons reported as residents by the NCHS survey to the total number of persons reported as being cared for by the state plans survey when multiple purpose facilities were reported by both of these surveys.

During 1971 the National Center for Health Statistics resurveyed residential facilities for the retarded. About 28,000 residents were reported as being in private facilities (about five times what the survey reported in 1967). The later survey is based on a more rigorously defined universe and should be reasonably comparable with the derived 1967 estimate in scope. Some facilities with under five residents were included in the later figure, but any reasonable adjustment for this difference would be of minor significance, probably of the order of 1%.

These estimates probably encompass most private facilities that were primarily concerned with providing residential care to the mentally retarded at the time of the surveys. It should be observed that this estimate includes nurseries as well as nursing homes and encompasses many facilities providing care to persons other than the retarded.

Based on a 1963 study of the status of special education directed by Romaine Mackie, the National Center of Educational Statistics estimated that in 1966 there were 7,900 pupils enrolled in public and private residential schools for the blind.[4] On the basis of the studies described in the previous chapter, it was estimated that 25% of these children were also retarded. No later figures were available.

In 1968 there were about 16,000 deaf pupils living in public and private schools for the deaf. In 1970 the comparable figure was a little over 13,000. In 1960 these schools reported that 4.6% of their pupils were mentally retarded[5] and that another 5.4% of the students were aphasic, blind, cerebral palsied, orthopedically handicapped, or brain injured. In 1970 the percentage reported as mentally retarded declined to 3.1%, but the percentage of multiply-handicapped students, in-

[4] Romaine Mackie, *Special Education in the United States* (New York: Teachers College Press, 1969), pp. 36, 41.

[5] *American Annals of the Deaf, Directory of Services for the Deaf in the United States* (May 1969): 622–23; (April 1971): 220. There were almost 20,000 pupils enrolled in residential facilities for the deaf in 1968. This figure was reduced by 4,000 because about 1,000 are blind students who, though not deaf, are enrolled in schools for the deaf and blind, and about 3,000 are day pupils only.

Table 13. Estimates of number of mentally retarded persons receiving 24-hour-a-day care, 1968 and 1970

Type of facility	No. of facilities	MR residents in facility	MR as percentage of total population in institution	MR admitted to facility for first time	MR as percentage of all first admissions for fiscal year
Public institutions					
June 30, 1968	170	192,520	100.0%	12,359	100.0%
June 30, 1970	190	186,743	100.0	12,075	100.0
Public mental hospitals					
June 30, 1968	312	33,994	8.5	4,143	2.4
June 30, 1970	315	30,339	9.0		
Private institutions and other private residential care					
1967	1,013	24,442[a]	100.0		
1971		28,304	100.0		
Private Mental Hospitals					
June 30, 1968	150	86	0.8	263	0.3
June 30, 1969	149	75	0.7	256	0.3
Public and private residential schools for the blind					
1966	55	1,975[a]	25.0		
Public and private residential schools for the deaf					

October 1968	74	1,280	8.0
October 1970	73	1,160	8.0
Residential Treatment Centers			
1968	188	2,390[a]	25.0
1969	261	3,370[a]	25.0
Other chronic disease hospitals			
1967		3,800[a,b]	7.0
Federal & state prisons			
1968		13,400[a]	7.0
1970		14,000[a]	7.0
General hospitals with psychiatric inpatient services			
1968		3,334[c]	0.9[d]
1970		4,354[c]	0.9[d]
Total			
1968		274,852[e]	
1970		268,799[e]	

[a] Estimated average daily population.
[b] Adults, age 18 to 64.
[c] Discharges during year.
[d] MR as a percentage of total discharges.
[e] When data were not available for the year of these estimates, the latest available figure was used. In the case of private institutions, estimates for 1968 and 1970 were interpolated from the 1967 and 1971 estimate. The number of discharges from general hospitals is not included in the total.

79

cluding the mentally retarded, was reported to be 10.8%.[6] In view of our previous discussion on the rate of retardation among the deaf-blind and cerebral palsied, it is likely that many, probably a majority, of these multiply-physically-handicapped children are also retarded. We will assume, therefore, that 8% of deaf pupils in residential schools are retarded.

Although NIMH collected data on patients in residential treatment centers for the mentally ill, information on the number who were mentally retarded was not available. However, NIMH personnel believed that between 25% and 50% are mentally retarded. Since the number of persons involved is small, it introduces no serious bias in our aggregate figures to use the lower estimate.

The great majority of institutionalized retardates are located in institutions for the mentally ill or mentally retarded. A few, however, are placed in other types of chronic disease facilities, such as those for tuberculosis patients, physical rehabilitation, etc. The only data on such facilities that is available is that obtained by the Social Security survey of institutionalized adults in 1967.[7]

Although there have been many exaggerated claims as to the number of mentally retarded prisoners, the only reliable national estimates are those published by Brown and Courtless for 1963.[8] In the first phase of this study, IQ scores were obtained for over 90,000 prisoners—over 40% of all inmates in state and federal prisons. About 9.5% of these prisoners had reported IQs below 70. Three hundred and ninety-five prisoners who were reported as retarded were selected for retesting. Of these, 74% were found on retest to have an IQ below 70. It was assumed, therefore, that 7% (9.5% X 74%) of the total state and federal prison population was retarded. About 200,000 persons were in these prisons.[9]

[6] *American Annals of the Deaf* (January 1961): 162–63; (April 1972): 237.

[7] Philip Frohlich, "Demographic Characteristics of Institutionalized Adults," Report Number 1, Social Security Survey of Institutionalized Adults: 1967, July 1971.

[8] Bertram S. Brown and Thomas F. Courtless, *The Mentally Retarded Offender*. Report prepared for the President's Commission on Law Enforcement and Administration of Justice (no date), pp. 29, 48.

[9] The U.S. Department of Justice, Bureau of Prisons. *National Prisoner Statistics, Prisoners in State and Federal Institutions for Adult Felons, April 1, 1972.* There is a small degree of under-reporting in the data. Prisons are included under residential care facilities because, distasteful as it may be, they are an important source of residential care for adult retarded persons, especially in the South. One out of every five prisoners in the southern states had an IQ below 70 according to the Brown and Courtless study.

Number served. At an average point in time during 1968, and 1970, a little less than 275,000 mentally retarded persons in the United States were in residential care in the facilities for which estimates are available. About 70% were in public institutions for the mentally retarded (hereafter referred to simply as public institutions). The total number receiving care during the course of the year would, of course, be greater because of admissions and releases. Some 208,000 persons were resident at some time in public institutions alone in 1968. In 1970 the comparable figure was 204,000.

Not all facilities providing residential care to retardates are included in Table 13, since we had no way to estimate the number of retarded in some types of facilities. The potential importance of some of these omitted facilities can be emphasized by noting their total residential population. In 1965 over 140,000 adults were incarcerated in *local* institutions and jails.[10] Also, in 1965, 208,000 children were in foster family care and another 79,400 were in institutions for neglected, dependent, and emotionally disturbed children.[11] In 1967 approximately 53,000 children were in public institutions for delinquent children.[12] There were almost 56,000 pupils in residential schools for the emotionally disturbed and socially maladjusted in 1963.[13] In 1964, 554,000 persons resided in nursing and personal-care homes.[14] In this regard, it is of interest to note that according to the state plans and NCHS surveys there were 1,650 mentally retarded persons living in county homes and hospitals in Wisconsin and 760 mentally retarded persons living in county homes in Iowa. Figures were not available for other states.[15]

About 16,000 mentally retarded persons are admitted to public institutions and public mental hospitals each year, about 7% of their total resident patient population of retardates. Although this information was not available for other facilities, these three facilities provide care to about 80% of all retardates receiving residential care in the facilities included in Table 13.

[10] The President's Commission on Law Enforcement and Administration of Justice, *Task Force Report: Corrections* (Washington, D.C.: USGPO, 1967), p. 163.

[11] USDHEW, Children's Bureau, *Foster Care of Children, Major National Trends and Prospects*, 1966, p. 10.

[12] USDHEW, Children's Bureau, *Statistics on Public Institutions for Delinquent Children*, 1967, p. 1.

[13] Mackie, *Special Education*, p. 36.

[14] USDHEW, NCHS, *PHS Publication 1000*, Series 12, No. 7.

[15] Some of the facilities in these omitted categories may be included in the estimates of retardates in private residential care facilities.

Demographic characteristics and trends. From 1950 to 1967 there was a small but steady increase in the number of first admissions and in the resident populations of public institutions. Between 1968 and 1970 the resident population slightly decreased each year, reflecting both a lower rate of admissions and a higher rate of releases.[16]

In contrast, the number of retarded in public mental hospitals has declined from a high of almost 55,000 in 1952 to around 30,000 in 1970. First admissions of the mentally retarded to public mental hospitals remained relatively constant over this period, so that an accelerated rate of release is responsible for this decline.

The number of retardates institutionalized per 100,000 population in public institutions rose from 85.3 in 1950 to 99.0 in 1967. In public mental hospitals this ratio fell from 35.0 to 18.4 over the same period. These trends have almost offset each other, so that the combined rate of institutionalized retardates showed a slight decline, from 120 to 117. In 1970 this combined rate fell further to 110. In part, this reflects a reduction in the number of institutionalized retardates and, in part, a shift from these facilities to community based private facilities.

In 1970, total admissions (first admissions plus readmissions) to public institutions were about 8% of the average daily resident population. Releases were at about the same rate and deaths were about 2% of the total. Thus, the public institution population can be described as relatively static. Once placed in these institutions, most retardates remained for a long period.

The turnover rate in public mental hospitals is considerably higher. The percentage of total admisssions to the resident population of retardates is about 30% and the percentage of releases must be even higher, since the number of retardates in public mental hospitals has declined in recent years.

Table 14 shows the distribution of patients in 24-hour care by sex and level of retardation in those facilities for which such information is available. These data are all based on information collected by NIMH or the Division of Developmental Disabilities (RSA, USDHEW) with the exception of the data on the severity of retardation of resident patients in public institutions, which was based on unpublished information collected by the AAMD for 196,000 residents during 1967. With the exception of private institutions, this information is based on 75% or more of the number of mentally retarded persons being cared for in each of these types of facilities. The only information that is available on the demographic characteristics of the retarded in private institu-

[16]Unless otherwise indicated, all data cited are based on statistics obtained from the National Institute of Mental Health.

tions is from a 1966 NIMH survey that obtained information on a little over 6,000 residents of these facilities.

One striking feature of the institutional population is the preponderance of males over females, in spite of our earlier conclusion that there are as many female retardates as male retardates and that among the severely retarded, females may slightly predominate. The preponderance of males over females was even more pronounced among first admissions.

The percentage of males varies inversely with the severity of retardation. In a study of over 23,000 residents in 19 public institutions located in western states, it was found that 54% of the profoundly retarded were males, as compared to 63% of the borderline retarded. NIMH data show a similar relationship for first admissions to public institutions in the United States:

Level of retardation	Percentage of males in 19 western institutions, by level of retardation, 1966[a]	Percentage of males among first admissions to public institutions, U. S., 1967
Borderline	62.6%	60.2%
Mild	58.6	60.5
Moderate	56.0	60.1
Severe	55.7	57.1
Profound	54.1	54.4

[a]Ronald C. Johnson, "On the Preponderance of Males among Individuals Diagnosed as Mentally Retarded," in *A Symposium, 1,500,000 Bits of Information . . . Some Implications for Action* (Boulder, Colorado: Western Interstate Commission for Higher Education, 1967), p. 23.

The preponderance of retarded males in residential care is concentrated among retardates under 35. Among retardates over age 35 in public institutions only 51% are males.

Almost four-fifths of the resident population of public institutions were moderately (IQ 40–54), severely (IQ 25–39), or profoundly (IQ less than 25) retarded. The proportions are approximately equally divided among these three groups. The mentally retarded in public mental hospitals appear to be less intellectually limited, but the large proportion of cases for which the level of retardation is unknown, as well as the lack of correspondence in diagnostic categories, makes a direct comparison difficult.

Over 60% of first admissions to public institutions had IQs below 55 in 1968. This proportion was apparently considerably lower for first admissions to public mental hospitals. In all cases first admissions are less severely retarded on the average than resident patients.

Table 14. Mentally retarded persons in residential care by sex and degree of retardation

Type of facility	sex		Level of retardation						
	Male	Female	None	Borderline	Mild	Moderate	Severe	Profound	Unspecified
Public institutions 1968									
First admissions	57.7%	42.3%	2.2%	6.9%	15.9%	18.3%	19.8%	24.4%	12.5%
Resident patients	55.7	44.3		4.6	13.9	22.3	27.9	28.9	2.4
Public mental hospitals 1968									
First admissions	63.0	37.0				71.9[a]		17.3[b]	10.8
Resident patients	57.2	42.8				53.7		24.1	22.2
1970									
Resident patients	57.8	42.2							
Private institutions 1966									
First admissions	58.9	41.1	2.6	16.4	18.3	20.8	16.7	19.0	6.2
Resident patients	54.0	46.0							
Private mental hospitals 1968									
Total admissions	52.6	47.4				55.5[a]		9.0[b]	35.5
Resident patients	52.9	47.1				60.8		21.6	17.6
General hospitals with psychiatric inpatient service 1968	53.1	46.9				39.1		10.0	50.9

[a] Includes mild and moderate retardation.
[b] Includes severe and profound retardation.

84

A number of studies have concluded that the proportion of the population served by public institutions that is severely retarded has been rising over time.[17] In New York State, for example, the percentage of "idiots" in state schools for mental defectives rose from 13% in 1935 to 20% in 1962, and the percentage of "imbeciles" rose from 35% to 49%. The proportion of "morons," conversely, declined from 52% to 32%.[18]

Table 15 shows the estimated distribution of the institutionalized mentally retarded by age and, when possible, by level of retardation. All of these data were supplied by NIMH or by the Division of Developmental Disabilities (RSA, USDHEW).

The mentally retarded in public institutions are considerably younger than those in public mental hospitals. In 1970 about half of the retarded in public institutions were under age 20. In contrast, in public mental hospitals about 10% were under 20 and their median age was 45. The median age of residents in private institutions was considerably younger than for public institutions, presumably because children are more apt to have parents able and willing to pay for their care. The median age of first admissions was only 12 years in public institutions and 24 years in public mental hospitals. The median age of admissions to public and private institutions declined as the extent of mental subnormality increased, except for persons who were diagnosed as borderline retarded or not retarded. Presumably, severe physical or behavioral disabilities were the primary problem of these latter two groups, not intellectual deficit.

In public mental hospitals, this relationship between admission age and level of retardation was slightly reversed. No significance can be attached to this fact, however, since most of the retarded in public mental hospitals were admitted as adults.

Among first admissions, 79% were under 20 in 1950 as compared to 90% in 1970. This trend toward younger admissions is related to the increasing proportion of the more severely retarded among first admissions. The same trend is apparent in public mental hospitals. In 1950 only 6% of first admissions among the mentally retarded were under age 15, as compared to 15% in 1968.

[17] Herbert Goldstein, "Population Trends in U.S. Public Institutions for the Mentally Deficient," *American Journal of Mental Deficiency* (1959): 599. Benjamin Malzberg, "Some Statistical Aspects of First Admissions to New York State Schools for Mental Defectives," *American Journal of Mental Deficiency* (1952): 27–37.

[18] New York State Department of Mental Hygiene, *A Plan for a Comprehensive Mental Health and Mental Retardation Program for New York State*, July 1965, p. 272.

Table 15. Percentages of mentally retarded persons in residential care, by age and level of retardation[a]

Type of facility	Under 5	5-19	20-54	55 and over	Median age
Public institutions					
Resident patients					
1968	1.9%	42.9%	48.3%	6.8%	23
1970	3.9	46.5		49.6[b]	20
First admissions					
1968	14.7	73.4	11.4	0.4	11
1970	13.8	73.7		12.5[b]	12
Level of retardation (1968)					
None	13.3	77.0	9.2	0.5	11
Borderline	4.5	81.7	13.0	0.7	15
Mild	5.2	80.0	14.3	0.5	14
Moderate	9.9	75.5	14.4	0.7	13
Severe	18.2	72.4	9.2	0.3	9
Profound	23.9	66.8	9.0	0.3	8
Unknown	16.2	71.3	12.2	0.3	11
Public mental hospitals					
Resident patients					
1968	0.1	7.2	61.6	31.2	46
1970	0.1	9.7	58.6	31.7	45
Level of retardation (1968)					
Mild and moderate	0.0	7.0	61.9	31.0	46
Severe	0.1	10.9	66.8	22.1	41
Unspecified	0.1	3.0	55.4	41.4	51
First admissions					
1968	0.7	37.4	55.4	6.5	24
Level of retardation (1968)					
Mild and moderate	0.2	37.4	56.7	5.6	24
Severe	1.7	42.7	49.2	6.3	23
Unspecified	2.7	28.3	56.6	12.4	27
Private institutions (1966)					
Resident patients	6.3%	59.4	26.9	7.4%	15
First admissions	23.0	66.3	9.6	1.1	11
Level of retardation:					
None	—	89.6	10.3	—	13
Borderline	0.5	95.2	4.3	—	14
Mild	2.4	86.0	8.6	2.9	13
Moderate	11.9	77.2	10.6	0.4	12
Severe	25.3	66.8	8.0	—	9
Profound	79.6	19.1	1.5	—	3
Unknown	35.7	48.6	5.7	10.0	9
Private mental hospitals (1968)					
Total admissions	0.0	37.9	58.3	3.8	25
Resident patients	0.0	19.6	41.2	39.2	45
General hospitals with Psychiatric inpatient service					
(1968)	14.4	38.4	40.1	7.1	19
(1970)	13.8	38.6	42.3	5.3	19

[a] All percentages sum horizontally.
[b] Includes all persons 20 years of age and over.

An important characteristic of the institutionalized mentally retarded is the high proportion of persons with multiple handicaps. Information collected by NIMH on over 9,000 first admissions to public institutions in 1968 indicated that:

16% had an impairment of the special senses
(primarily sight and hearing)
25% had a convulsive disorder
16% had a psychiatric impairment
28% had motor dysfunction

A 1968 survey of over 24,000 residents of 22 public institutions located in western states reported a high level of sensorimotor difficulties as seen in Table 16. These may well be underestimates, especially for vision and hearing, since these figures are based on institutional records and not clinical examination. Data on psychological handicaps were not provided, but it is noteworthy that the survey reported that almost 40% of the resident population was hyperactive. As would be expected, the percentages of multiply-handicapped retarded are greater among the resident population of institutions than among first admissions.

Table 16.   Percentage of patients with sensorimotor difficulties in 22 western institutions for the mentally retarded[a]

Items	% with difficulty
Cannot walk	25%
Impaired vision	17
Impaired hearing	9
Impaired arm-hand use	24
Impaired speech	65
Impaired comprehension of speech	33
Chronic enuresis	32

[a]*Source:* Don Payne, Ronald C. Johnson, and Robert B. Abelson, *A Comprehensive Description of Institutionalized Retardates in the Western United States.* (Boulder, Colorado: Western Interstate Commission for Higher Education, 1969), p. 22.

These complicated and interrelated characteristics of the institutionalized retarded may be summarized as follows. A majority of resident patients are male, severely retarded, and multiply-handicapped. The concentration of males is primarily among children and young adults. First admissions follow the same pattern except that the excess of males is more pronounced, and the excess of the severely retarded and multiply-handicapped retarded is less pronounced. It follows that males, the mildly retarded, and the nonmultiply-handicapped retarded are more likely to be released than other admissions (otherwise the resident population would have the same characteristics as admissions). The smaller excess of males among the severely retarded indicates that, on the average, males are less severely retarded than females at admission, which may explain much of their higher release rate. These conclusions are supported by a study of admissions to the Pacific State Hospital, where Tarjan et al. concluded that the younger, more severely retarded admissions have higher death rates and lower chances of release than older, less retarded admissions, who, more often than not, were released within four years of admission.[19]

Public mental hospitals admit much older and generally less severely retarded persons than public institutions. In fact, after about age 40, a mentally retarded person who is being institutionalized is more likely to go to a public mental hospital than a public institution. Over time, there has been a tendency for admissions to public institutions and public mental hospitals to be younger and, at least in the case of the former, to be more severely retarded.[20]

Reasons for institutionalization. Although many variables are associated with the probability of institutionalization, most can be subsumed under one or more of the following interrelated categories: (1) the difficulty of providing adequate care in the home; (2) illegal, immoral, or otherwise undesirable behavior; or (3) lack of alternative living arrangements in the community.

1) The degree of mental subnormality and the extent of associated physical and psychiatric disabilities are the major factors influencing the difficulty of caring for the retarded.

a) Severity of retardation alone would probably be sufficient ultimately to cause the institutionalization of almost all of the profoundly retarded, most of the severely retarded, and many of the moderately retarded.

Earlier, we estimated that there were approximately 200,000 persons with IQs below 25 in the United States in 1970. The number of these individuals in residential care is difficult to estimate because of the substantial number of institutionalized persons for whom no IQ was specified, the NIMH practice of combining the severely and profoundly

[19] George Tarjan et al., "The Natural History of Mental Deficiency in a State Hospital. I. Probabilities of Release and Death by Age, Intelligence Quotient, and Diagnosis," *A.M.A. Journal of Diseases of Children* (July 1958): 64–70.

[20] Goldstein, "Population Trends in U.S. Public Institutions," p. 599. Malzberg, "Some Statistical Aspects of First Admissions," pp. 27–37.

retarded into one category, and the fact that profound retardation is usually diagnosed on the basis of an IQ below 20 rather than 25. However, the total number of persons diagnosed as profoundly retarded in institutions appears to be between 65,000 and 70,000—a little over one-third of the number of persons with IQs below 25. Because of the inexact convergence of these categories, the actual proportion of persons with IQs below 25 who are institutionalized may be slightly higher.

We estimated that there were almost 490,000 persons with IQs between 25 and 50 in the United States. In institutional care there are between 125,000 and 135,000 persons classified as severely or moderately retarded. Unfortunately, these two groupings are not strictly comparable since the latter group encompasses persons with IQs between 20 and 55. If they were equivalent, it would indicate that a little over one-fourth of the moderately and severely retarded are in institutions. As it is, a proportion of about one-fifth is probably more accurate.

We also estimated that almost 5,310,000 persons in the United States had IQs between 50 and 70. A liberal estimate of persons with IQs between 55 and 70 (the NIMH definition of mild retardation) in institutions would be less than 75,000. Adding another 25,000 to allow for persons with IQs between 50 and 55 would indicate that less than 2% of persons with IQs in the 50 to 70 range are in institutions.

b) In addition to severity of retardation, physical and psychiatric handicaps and behavioral problems complicate home care of the retarded. A recent (1966) study in New York State concluded that continued institutionalization was appropriate for 70% of the resident population of the state schools for the mentally retarded. Of these, three-fourths were severely or profoundly retarded, four-fifths required special care for physical disabilities, and nine-tenths required special care for emotional or behavioral conditions. In the majority of cases, the amount of special care needed was well beyond what the average family could provide.[21]

Many studies have reviewed the behavioral and emotional problems of the institutionalized mentally retarded. In the WICHE study of public institutions in western states, it was reported that almost one-third of the residents of these institutions constituted a danger to other persons. Apparently, almost one-fifth would physically attack children,

[21] Arthur D. Rosenberg, study director, *Appropriateness of the Continued Institutionalization of the State School Population in New York State* (New York: Department of Mental Hygiene, 1969), pp. 34, 50.

employees of the institutions, or other residents. Many other aggressive and destructive tendencies were noted.[22]

In a study of 326 female admissions to an English institution (average IQ 50), 11% were psychotic (mostly schizophrenic), and 46% had a less severe mental illness or presented behavioral problems.[23] In another study of 30 institutionalized and 24 noninstitutionalized female retardates between the ages of 14 and 18 with IQs between 50 and 80, it was concluded that the institutional group tended to be more dominated by their needs and were more negative about their personal worth. The investigators felt that these attitudes played "a significant role in the failure of these girls to adjust to society's demands."[24]

A study at Laurelton State Village (Pa.) compared 49 girls who were being considered for parole with 32 girls who had never been considered for parole. The mean IQs of the two groups were almost identical. The investigator found that those who were never considered for parole exhibited about the same degree of independence in dressing, eating, and bathing as those being considered for parole, and, in addition, equaled or surpassed their level in socialization, locomotion, and self-direction. The basic differences between the two groups were that those who were never considered for parole often suffered from deep-rooted emotional maladjustment which led to persistent delinquent behavior—pilfering, fighting, homosexual activity, destructiveness, disobedience, etc.[25]

Physical and psychiatric handicaps and behavioral problems are evidently the *major* factors in the institutionalization of the *mildly* retarded. Tarjan et al., in a study of 724 first admissions to Pacific State Hospital, found that behavioral difficulties were far more common among older admissions than younger admissions.[26] As we have noted, older admissions tend to be less severely retarded. Saenger found that 90% of a sample of mildly retarded persons (N=84) age 6 to 24, in New York State schools for the mentally retarded had behavioral problems, as compared to 26% of a sample of high-grade retardates (N=85) living

---

[22] Don Payne, Ronald C. Johnson, and Robert B. Abelson, *A Comprehensive Description of Institutionalized Retardates in the Western United States* (Boulder, Colorado: Western Interstate Commission for Higher Education, 1967), p. 25.

[23] M. C. Liu, "Changing Trends in the Care of the Subnormal," *American Journal of Mental Deficiency* (1963): 345–53.

[24] George M. Guthrie, Alfred Butler, and Leon Gorlow, "Personality Differences between Institutionalized and Non-institutionalized Retardates," *American Journal of Mental Deficiency* (1963): 547–48.

[25] Marina A. Whitcomb, "A Comparison of Social and Intellectual Levels of 100 High-Grade Adult Mental Defectives," *American Journal of Mental Deficiency* (October 1945): 247–52.

[26] Tarjan et al., "The Natural History of Mental Deficiency," pp. 56, 58.

in New York City. The comparable percentages for the low-grade retarded (IQ = 20–49) were 61% (N=57) and 28% (N=53).[27] Surprisingly, Saenger reported (p. 51) that the *only* physical handicaps to have a significant effect on the probability of being institutionalized were severe difficulties of coordination, severe epilepsy, and spastic conditions. This unexpected result probably stems from his failure to consider the mentally retarded who are placed in residential facilities for the physically handicapped (e.g., for the blind or for the deaf).

Behavioral problems probably also explain the excess of males in public institutions, since males tend to be more aggressive than females. In addition, the decreasing ratio of males to females among the more severely retarded evidently reflects the increasing importance of severity of retardation as a reason for institutionalization among the severely retarded as compared to the midly retarded. The decreasing ratio of males to females among older retardates is probably the result of less boisterous behavior among older retardates, enabling more to be released from residential care.

c) A final factor that should be mentioned under the heading of difficulty of care is the unavailability of community services. Home care for the retarded, especially the more severely retarded and the physically and psychiatrically handicapped, can be a trying experience. Without supportive help, many families find home care beyond their capability. In this regard, it is worth noting that it is generally believed that the development of special education classes and other community services is a major factor in the declining proportion of midly retarded persons in institutions in recent years. (Declining death rates and a lowering of the age at which the retarded can be institutionalized are also contributing factors to this trend.)[28]

2) Illegal, immoral, or otherwise undesirable behavior is another broad category of reasons for the institutionalization of the retarded.[29] It should be noted that the distinction between behavioral problems and illegal and immoral behavior is tenuous. Perhaps it is best to consider the former category as relating primarily to children and the latter

[27] Gerhart Saenger, *Factors Influencing the Institutionalization of Retarded Individuals in New York City* (New York: New York State Interdepartmental Health Resources Board, January 1960), p. 60.

[28] Goldstein, "Population Trends in U.S. Public Institutions," p. 599; Malzberg, "Some Statistical Aspects of First Admissions," pp. 27–37; Betty V. Graliker and Richard Koch, "A Study of Factors Influencing Placement of Retarded Children in a State Residential Institution," *American Journal of Mental Deficiency* (1965): 553–59.

[29] Mary T. Hobbs, "A Comparison of Institutionalized and Non-institutionalized Mentally Retarded," *American Journal of Mental Deficiency* (1964): 206–10.

category to adults. The aggressiveness of many institutionalized retardates was pointed out above as a factor increasing the difficulty of their care. Among adults, aggression is, of course, illegal when it threatens others.

Among adult retarded women a major concern is sexual misdemeanors. In the study of female admissions to an English institution cited above, about one-sixth of these admissions were involved in sexual misdemeanors.[30] Saenger (p. 60) reported that 17% of the high-grade retarded and 14% of the low-grade retarded in institutions had committed a sex offense in the community. In contrast, *none* of the mentally retarded in the community had been detected in a sexual offense.

The explanation of why more retarded adults are admitted to public mental hospitals than to public institutions is apparently that most are mildly retarded persons who are institutionalized because of unacceptable social behavior. The impetus for institutionalization is thus more likely to originate with law enforcement authorities than concerned parents. If a mental problem is suspected, the long waiting lists of most public institutions, plus the lack of expertise of the police in distinguishing mental illness from mental retardation means that the person will probably be sent to a public mental hospital. It is noteworthy that in a study of 81 retarded patients (54 were men) under the age of 40 at St. Elizabeth's Hospital (a public mental hospital), it was found that 50 were admitted because of destructive, hostile or unmanageable behavior.[31]

3) A third major reason for the institutionalization of the retarded is that they often have no acceptable place to reside in the community. Tarjan et al. reported that one in four of the families of children under 10 years of age admitted to Pacific State Hospital considered their retarded children a financial burden. Among admissions age 14 to 17, the corresponding proportion was one in ten.[32] Rejection may also be motivated by parents or siblings who are ashamed of a retarded child or are unwilling to continue the extra physical burden of providing adequate care.

In some cases, parents institutionalize a child because of concern for the safety of younger children. Tarjan et al. reported that almost one in four of the admissions in their sample were aggressive toward their siblings. Graliker and Koch, in a study of 143 retarded children at the Child Development Clinic of Children's Hospital (Los Angeles), con-

[30] Liu, "Changing Trends," pp. 345–53.

[31] Margaret Mercer, "Why Mentally Retarded Persons Come to a Mental Hospital," *Mental Retardation* (June 1968): 8–10.

[32] Tarjan et al., "The Natural History of Mental Deficiency," pp. 56, 58.

cluded that the earlier a child appears in the birth order, the greater the probability of its being institutionalized. This would seem to reflect a concern for younger siblings.[33]

A recent study by Hammond et al. provides stunning evidence of the unwillingness of the parents of institutionalized retardates to accept their children back into their homes. Letters were sent to the parents of almost 5,400 patients resident in Willowbrook State School (New York) in December 1967, inviting them to discuss the patient's progress and the possibility and advisability of removing their child from the institution. Only 749 replies were received (285 letters were returned as undeliverable). Five hundred and fifty-two of the respondees expressed a desire to discuss their child's current institutionalized situation, but only 77 indicated a wish to discuss the *possibility* of having the child return home. In short, less than 11% of the parents of patients at Willowbrook desired to discuss their child's program and only 1½% were willing to consider having the child return home, most of whom were parents of moderately or mildly retarded children. Not one parent of a physically handicapped retardate expressed an interest in discussing the patient's program or possible release.[34]

Some families are inherently unable to provide proper care for their retarded child even if willing to do so. Hobbs, in contrasting institutionalized (N=27) versus noninstitutionalized (N=23) retardates in Tennessee, found that the former were more likely to come from broken homes or homes where the families were frequently quarrelsome, unemployed, or in other ways failed to conform with societal standards.[35] Liu, in the previously cited study, described the homes of 71% of these admissions as dysmorphic, i.e., "broken homes with poor or absent parental relationships to the child." Only 16% came from homes rated average or better.[36] Saenger reported that 71% of the retarded children who came from families where the parents were considered to be inadequate or where there was a high degree of social deprivation were institutionalized, as compared to 29% of the retarded where the parents were competent and did not suffer from deprivation.[37] Poor health on the part of parents also inhibits adequate home care of the retarded. Saenger found that 18% of the mothers and 15% of the fathers of

[33] Graliker and Koch, "A Study of Factors Influencing Placement," pp. 553–59.

[34] Jack Hammond, Manny Sternlicht, and Martin R. Deutsch, "Parents' Interest in Their Institutionalized Children" (mimeograph).

[35] Hobbs, "A Comparison of Institutionalized and Non-institutionalized Mentally Retarded," p. 210.

[36] Liu, "Changing Trends," pp. 345–53.

[37] Saenger, *Factors Influencing Institutionalization*, p. 77.

institutionalized retardates in his sample had major physical limitations. In contrast, the corresponding figures for retardates in the community were 7% and 7% (p. 159).

Even adequate and well-intentioned parents may institutionalize their retarded children before death in order to ensure their future security. After the death of parents, unless other relatives are willing to take them in, there is little alternative for the more severely retarded but to be institutionalized.

Earlier, we cited a New York study that concluded that 30% of the resident population in state schools for the mentally retarded could be returned to the community if appropriate services were available. Almost two-thirds of these individuals could not be placed because their families were unsuitable and alternative living facilities were not available.[38]

One unsettling aspect of public institutions is that they contain a small number of patients who are not retarded. In 1970, 2.2% of all first admissions to public institutions in the United States had IQs of 85 or more. In the WICHE survey, it was found that 1.5% of the resident population had IQs above 80, and almost 0.4% had IQs above 90.

Garfield and Affleck studied 24 nonretarded residents of institutions and found that most had one or more of the following additional difficulties: emotional or social problems, poor educational achievement, physical disability, a disturbed home situation, or a deceased parent. Their IQs ranged from 71 to 96; six persons had IQs exceeding 90 and fifteen had IQs between 80 and 90. In most cases, precommitment examinations had found IQs within the retarded range and it was only subsequent testing that demonstrated the error. The investigators felt that the precommitment mental tests were poorly done and complicated by emotional problems on the part of the testee. It appeared that the community or parent or guardian frequently seized the opportunity to dispose of an unwanted person.[39] Saenger reported that a small number of nonretarded persons are sent to state schools in New York because of delinquent behavior, but that they are soon released.[40]

However, almost half of the nonretarded first admissions to public institutions in 1967 were under the age of 10 so that delinquent behavior could hardly be the reason for commitment. Moreover, not all of the nonretarded are quickly released. In the Garfield and Affleck study,

[38] Rosenberg, *Appropriateness of Continued Institutionalization*, p. 31.

[39] Sol L. Garfield and C. C. Affleck, "A Study of Individuals Committed to a State Home for the Retarded Who Were Later Released as Not Mentally Defective," *American Journal of Mental Deficiency* (1960): 907–15.

[40] Saenger, *Factors Influencing Institutionalization*, p. 142.

the length of time in institutional care ranged from 20 months to 58 years. Only 3 persons had been committed for fewer than 5 years. In the WICHE survey, the mean length of stay for residents with IQs above 80 was 11.4 years *at the time of survey.*

Payne et al. studied those persons with IQs above 80 located by the WICHE survey.[41] Almost 75% of these persons had one or more physical difficulties. A careful evaluation was made of 59 of the 74 patients with IQs above 80 but without physical handicaps. They were found to be almost completely self-sufficient in dressing, eating, grooming, and toilet use, of normal height and weight, receiving minimal medication, and on the whole were relatively well-behaved.

On further investigation, the WICHE researchers found that these self-sufficient normal persons were most frequently found in institutions with the lowest average cost per resident patient and that 95% were used as ward helpers. They surmised that hospitals were unwilling to release such valuable sources of labor. They found no apparent reason for continued institutionalization.

Cost of residential care—sources and methods. Table 17 shows the estimated cost of residential care for the retarded. Several steps were required to develop these estimates.

1) The initial step was to estimate total current expenditures on the retarded (excluding expenditures on construction, training, and research). Information on the maintenance expenditures of public institutions, public and private mental hospitals, and residential treatment centers for the emotionally and mentally ill was available from NIMH or from the Division of Developmental Disabilities (USDHEW). Four assumptions were made. (1) It was assumed that the average costs of caring for the retarded were the same as for the mentally ill in the case of facilities serving both types of residents. (2) Because of the substantial outpatient program of residential treatment centers, it was assumed that inpatient care in these facilities was twice as costly as outpatient care.[42] (3) Since cost data for 1970 were not available for private mental hospitals or residential treatment centers, it was assumed that average maintenance costs increased in these facilities by the same percentage as in public mental hospitals. (4) Since the latest year for which the number of retardates in residential treatment centers or private mental hospitals is available is 1969, it was assumed that this number did not change in 1970.

[41] Payne, Johnson, and Abelson, *A Comprehensive Description*, pp. 52–59.

[42] This adjustment was not necessary in the case of public institutions or public mental hospitals since they are instructed to exclude the costs of outpatient care in their reports (as well as the costs of construction, research, and training.)

Table 17. Estimated costs of residential services for the mentally retarded, 1968 and 1970

Type of facility	Total maintenance expenditure	Average yearly maintenance expenditure per resident	Value of additional resources in care of retarded			Total cost of care	Average yearly total cost of care per patient
			Unpaid patient help	Volunteer help	Rental value of buildings, land, and equipment		
Public institutions							
1968	$ 672,736,000	$ 3,472	$ 970,000	$1,550,000	$200,000,000	$ 875,256,000	$ 4,546
1970	870,890,000	4,635	1,050,000	1,960,000	221,400,000	1,095,300,000	5,865
Public mental hospitals							
1968	134,099,000	3,831	190,000	310,000	35,300,000	169,899,000	4,998
1970	164,892,000	5,435	200,000	370,000	36,000,000	201,462,000	6,640
Private institutions, residential schools, and other private residential care							
1968	104,118,000	4,098			19,100,000	123,218,000	4,850
1970	149,533,000	5,470			23,400,000	172,933,000	6,326
Private mental hospitals							
1968	1,318,000	15,695			60,000	1,378,000	16,023
1970	1,670,000	22,265			60,000	1,730,000	23,067
Public and private residential schools for the blind (based on 1966 resident population)							

Category	Year					
	1968	8,739,000	4,425	2,100,000	10,839,000	5,488
	1970	10,606,000	5,370	2,300,000	12,906,000	6,535
Public and private residential schools for the deaf	1968	4,928,000	3,850	1,300,000	6,228,000	4,866
	1970	5,417,000	4,670	1,400,000	6,817,000	5,877
Residential treatment centers	1968	9,309,000	3,895	1,800,000	11,109,000	4,648
	1970	18,619,000	5,525	2,900,000	21,519,000	6,385
Other chronic disease hospitals (based on 1967 resident population)	1968	36,784,000	9,680	3,900,000	40,684,000	10,706
	1970	46,778,000	12,310	4,500,000	51,278,000	13,494
Federal and state prisons	1968	28,274,000	2,110	13,900,000	42,174,000	3,147
	1970	32,970,000	2,355	16,600,000	49,570,000	3,541
General hospitals with psychiatric inpatient wards	1968	3,484,000		160,000	3,644,000	
	1970	5,769,000		170,000	5,939,000	
Total	1968	$1,003,789,000	$1,160,000	$1,860,000	$277,620,000	$1,284,429,000
	1970	$1,307,144,000	$1,250,000	$2,330,000	$308,730,000	$1,619,454,000

97

There has been no compilation of the aggregate costs of operating private institutions. There are, however, several reasons why the average cost of care in private institutions would be expected to be greater than in public institutions. To begin with, there is a presumption that private institutions provide, *on the average*, higher quality care than public institutions. In addition, private institutions serve a much younger population. This reduces the proportion of residents who can supplement the institutional staff and increases the proportion who require more expensive developmental services.

The AAMD, in its directory of residential facilities, listed the charges made by private facilities in 1967. These charges should approximate the actual average costs of providing care in these facilities. Excessive profits are practically unheard of and, unless generously endowed, private facilities could not operate continuously at a loss and, in any case, would attempt to restrict subsidies to those unable to afford their services.

Annual charges in private institutions (based on the highest listed charge when a range of charges was provided) varied between $1,000 and $9,000 and averaged $3,300. The actual average charge is somewhat higher, probably of the order of $3,500, since many private institutions listed only their base rates, with provisions for additional charges if special services were required. It was assumed that the cost of maintenance in private institutions increased at the same rate as in public institutions between 1967 and 1970.[43]

On the assumption that the per patient expenditures in private residential schools for the deaf are equivalent to those in public residential schools for the deaf, total expenditures in both types of schools would be of the order of $71 million for the 1967–68 school year and $78 million for the 1969–70 school year.[44] Part of this total, however, was expended for blind pupils (some schools were for the deaf and blind) and part for day students. Approximately 5% of the pupils in these facilities were blind and 15% were day students.

Residential care for the blind is evidently somewhat more expensive than residential care for the deaf. In 1966 Mackie reported that the student-to-teacher ratio was 6.4 in residential schools for the deaf compared to 5.6 in residential schools for the blind.[45] If costs are roughly

[43]This estimate is not, strictly speaking, comparable to average per-resident costs in public institutions, since most private institutions required parents or guardians to provide medical care and clothing, services which are usually included in the costs incurred in public institutions.

[44]Based on data provided in *American Annals of the Deaf* (1969): 621 and (1971): 220.

[45]Mackie, *Special Education*, pp. 37, 48.

in proportion to these ratios, then the average cost for the blind is about 15% higher than the average cost for the deaf. Thus, about 5¾% (5% × 1.15) of the cost of operating these residential institutions for the deaf should be allocated to serving the blind.

Another 7½% of the total cost of residential facilities for the deaf are allocated to day pupils on the assumption that expenditures on day pupils are one-half of those of resident pupils. From this we estimate that the average cost of serving deaf students in residential schools for the deaf was about $3,850 per year per pupil in 1968 and $4,670 in 1970.

Presumably, the cost of serving deaf mentally retarded pupils in these facilities is higher than this average cost. However, we have no basis for estimating this additional cost. Because of the low teacher-pupil ratio, such an adjustment would probably be small.

The cost of serving the blind in public residential schools for the blind was approximated by adding 15% to the average per capita cost of serving the deaf in residential facilities. As before, it is conservatively assumed that the cost of serving blind mentally retarded pupils is the same as the average cost of serving all of the blind in these facilities.

If mentally retarded persons treated in psychiatric wards of general hospitals have about the same average length of stay as other psychiatric patients (17 days) and if they incur the same average daily cost as short-term patients in general and special hospitals, then the average cost of a course of treatment for the mentally retarded in general hospitals in 1968 was about $1,045, and in 1970, $1,325.[46]

The President's Commission on Law Enforcement and Administration of Justice, in a survey of correctional agencies and institutions operated by states and communities throughout the United States, reported that the average daily cost per person was $5.24 in 1965, a little over $1,900 per year.[47] A rough estimate of the cost in 1968 and 1970 was made by increasing the 1965 cost by the change in the consumer price index. This underestimates the true expense of imprisonment, since it does not take account of the cost of apprehension, conviction, or subsequent probation.

2) Patient work is a significant resource in many institutions providing residential care. In a study at Polk State School (Pennsylvania), circa 1959, it was found that 12% of the severely retarded, 58% of the moderately retarded, and 85% of the mildly retarded were working

---

[46]Carl Taube, *Average Stay per Discharge in General Hospital Inpatient Psychiatric Units, 1968*, Statistical Note 21, Biometry Branch, NIMH; *Statistical Abstract of the United States, 1971*, p. 71.

[47]The President's Commission on Law Enforcement and Administration of Justice, *Task Force Report: Corrections* (Washington: USGPO, 1967), p. 194.

without remuneration for the institution. Hours of work ranged from 3½ to 80 per week. Patient-workers outnumbered full-time paid employees by a ratio of almost 2 to 1. These patient-aides worked 45% more hours than all of the paid employees of the institution.[48]

In the WICHE survey of patients in western institutions it was reported that 27% of the patients were ward helpers (another 12% were possible candidates for ward helpers). In addition, 21% of the patients were involved in other institution work projects (another 9% were considered possible candidates for such activities). These figures are not additive since some patients were employed on both types of projects.

Fifty-four percent of the resident population in these western institutions was 20 years of age or older. Recognizing that the number of patients gainfully occupied in the institutions exceeded 27%, it would appear that at least one in every two adults was involved in a work program. In comparison, if we divide the number of patient-workers reported by the Polk State School study by the resident population age 15 or over in that institution, the resulting percentage is 53%.[49]

Since the age distribution of the resident population encompassed in the WICHE survey is almost identical with that of residents of all public institutions in the United States, it is reasonable to believe that the proportion of residents who are ward helpers is also approximately the same. In 1968 this would have amounted to almost 52,000 patient-aides and in 1970, 50,000 patient aides. The value of their work depends upon the number of hours worked by the patients and the efficiency with which they perform their tasks. In the Polk State School study, average hours of work were 34. If this were the average for all ward helpers in the country, then these patients would have worked 1,768,000 hours in 1968 and 1,700,000 hours in 1970.

The table on the opposite page shows the rating of the work performance of the patient-helpers in the Polk State School study. It will be assumed that the efficiency of the hours of work performed by all patient-aides parallels the work performance ratings of patient-aides at Polk State School.[50]

Conservatively, in 1968 patients' hours of work rated as excellent will be valued at $1.50, those rated as good at $1.00, those rated as fair at $.50, and those rated as poor at $.00. The therapeutic value of such work is, of course, additional to these assigned values. In 1970 these

---

[48]Sidney Kaplan, "The Growing Importance of the Trainable in an Institution Setting," *American Journal of Mental Deficiency* (1961): 394–98.

[49] Ninety-two percent of the resident population at Polk State School was 15 years of age or over in 1966. It was assumed that this same ratio existed in 1959.

[50] Presumably this underestimates the average quality of patients' work, since the more efficient probably work longer hours than the less efficient.

| | Patient workers at Polk State School | | | | |
| Degree of retardation | Percentage of patient-workers by level of retardation | Work performance rating of aides by level of retardation | | | |
		Excellent	Good	Fair	Poor
Mild	29.5%	14.8%	45.0%	27.6%	12.6%
Moderate	63.5	2.5	24.8	42.7	29.9
Severe	7.0	1.0	9.7	28.2	61.2
All	100.0	6.1	29.7	37.3	27.0

assumed values were increased by the increase in average hourly earnings of workers on private payrolls (13%). On the basis of these speculative figures, the average hourly value of patient work is slightly less than $.60 in 1968 and slightly over this amount in 1970. The average weekly value is around $20. The total value of patient labor is a little over $1 million in both years.

To estimate how much of this value should be added to the operating expenditures of public institutions, we must determine the extent to which the efforts of patient-aides are not compensated. In a 1967 survey, it was reported that 26 out of 45 reporting states provided some reimbursement to patient-workers in public mental hospitals or public institutions.[51] Not all of these states provided reimbursement to workers in both types of facilities. Moreover, some states restricted payment to certain types of patient-workers, such as those in sheltered workshops, or those in laundries or kitchens. Almost without exception, pay rates were minimal. For the mentally retarded they ranged between $.60 and $5.00 per *week* in 12 states providing this information. The average reimbursement appeared to be of the order of $1.25 per week.

Taking account of the states which do not remunerate patient-workers, it appears that patient-workers are reimbursed no more than 5% of the value of their efforts. The total value of *unpaid* patient labor would therefore be of the order of $970,000 in public institutions in 1968 and $1,050,000 in 1970.

We would expect that the mentally retarded in public mental hospitals are more likely to be utilized as patient-workers and that their services are of higher quality than the mentally retarded in public institutions, because they tend to be less severely retarded. Unfortunately,

[51] National Association of State Mental Health Program Directors, *Rate of Pay for Patient Labor*, Study #26, February–March 1968.

Table 18. Unpaid patient labor in public institutions for the mentally retarded, 1968 and 1970

Performance rating of aides	Estimated aggregate hours of work		Assumed value of each work hour		Estimated total value of patient labor	
	1968	1970	1968	1970	1968	1970
Excellent	108,000	104,000	$1.50	$1.69	$ 162,000	$ 176,000
Good	526,000	505,000	1.00	1.13	526,000	571,000
Fair	659,000	634,000	0.50	0.56	330,000	355,000
Poor	477,000	459,000	0.00	0.00	—	—
					Total $1,018,000	$1,102,000

there is no data to verify this hypothesis. Therefore, it is assumed that the ratio of the estimated value of unpaid help to total current expenditures is the same in public mental hospitals as in public institutions.

It was not possible to estimate the value of unpaid patient help in other facilities. However, because of the youth of the residents in most other facilities, the value of any patient-help performed would be small.

3) In 1964, 108 schools and institutions serving the retarded reported that volunteers contributed almost 55,000 hours per month to their operations.[52] To estimate volunteer hours contributed to institutions in 1968 and 1970 this earlier figure was increased by 57% and 76% to adjust for the greater number of known public institutions in the later years. This comes to an estimated 1,000,000 volunteer hours provided to public institutions in 1968, and 1,150,000 volunteer hours contributed in 1970.

These volunteer hours will be valued at $1.50 each in 1968 and $1.69 in 1970. Although a small proportion of volunteers are highly trained professionals (14% graduated from college), most are lay persons who assist in providing routine care for retardates.

As in the case of unpaid patient-help, it is assumed that the value of volunteer help to total current expenditures is the same in public mental hospitals as in public institutions. Again, it was not possible to make estimates of this category of cost for other facilities.

4) It is unfortunate that there is little basis on which to estimate so important a component of cost as the fair rental value of the land, buildings, and equipment used for the care of the institutionalized mentally retarded. This element of cost is almost always omitted from operating expenditures, since these assets are usually owned by the state or operating agency rather than rented.

No survey has been undertaken of the value of the capital employed in residential care. As an indication of this value, the California Department of Mental Hygiene estimated in 1965 that it would cost between $6,000 and $20,000 per bed to construct a 500-bed residential facility, with an average cost of $15,000 per bed.[53] If this were, in fact, the actual average cost per residential bed in public institutions throughout the country in that year, the capital value would have been of the order of $2.8 billion. In 1968 increased price levels and a rising resident population would increase this value to $3.2 billion.

[52]Thomas A. Rich and Alden S. Gilmore, "Volunteer Work with the Retarded," *Mental Retardation* (August 1964): 231–34.

[53]Report of the Assembly Interim Committee on Ways and Means, Subcommittee on Mental Health Services, Assembly of the State of California, *A Redefinition of State Responsibility for California's Mentally Retarded*, March 1965, p. 46.

Of course the institutions being contemplated are of a higher quality than generally prevail. A more reasonable estimate of the capital value of public institutions would be of the order of $2 billion in 1968, a little over $10,000 per bed. As a rough check on this figure, in 1961 the value of buildings and grounds for public residential schools for the deaf in the United States was $9,400 per pupil in attendance.[54] If we adjusted this figure to allow for the fact that building values were lower in 1961 and that some of the pupils were day students only, we would undoubtedly find that the capital investment per resident student in these facilities was well above $10,000 in 1968.

In 1960 Schultz estimated that fair rental value of the physical property of educational facilities would be 8% of their capital value.[55] This was based on an interest rate of 5.1% and depreciation of 2.9%. It does not seem likely that the rate of depreciation of the physical assets of residential facilities would differ significantly from those of educational institutions. For reasons to be discussed in Chapter VI, however, we will use a 7% rather than a 5% interest rate. The annual rental value of residential facilities will, therefore, be estimated at 10% of their capital value, a little over $1,000 per year per resident in 1968.

There is almost no basis on which to estimate capital costs for other residential facilities. It will be assumed that capital costs for the mentally retarded in other public or predominantly public facilities—public mental hospitals, residential schools for the deaf, residential schools for the blind,[56] general hospitals,[57] and federal and state prisons—are the same per patient as in public institutions.

Private residential facilities usually have a lower per-patient capital investment than public residential facilities, partly because they tend to be located in areas where they are able to utilize community services (hospitals, laundries, repair shops, etc.), and partly because they tend to utilize less expensive construction methods.[58] For example, as of the end of 1968, 11 new community residential facilities serving 606 patients had been funded under the Mental Retardation Facilities and Community Mental Health Centers Construction Act of 1963. The aver-

[54] *American Annals of the Deaf* (January 1961): 137.

[55] Theodore W. Schultz, "Capital Formation by Education," *Journal of Political Economy* (December 1969): 578–79.

[56] The patient populations of residential schools for the deaf and for the blind are predominantly in public institutions.

[57] The per-patient capital cost in general hospitals is unquestionably much higher than in other residential facilities. To a large degree, this is due to the very expensive medical equipment which must be maintained. The per-patient capital costs of psychiatric wards may, however, be below average, since much of this medical equipment would not be required for mental patients.

[58] *A Redefinition of State Responsibility*, p. 24.

age capital investment per patient was just slightly over $9,000.[59] Although most of these facilities were under public auspices, these data illustrate the lower costs involved in locating facilities in community settings and the possibility of utilizing lower-cost construction.

Since these are new, and presumable high-quality facilities, we may expect that the average capital investment per patient in these facilities would be greater than for all private residential facilities. We will assume an average capital investment per patient in private residential facilities of $7,500 per year in 1968 and, therefore, an implicit rental value of $750 per year per patient for the following facilities: private institutions, private mental hospitals, and residential treatment centers (which are almost all private).

The fair rental value of buildings, land, and equipment in 1970 was estimated by adjusting the estimates of the fair rental values per patient of these assets in 1968 upward by the percentage change in the housing component of the consumer price index between these two years.

Cost of residential services: Residential care for the mentally retarded is costly. Average yearly maintenance expenditures on patients in public institutions were just slightly less than $3,500 in 1968 and rose to over $4,600 in 1970. Annual maintenance costs in other residential institutions were higher (other than the special case of federal and state prisons), in part because most of these other facilities were predominately oriented toward developmental services—residential schools for the blind, deaf, and emotionally and mentally ill, and most private institutions. In evaluating these differences, it should be emphasized that the figure for the cost of maintenance in public institutions is the only one that is based on a direct accounting of expenditures on the retarded. All other estimates were based on inferences from various data sets. When allowance was made for unpaid patient help, volunteer help, and the implicit rental value of land, buildings, and equipment, annual per patient costs rose sharply—by almost one-third in the case of public facilities and by about one-fourth in the case of most private facilities. Capital costs account for almost all of this increase.

If we add together maintenance expenditures for all forms of facilities, we find that these expenditures totaled $1 billion in 1968 and $1.3 billion in 1970. If we sum the value of all resources used for residential care of the retarded, the totals rise to $1.3 billion and $1.6 billion.

Average per resident maintenance costs in public institutions increased 33% between 1968 and 1970 due to the combined influence of improvements in the quality of care and to inflation. During this same

[59] USDHEW, Secretary's Committee on Mental Retardation, *Mental Retardation Construction Program* (March 1969): 41–56.

period, the number of full-time staff per 100 residents in these facilities grew by 18%. If we use this as an index of changes in the quality of care, then we can estimate that 60% of the increase in expenditures was used to improve the quality of care. One justification for this procedure is that if we multiply this index of change in the quality of care times an index of price level change (using the consumer price index) between the two years (1.18 X 1.12), the product 1.32 is almost exactly equal to the ratio of maintenance costs in 1970 to maintenance costs in 1968.

EDUCATION

Data on the educational status of retarded children who are not in institutions are summarized in Table 19. One point must be emphasized. The mentally retarded are enrolled in a wide variety of educational programs, special classes for the retarded, regular academic classes, special classes for the deaf, special classes for the blind, etc.

Number served: Between 1952 and 1966 enrollment in special education programs for the mentally retarded (hereafter referred to as special education programs) conducted by local public school systems grew from 113,000 to 495,000.[60] On the basis of reports from individual states, the U.S. Office of Education estimated that 689,000 pupils attended special education programs during the 1967–68 school year. This last estimate is not comparable to the 1966 figure, since the states were asked to estimate the number of retarded children in private day school clasess and in public and private residential schools, as well as in local public school systems. Information was not provided on the number of children in each type of system.

In 1968, 48,700 mentally retarded pupils were enrolled in state-operated school systems which were partly financed by federal funds (PL 89-313). In that year, almost all systems which received funding under this act were in state operated residential facilities. (Since then, increasing amounts of these funds have been used to support community programs.) Undoubtedly, this includes most retarded children enrolled in special education programs in public institutions, since states are reimbursed on the basis of the number of children attending school and would have no reason to understate their number. In addition, there were about 15,000 mentaly retarded children, age 5 to 19, in *private* residential care, most of whom were in some form of special education program. It is doubtful, however, if, in reporting to the Office of Education the states took full account of retarded children in

[60]USDHEW, Office of Education, *Digest of Educational Statistics, 1968* (prepared by Kenneth A. Simon and W. Vance Grant), p. 35.

school programs in private residential facilities, partly because of the difficulty of obtaining this information, and partly because it would not affect federal funding. If both of these figures are subtracted from the total number in special classes, therefore, we obtain a conservative estimate of the number of persons who attended special education programs for the retarded sponsored by *local* public or private school systems in 1968, 626,000.

The number of these children being served in private school systems cannot be reliably estimated. This much can be noted however. Only about one out of every fifteen private schools offering regular academic programs offered special education of any type during the 1965–66 school year.[61] Only ½ of 1% of the students enrolled in these schools were in ungraded classes (33,500 pupils). Many of these special-class enrollees were so placed because of physical handicaps or behavioral problems rather than retardation.

Private educational efforts on behalf of the retarded should not, however, be dismissed as inconsequential. Many private day schools are operated specifically for the retarded and would not be included in the data contained in the preceding paragraph. To a large extent these schools provide educational service to children who are ineligible for public classes because of the severity of their retardation or associated handicaps, or who live in school districts that do not operate special classes.

Special education in the community may be divided into roughly four categories: classes for the educable retarded, classes for the trainable retarded, homebound instruction, and day development classes.[62] This last category requires further explanation. Traditionally, when children have been too severely retarded to be enrolled in classes for the educable or trainable retarded, any care they received outside the educational system has been classified as "day care." Since most of these programs are developmental, this is misleading. It is preferable to describe these programs as "day development" classes.

The great majority of special-education pupils attend classes for the educable retarded. The Office of Education (unpublished data) reported that in 1968, 555,000 persons were enrolled in programs for the educable (including those in residential care), 94,000 in programs for the

---

[61] USDHEW, Office of Education, *Statistics of Nonpublic Elementary and Secondary Schools, 1965–66*, p. 40.

[62] Some retarded pupils spend part of their time in special classes (or in receiving individualized instruction) and part in regular classes. In 1963 almost 10% of students in special classes maintained this schedule. In 1970 this ratio rose to over 25%, reflecting changes in attitudes and philosophies.

Table 19. Community services provided to the mentally retarded, 1968 and 1970

Services	Number of retarded served	Proportion of total population served who are retarded	Operating cost/year/person	Total operating cost	Volunteer services	Rental value of buildings, land, & equipment	Total measurable cost	Average total measurable cost
Children's educational programs								
Special education in public and private day classes								
1968								
Classes for the educable retarded	552,000	100.0%						
Classes for the trainable retarded and day development classes	76,000	100.0%						
Classes for the deaf	2,200	9.2%						
Total	630,200		$1,274[a]	$ 802,900,000	b	$252,100,000	$1,055,000,000	$1,674
1970								
Classes for the educable and trainable retarded and day development classes	686,000	100.0%						
Classes for the deaf	1,900	9.2%						
Total	687,900		1,625[a]	1,117,800,000	b	340,200,000	1,458,000,000	2,119
Residential treatment centers (outpatients)								
1968	1,220	25.0%	1,948	2,400,000	b	500,000	2,900,000	2,348
1970	1,720	25.0%	2,762	4,800,000	b	800,000	5,600,000	3,256
Regular academic programs								
1968	738,000		658	485,600,000	b	162,400,000	648,000,000	878
1970	724,000		783	566,900,000	b	181,700,000	748,600,000	1,034

Program / Year	Number served	Percent	Measurable operating cost	Cost recovered	Capital cost	Total cost	
Not in school (5 to 19 years old)							
1968	461,000						
1970	451,000						
Clinical services							
Mental retardation clinics							
1968	66,400	100.0%	13,300,000		b	13,300,000	f
1970	97,600	100.0%	26,100,000		b	26,100,000	f
Outpatient psychiatric clinics							
1968	41,400	3.4%	10,400,000		b	10,400,000	f
1970	66,100	3.8%	22,100,000		b	22,100,000	f
Community mental health centers							
1968	7,800	2.9%	2,300,000		b	2,300,000	f
1970	15,300	3.0%	6,200,000		b	6,200,000	f
Employment programs for adults							
Vocational rehabilitation							
1968	22,247c	10.7%	54,600,000		b	54,600,000	f
1970	31,503c	11.8%	89,200,000		b	89,200,000	f
Sheltered workshops and activity centers							
1968	26,000d	30.1%	19,800,000e	$600,000	b	20,400,000	785
1970	34,000d	30.1%	34,700,000e	$900,000	b	35,600,000	1,047
Totals							
1968			$1,391,300,000	$600,000	$415,000,000	$1,806,900,000	
1970			$1,867,800,000	$900,000	$522,700,000	$2,391,400,000	

a Represents average cost for students in classes for the educable retarded, trainable retarded, and deaf.
b Not available.
c Represents the number rehabilitated, not the number served.
d Based on number of clients in average daily attendance.
e Represents the part of workshop costs not recovered through business operations.
f Average total measurable cost is equal to operating cost per year per person.

109

trainable, and 40,500 were in an unknown status. If this latter group is allocated between the educable and trainable programs in proportion to the known number enrolled in each type of program, the two estimates would be raised to 590,000 and 100,000. It is probable, for reasons to be described below, that this latter figure includes most of the children in "day development" classes. Children in homebound programs would also be encompassed in these figures. In 1963 less than 2% of the total special-class enrollment were in homebound programs.

These estimates of the number of children in special education programs for the educable retarded and trainable retarded include both those in institutions and in the community. In 1968 there were more mildly and borderline retarded persons admitted to institutions than were moderately retarded, by a factor of 3 to 2. Moreover, the ratio of mild to moderate retardation was higher in the past and would be higher among admissions of children. It is probable, therefore, that more children attend classes for the educable retarded than for the trainable retarded in institutions, because of the relatively high rate of mild mental retardation among young residents of institutions. We will assume that 60% of institution residents in special education programs attend programs for the educable retarded. We estimate, therefore, that there were about 74,000 persons in classes for the trainable retarded (including some in day development classes) and 552,000 persons in classes for the educable retarded who were enrolled in local public or private school systems in 1968.[63]

Stohrer recently reported that there were 934 community day care and child development centers for the retarded that received a direct state subsidy in 1968. Since not all of these facilities are subsidized, he believed that there must have been over 1,200 such programs.[64]

Information on 370 day facilities for the mentally retarded from 10 states indicates that an average of 37 persons are served per facility.[65] If this average is valid for all 1,200 such facilities, then there are about 44,000 persons in community day care or child development centers serving the retarded.

The number of retarded children in "day development" classes would be far less than this total. Fragmentary information on the 370 day facilities previously described indicated that about one-third of

[63] In 1963, 30,000 children were enrolled in classes for the trainable retarded in local public school systems (Mackie, *Special Education*, p. 44).

[64] John F. Stohrer, New Hampshire Office of Mental Retardation, "The Trend toward State Support of Community Mental Retardation Day Activities," September 1968 (unpublished manuscript).

[65] For nine states (California, Colorado, Georgia, Illinois, Iowa, Maryland, Michigan, New York, and Pennsylvania) the information was obtained by the Council of

these clients were adults and about one-third were emotionally or physically handicapped rather than retarded, so that the number of retarded children served by all such facilities would have been of the order of 20,000. Some of these were educable and the majority were in the trainable range.[66] It would be surprising if the number of children below the trainable level, and thus of a level that would be appropriate for "day development" classes, exceeded 5,000.

Since the majority of day facilities receive a state subsidy, most of the children in these facilities must have been included in the state estimate of the number of children in special education. It is certainly true for children in the educable and trainable ranges, and is probably true for a majority of those on a lower level of educability (who would be reported as trainable or in an unknown status).

Because of the difficulty of making a meaningful empirical distinction between classes for the trainable retarded and "day development" classes, these categories are combined in Table 19. It was assumed that about 2,000 students in "day development" classes were not included in the state estimates of the total number of children in special education classes. This figure was added to our earlier estimate of 74,000 pupils in public and private day classes for the trainable retarded, so that the final estimate for this group is increased to 76,000.

In the spring of 1970, the National Center for Educational Statistics (Office of Education, USDHEW) undertook a survey of special education programs in local public school districts. The schools reported that 936,000 retarded pupils had been identified. Of these, 208,000 were reported as not receiving any type of specialized instruction. Of the remaining 728,000, 499,000 were reported as being in separate special classes for all of their instruction, and the remaining 229,000 were in special classes part-time, or were receiving individualized instruction or assistance either from a specialized professional or in a regular classroom from a regular teacher.

Regardless of what school systems may report, individualized instruction in regular classrooms by regular teachers is unlikely to be either individualized or special and does not qualify as a special education program. The survey reported that 99,000 retardates were receiving special education programs in regular classrooms staffed by regular teachers. Some of these, however, were in regular classrooms only part-time, the rest of the time being spent in special education classes or in

---

State Governments (unpublished). Data from Wisconsin was provided by the Division of Mental Hygiene of that state.

[66] Not all school systems operate special classes for the trainable retarded. Often school systems purchase care from outside the system.

being tutored by professional personnel and, thus, can be considered as being in a special education program.

It was not possible to determine directly how many of the retarded students who were reported as receiving special instruction in regular classrooms by regular teachers received all of their instruction in this manner, since students who received more than one type of instruction were recorded twice in the distribution of retarded children in special education programs by type of instruction. Thus, 283,000 students were reported as being in special classes part-time or receiving special instruction by professional personnel or by their regular teacher. It can be observed, however, that double counting could have occurred in only 54,000 cases (283,000–229,000). If it is assumed that all of these cases occurred among retarded pupils receiving part of their instruction in regular classrooms, then only 45,000 of these students (99,000–54,000) could have received full-time instruction from a regular teacher and the number of retarded students in special education programs in local public school districts in 1970 would have been 674,000. This appears to be a reasonable assumption, since the alternative would have been for some retarded pupils to receive part of their education in special classes and part from specialized professionals, a circumstance which is not likely to occur often, and even when it does occur it is unlikely that schools would bother to make a distinction. Schools that place retardates in regular classes, however, would find it important to point out that these students do receive specialized instruction.

To estimate the total number of retarded students in special education programs in 1970 we assume that 10,000 were in special education programs in private school systems and another 2,000 were in day development classes and not reported by the local school districts. Altogether, we estimate that 686,000 retarded students were in special education programs for the retarded in public or private school systems or in day development classes. No information was available on the distribution of these pupils between programs for the educable and trainable.

Many multiply-handicapped retarded children are in special classes for the emotionally or physically handicapped. In 1968 an estimated 23,700 children were enrolled in special day classes for the deaf and hard of hearing. During October 1970, the comparable figure was 20,433.[67] The great majority (about 85%) were enrolled in public schools. Almost one-third were in preschools.

_____

[67]*American Annals of the Deaf* (May 1969): 624 and (April 1971): 214. The Bureau for the Education of the Handicapped (Office of Education) reported that in 1967–68, almost 62,000 deaf and hard-of-hearing children were in special educa-

In 1960 (the last year in which this information was collected) it was reported that 4.6% of deaf children in special day classes were also mentally retarded. Another 9.2% were asphasic, blind, cerebral palsied, orthopedically impaired, or brain injured.[68] It can be assumed that at least half of these multiply-physically-handicapped children were also retarded, so that at least 9.2% of the children in classes for the deaf and hard of hearing are also mentally retarded—about 2,200 pupils in 1968 and 1,900 in 1970.

The Office of Education reported that 24,600 visually impaired children, 105,000 emotionally disturbed children, 69,000 crippled children, 24,000 multiply-handicapped children, and 138,000 children with other health impairments were enrolled in special education programs in the 1967–68 school year. Most were in local public school systems. Unfortunately, with one minor exception, we are unable to estimate the number of these children who are retarded. For reasons previously mentioned, it was assumed that 25% of the children who were outpatients in residential treatment centers for the emotionally and mentally ill were mentally retarded. Information was not available on the number of outpatients in residential treatment centers for any year past 1968. It was assumed that outpatients increased at the same rate as inpatients between 1968 and 1969 in these facilities and the 1969 estimate is assumed to be valid for 1970.

In 1968 and 1970 there were approximately 1,936,000 and 1,975,000 children who were 5 to 19 years of age with IQs below 70. We have estimated that about 631,000 and 690,000 were in special education programs. On the basis of previously computed information, it is estimated that the number in institutional care is 108,000 in 1968 and 110,000 in 1970. This leaves about 1,197,000 who must have been in regular academic classes or not in school in 1968, and 1,175,000 in 1970, a slight decrease.[69]

Most retarded children who are not in special classes or in residential care attend regular academic classes. Of over 11,000 school-age children identified as mentally retarded in New Jersey in 1953, 41% were in

---

tion programs (including residential programs). Subtracting the number of children in residential care would indicate that almost 42,000 are being served on less than a 24-hour basis, almost twice the above estimate. The discrepancy is evidently due to a large number of deaf and hard-of-hearing children being provided clinical services by local school districts, but who are retained in regular academic programs.

[68] *American Annals of the Deaf* (January 1961): 162.

[69] The actual number may be even larger since many special classes accept students with IQs above 70, sometimes as high as 85. On the other hand, there is an offsetting bias in that we have no estimate of the number of retarded children in certain types of residential facilities and special classes.

special education classes, 49% were in regular classes, and only 10% were not attending school. In the 1970 survey of special education programs conducted by the National Center for Educational Statistics, an estimated 28% were attending regular classes on a full-time basis. Undoubtedly in both cases many more retarded children attended regular classes but were not identified as retarded.[70]

In 1957 Levinson concluded that about 1/3 of 1% of the school-age children in Maine living at home were excluded from school and had an IQ below 50. Less than one-third of these were known to school systems.[71] On this basis, there would have been almost 200,000 such school-age children nationwide.

In view of the enormous increase in classes for the trainable mentally retarded since 1957, this figure is surely too high. Of the 237,000 children aged 5 to 19 in the United States with IQs below 50, in 1968, we estimate that about 70,000 were in residential facilities (this assumes that institutionalized school-age children have the same proportion of persons with IQs below 50 as exists in the entire institutional population). Most of the 76,000 students in classes for the trainable retarded and day development classes have IQs below 50. Thus, we estimate that about 91,000 school-age children with IQs below 50 were living at home and did not attend any educational facility in 1968. Not all of these children are denied educational opportunity, since many enter school several years beyond the normal age of enrollment and most leave before age 19.

We would not expect to find appreciable numbers of mildly retarded children totally excluded from school unless severely physically handicapped. Of an estimated 1,699,000 mildly retarded children between the ages of 5 and 20 in the United States in 1968 approximately 38,000 were in residential facilities and about 553,000 were in classes for the educable mentally retarded or residential treatment facilities. Apparently, almost 1.1 million mildly retarded children were either in regular academic programs, had terminated their educational programs, or were waiting to begin their educational programs. After age 16, school enrollment as a percentage of the population in each successive age level

---

[70] New Jersey Department of Education, *Found, A Report of the Committee to Study the Education of Handicapped Children* (no date), p. 22.

[71] This estimate was based on a study of two New Hampshire communities which Levinson felt would be typical of Maine. Six-tenths of 1% of the children in these communities were excluded from school. Of these Levinson estimated that one-half had IQs below 50 and adjusted the results upward by 0.05% to compensate for the lack of a canvass (E. J. Levinson, *Retarded Children in Maine* [Orono, Maine: University of Maine Press], p. 147).

declines rapidly,[72] and it can be assumed that the mildly retarded in regular academic programs are heavy casualties of this trend. It also seems probable that many of the mildly retarded would delay school entrance for a year or more beyond the age they can legally enter school. It is a reasonable surmise that about two-thirds of the mildly retarded who are not in residential care or special education programs in the age range 5 to 19 were in regular academic programs—about 738,000 persons. A small number would be in types of special education classes for which we have no estimate of the number of retardates.

In 1970 there were an estimated 1,975,000 retarded children in the United States (all IQ ranges) of whom 110,000 were in residential facilities and 690,000 were in special education programs, leaving 1,175,000 who were in regular academic programs or not in school. Between 1968 and 1970, the number of retarded children of school age rose by 39,000, while the number of retardates in special education programs increased by 59,000, which should have the effect of reducing the percentage of retarded children who are not in school. However, the development of special education programs usually results in the transfer of some students in regular academic classes to special education classes. Nevertheless, the emphasis in recent years on the development of school programs for the trainable retarded and on high school programs for the retarded leads one to expect that a substantial part of the growth of special education has resulted in reducing the number of out-of-school retarded children. We will assume that this group fell from 461,000 in 1968 to 451,000 in 1970, and that the number of retardates in regular academic classes fell from 738,000 to 724,000. It is worth noting that had the percentage of school-age retardates not in school remained constant between these two years, the number not in school would be almost 19,000 higher than our estimate.

These estimates, although subject to a considerable margin of error, are sufficiently accurate to permit the following generalizations.

1) Probably no more than 3 to 4% of noninstitutionalized retarded children are denied any form of educational training. This seemingly optimistic statement must be tempered by the observations that the effects of total exclusion from educational programs are catastrophic, and that there is no assurance that educational services provided to the retarded are of sufficient duration or are appropriate to their needs.

2) More retarded children are in regular academic programs than in special education programs. Moreover, it is probable that a majority of retarded children in regular academic programs are not identified as

[72] Simon and Grant, *Digest of Educational Statistics*, p. 4.

retarded. In the Alamance County survey cited in the previous chapter, the schools reported that only 2.1% of the school population was mentally retarded, although the clinically determined rate was 9%.

3) The rapid growth of special education programs has probably had a greater effect in shifting children to special classes from regular classrooms than it has had in enabling increased numbers of retarded children to be enrolled in educational programs.

Demographic characteristics and reasons for special-class placement: There are a number of interrelated, and sometimes surprising, factors which determine which retardates will be placed in special classes and which will be left in regular classes. Severity of retardation is the most obvious of these considerations. Kirk has reviewed studies comparing mentally retarded children in regular and special-class programs and concluded that the former are, "on the whole, superior academically to the children assigned to special classes."[73]

IQ alone is not always sufficient to predict special-class placement. Physical handicaps and social adjustment must also be considered. Blatt, in a 1958 study, found that the retarded in special classes (N=75) had more uncorrected or permanent physical handicaps than those in regular classes (N=50).[74] Surprisingly, Kirk felt that the existing studies showed that children in special classes were superior in social adjustment to those left in regular classes. However, special classes lay greater stress on improving social adjustment and motivation than regular classes, which probably explains this finding.

Several studies have found that significantly more males are enrolled in special education programs than females. In a survey of students who graduated from special education programs in New York City during 1960 and 1963, females constituted about 38% of the total sample. When the sample was broken down into two IQ groups—65 or under and 66 or over—the percentages of females were 44% and 34% respectively.[75] A 1954 nationwide survey of classes for severely retarded

[73] Samuel A. Kirk, "Research in Education," in *Mental Retardation, A Review of Research*, Harvey A. Stevens and Rick Heber, eds. (Chicago: The University of Chicago Press, 1964), p. 63.

[74] Burton Blatt, "The Physical, Personality, and Academic Status of Children Who Are Mentally Retarded Attending Special Classes as Compared with Children Attending Regular Classes," *American Journal of Mental Deficiency* (March 1958): 813.

[75] Jack Tobias, Ida Alpert, and Arnold Birenbaum, *A Survey of Employment Status of Mentally Retarded Adults in New York City* (New York: Association for the Help of Retarded Children, April 1969), p. 11.

children (IQ below 50) reported that 43% of the students were females.[76]

One reason why males are more likely than females to be enrolled in
special education programs is that young males are more prone to dis-
ruptive classroom behavior than females, which is often a consideration
in the decision to transfer a student to a special education program.
Another, and perhaps more important reason is that scholastic achievement among retarded females tends to be considerably higher than
among comparably retarded males, perhaps for attitudinal reasons. In
the New York survey females were two to three months more advanced
in arithmetic achievement than males and four to five months more
advanced in reading achievement. Bensberg has made a similar observation.[77] Few children with IQs below 65 are capable of satisfactory
progress in a regular classroom which explains the smaller excess of
males in this IQ range.

In the New York City survey, the proportion of Negroes in special
classes corresponded roughly to the proportion of Negroes in the total
school population; the population of Puerto Ricans was about double;
and the proportion of whites was about half of the expected frequency.
Data from Texas and California also affirm that the proportion of
children with Spanish surnames enrolled in special classes is twice their
proportion in the total school population—a fact which in California
was also true for Negroes.[78]

What is surprising is not the over-representation of these minority
groups in special education programs, but that their numbers are not
even higher. Perhaps the essentially segregated nature of much of the
educational system makes it possible for the retarded among minority
groups to remain in regular classes, while the same level of achievement
in a class of white children would result in a transfer to special classes.

One other factor must be considered. Recently, students of Mexican
descent who were enrolled in educable mentally retarded classes and
who had evidenced a problem in using the English language were tested
with a Spanish version of the Wechsler Intelligence Test for Children

[76] Elizabeth M. Boggs, "Day Classes for Severely Retarded Children," *American
Journal of Mental Deficiency* (January 1954): 360.

[77] E.g., Gerald J. Bensberg, "The Relationship of Academic Achievement of
Mental Defectives to Mental Age, Sex, Institutionalization, and Etiology," *American Journal of Mental Deficiency* (October 1953): 328.

[78] Jane Case Williams, *Improving Educational Opportunities for Mexican-Ameri-
can Handicapped Children*, Bureau of Education for the Handicapped, U.S. Office
of Education, April 1968, p. 5.

(although a few students preferred to use the English version). They achieved a mean IQ of 82 compared to a previous mean of 69 based on the English version. Slightly over one-sixth of the children scored 90 or above. Their average IQ on the performance scale was 87 points, and 44% scored 90 or above.[79] Had these children been enrolled in schools taught in Spanish, so that they might gain greater proficiency in the use of the written version of their language, it can be assumed that their scores would have been even higher. It is probable that lack of facility with English also constitutes a learning handicap for some Negro children.

Relatively few retarded children are identified as retarded upon initial entrance to school. Many do well enough to remain in regular classes for several years before the accumulated deficits of their academic history and the increasingly abstract nature of the material they are called upon to learn precludes continuing in regular classrooms.

In the New York study (Tobias et al.), about one-third of the white children in special classes were so placed while they were 6 to 7 years old, and about one-fourth were not so placed until they were 12 to 13 years old. The proportion of Puerto Rican and Negro children in special classes who were identified as retarded when 6 to 7 years old was significantly lower than for whites, but little importance can be attached to this observation because of the larger number of these children who migrated to New York after they became of school age.[80] What is of interest is that a significantly higher proportion of special-class children with IQs above 65 were identified as retarded before age 10 than were special-class children with IQs 65 or lower. This was true for all ethnic groups. Possibly, lower-IQ retarded children are more tractable in their behavior than the higher-IQ retarded children and regular classroom teachers are less anxious to remove them from the classroom.

In one large metropolitan area it was observed that a circumscribed census tract area which had the highest rate of dilapidated housing, the lowest median educational level, and the lowest median income, contributed over 33% of the enrollment in the city's special classes, although these census tracts contained only 2.5% of the city's popula-

---

[79] John T. Chandler and John Plako, *Spanish-Speaking Pupils Classified as Educable Mentally Retarded*, California State Department of Education, 1969.

[80] These data were provided only for males with the comment that females "showed no consistent or notable variation from the boys in their corresponding IQ or ethnic groups."

tion.[81] This is readily explainable by the high prevalence of mental retardation among low-income nonwhites.

In sum, placement in special classes depends upon level of retardation, other physical handicaps, and behavior. Males are more likely to be placed in these classes than females of comparable intellect. The proportion of poor and nonwhite students in these classes is above average, which is apparently caused by the relatively higher frequency of retardation among these groups.

Costs: In the 1967–68 school year, the student-teacher staffing ratio (full-time equivalent) for all retarded children in special classes was 14.8. Although these data include children attending special classes in residential facilities, it is unlikely that this overall ratio differs significantly from the student-teacher ratio in local public school systems.[82] At the beginning of the 1967–68 school year the number of students per room in public elementary and secondary schools in the United States was 26.1. Since it required 1.8 times as many classrooms and teachers to serve the same number of students in special education programs as in regular academic classrooms (26.1/14.8), it can be assumed that the average per capita cost of the former was at least 1.8 times that of the latter.[83]

During the 1967–68 school year current operating expenditures for all public elementary and secondary schools in the United States averaged $658 per pupil.[84] The equivalent figure for retarded special education students therefore would be at least $1,185 per pupil. This figure understates the actual current costs of special education for several reasons.

[81] Herbert J. Prehm, "Concept Learning in Culturally Disadvantaged Children as a Function of Verbal Pretraining," *Exceptional Children* (May 1966): 600.

[82] In 1963 the student-teacher ratio for special education classes conducted by local public school systems for the retarded was 15.6. The decline between 1963 and 1968 probably resulted from the increasing number of classes for the trainable retarded, which are generally smaller than classes for the educable retarded.

[83] Had we compared the student-teacher staffing ratio for all students with that for the retarded, our estimate would have been slightly lower, since the overall student-teacher staffing ratio was of the order of 24 to 1. However, the above comparison is probably more accurate, since the overall student-teacher ratio would include some specialized instructors, such as music teachers, who may serve both the retarded and nonretarded and a portion of whose time should be allocated to the retarded.

[84] These expenditures ranged from $982 per pupil in New York to $346 in Mississippi. In part, these differences reflect differences in teacher salaries and not differences in the quality of classroom instruction. These and succeeding data are

The mentally retarded in special classes probably require more extra-classroom services than regular academic students. We will allow $15 per student to adjust for this variable, although there is little tangible evidence to justify this figure.

Transportation costs are above average for the mentally retarded, due to their decreased ability to utilize regular transportation facilities and because special education programs are frequently consolidated over several school districts. The average transportation cost of students enrolled in classes for the trainable retarded was $318 during the 1964–65 school year in California.[85] For all students in the United States it was only $20 during the following year.[86] Thus, excess transportation costs for the trainable retarded appear to be of the order of $250 to $300.

The excess transportation costs of students in classes for the educable would be lower, because of the greater ability of these children to use normal transporation facilities and the greater number of such classes. We will assume that it is $50.

Still other elements of current costs for special education are the forgone earnings of students, the value of volunteer help, and the value of privately provided transportation to and from school, school supplies, and additional costs of clothing required for school attendance. Because of lack of data, we will not attach a value to these variables.

An estimate of the current cost of special education for the retarded in 1968 was derived by multiplying the total number of students in special classes (all levels) by $1,200, the number of students in classes for the educable retarded by $50, and the number of students in classes for the trainable retarded and "day development" classes by $250 (using the lower range of our estimate for excess transportation costs) and summing. It was assumed that these costs were applicable to both public and private classes for the retarded and for those retarded in classes for the deaf. Student-teacher ratios are comparable between public and private school systems.

Current operating costs for retarded students in *regular* academic programs were assumed to be the same as the average for all students. In the case of residential treatment centers for the emotionally and mentally ill, outpatient care costs were assumed to be one-half of the

---

derived from Simon and Grant, *Digest of Educational Statistics* (1971): 59, and (1968): 24, 31, 38, 39.

[85] Based on data in Flora M. Daly, "The Program for Trainable Mentally Retarded Pupils in the Public Schools of California," *Education and Training of the Mentally Retarded* (October 1966): 111.

[86] Simon and Grant, *Digest of Educational Statistics,* p. 47.

costs of residential care in these facilities. The operating cost for out-patients in residential treatment centers in 1969 was adjusted to a 1970 basis as described in the section on residential care costs for inpatients.

At the beginning of the 1970 school year, the number of students per room in public elementary and secondary schools fell somewhat to 24.6. The survey, conducted by the National Center for Health Statistics, found that the ratio of retarded students who received part or all of their instruction in separate (special) classes to the number of full-time equivalent professional staff was 12.6. On this basis, it cost 1.95 times as much to provide special education programs for retarded children in 1970 as education cost for a nonretarded student. The increase since 1968 is consistent with increased educational services to the severely retarded and expanded special education programs in secondary schools.

During the 1969–70 school year, average operating expenditures for public elementary and secondary students in the United States were estimated at $783.[87] The average annual operating cost per student in special education was estimated by: (1) multiplying $783 by 1.95; (2) adding $15 for extra classroom services; and (3) approximating the transportation cost component by increasing the average transportation cost for retarded students in special education programs in 1968 by the percentage increase in transportation cost per student transported between 1968 and 1970 (12%). The estimated average cost of special education increased over 25% over the two years to over $1,600 per year.

The fair rental value of the capital goods used for education programs is a major element of educational costs that must be taken into consideration. Data from thirty-seven states indicated that the average value of land, buildings, and equipment owned by local units charged with administering the education systems was $1,491 per pupil in average daily attendance during the 1967–68 school year.[88]

The problem is that the principal basis for determining 'value" was original cost plus the cost of all additions and alterations, rather than the current market or replacement value of these assets. Since their replacement values are undoubtedly greater than their original costs, we will increase the original cost estimate by 50%.

On this assumption, and using 10% of market value as a measure of fair rental value, the capital costs of regular education would be $220

[87] Simon and Grant, *Digest of Educational Statistics, 1971*, p. 59.

[88] USDHEW, Office of Education, *Statistics of State School Systems*, 1967–68, pp. 66.

and of special education $400 ($220 times 1.8) per year per pupil in 1968. It is assumed that these amounts apply to both public and private facilities. The figure was also imputed to retarded children receiving day care in residential treatment centers. In 1970 these estimates were increased by the percentage change in the housing component of the consumer price index and adjusted to reflect the smaller number of retardates in each special class ($400 X 1.27 X 1.95/1.80 = $494) per special education student.

The results of these calculations are summarized in Table 19. The following conclusions are drawn: (1) The total value of educational resources being utilized for the retarded was $1.7 billion in 1968 and increased to almost $2.2 billion in 1970, an increase of 28%. Over three-fifths of these amounts was utilized for special education programs. (2) On a per pupil basis, special education programs are twice as expensive as regular academic classes. It should be noted, however, that they are about one-third of the cost of residential care.

CLINICAL SERVICES

Number served: For the most part, clinical services consist of diagnosis, evaluation, and counseling, with subsequent referral to agencies where needed services can be obtained.[89]

In 1968 slightly over 40,000 children were served in 142 out of 235 mental retardation clinics (hereafter referred to as MR clinics) in the United States known to the Children's Bureau.[90] If the nonreporting clinics have the same average number of clients, the total number of persons served would be a little over 66,000. A comparable estimate in 1970, based on 145 reporting clinics out of 250, yielded an estimate of over 97,000 clients served. Not all of these children were retarded, since one function of these clinics is to determine whether retardation exists. Of 13,000 new patients in 118 MR clinics in 1970 about 40% were borderline retardates (IQ between 69 and 84).

In 1968 NIMH reported that the cases of 20,500 retarded patients were terminated at outpatient psychiatric clinics (hereafter referred to as OPCs). In 1970 the number of retarded clients who were terminated

---

[89] Although many clinics provide educational services, the children in these classes have already been accounted for in our estimate of children in classes for the trainable or in day development classes.

[90] The 142 clinics were those which were wholly or partially supported by federal grants under title V of the Social Security Act. USDHEW, Social and Rehabilitation Service, National Center for Social Statistics, *Statistical Summary of Patients Served in Mental Retardation Clinics, Fiscal Year 1968*, and unpublished data for 1970.

was 32,703. In 1967 (the last year for which this information was available) the ratio of patients treated in OPCs (cases terminated and cases remaining in treatment) to patients terminated was slightly over 2 to 1.

Assuming a similar proportional relationship among retarded clients in 1968 and 1970, the total number of retarded served would have been slightly over 41,000 and 66,000 in the two years. This is probably an understatement, since some patients with psychiatric diagnoses and some of the almost 20% who had no reported diagnosis were undoubtedly retarded.

Community mental health centers (CMHCs) are a rapidly expanding form of mental health care. Estimates based on NIMH data indicate that 4,675 mentally retarded persons were admitted to care in 1968, and 10,036 in 1970. Less than 10% of these persons were admitted to 24-hour care and would perhaps be more appropriately included in the section on residential care. However, since most inpatients are quickly switched to outpatient status, such a distinction does not seem warranted.

NIMH has estimated that there were almost 272,000 persons under care in CMHCs during 1968 and 512,000 in 1970. If we assume that the proportion of mentally retarded among the total patient population is the same as among those admitted to care during the year (slightly less than 3%), about 7,800 retarded persons were treated in these facilities in 1968 and 15,300 in 1970.

In sum, about 115,000 persons were provided clinical services in 1968 in these three types of facilities, and 180,000 in 1970. The total number was undoubtedly even larger, since it is unlikely that the Children's Bureau was aware of all MR clinics. In addition, we have no estimate of the number of retardates served in clinical programs for the physically disabled or in clinics in general hospitals with specialized mental retardation programs.

Demographic characteristics: Almost 75% of the mentally retarded served in OPCs were under age 18 in 1970. For all practical purposes, all of the clients of MR clinics were children. Their median age was 7.1 years and almost half were 5 to 9 years old. About half of the retarded persons served in CMHCs were over age 18.

About three-fifths of the retarded provided clinical services were males. In view of the greater maturity and less boisterous behavior of female children, and the youth of the retarded being served in these facilities, this should occasion no surprise.

Costs: Information from 665 OPCs (about two-thirds of the number surveyed) indicated that the average annual cost (excluding capital expenditures) for all patients under care was $178 in 1968. In 1967 clinics which served children only reported an average cost over half again as high as the average for all outpatient clinics.[91] In view of the preponderance of children among the mentally retarded receiving OPC services, the last figure is more relevant for our purposes.

We will assign a cost of $250 for each retarded person receiving care in an OPC in 1968. This represents a small downward adjustment of the average cost incurred for all children under treatment to compensate for the fact that about 25% of the retarded who are served are adults and assumes that the average cost of serving the mentally retarded in OPCs is the same as for all patients served by these clinics.

It is probably less costly to serve children in MR clinics, since they are less likely to provide psychiatric care, other than diagnosis and evaluation. Therefore, in 1968 we will assign an average cost of $200 per year for these children. Since the average number of visits to a MR clinic per child under treatment is about four per year, this estimate could not be greatly in error. Estimates for retarded clients in outpatient clinics and MR clinics in 1970 were calculated by assuming that costs in these facilities increased at the same rate as for residents in public institutions.

On the basis of NIMH data, it was estimated that average operating cost per year per patient under treatment in community mental centers was $402 in 1970. We will assume that this figure is also applicable to the mentally retarded served in these facilities. To calculate the cost for 1968, it was assumed that the costs increased at the same rate as for public institutions.

In all, an estimated $26 million was expended in 1968 on the provision of clinical services to the mentally retarded or those suspected of being mentally retarded, a figure that rose sharply to $54 million in 1970. This does not include the value of volunteer help or the rental value of buildings, land, and equipment. There is no basis for estimating these cost factors, which, however, are unlikely to loom large.

Long-term care: Clinical services encompass the initial diagnosis and evaluation and long-term follow-up. Long-term follow-up will require that most clients return to the clinic at least once a year, about twelve additional times after the initial evaluation and before adulthood.

A 1959 study of two MR clinics in New York City estimated that the total cost for a diagnostic evaluation was $310 (which included the

---

[91] USDHEW, NIMH, Biometry Branch, *Statistical Note 4, Expenditures per Patient in Free Standing Outpatient Psychiatric Clinics—1967.*

value of services by both professionals and nonprofessionals.[92] Inflationary pressures would have increased this to about $430 in 1968 and about $575 in 1970 (assuming the same rate of increase of costs between 1968 and 1970 as assumed above).

If the average annual cost of follow-up services is estimated at $50 in 1968 and $67 in 1970, it becomes clear that clinical services are not an insubstantial part of the services provided to retardates.[93] In 1967 the average cost per *terminated* patient in OPCs serving children only was $562. It should be emphasized that this figure, or a similar figure for MR clinics, cannot be used as an estimate of the total cost of clinical services over time for retarded children. For one thing, the caseload of OPCs is increasing, so that the services received by terminated clients in previous years will be less than the services received by current clients in future years. In addition, in a labor-intensive activity such as clinical care, rising salaries (due to productivity charge in manufacturing) will cause the costs of clinical care to rise, so that average annual cost will increase over time.

Finally, many of the terminations will not receive the full range of clinical services, since some will be diagnosed as not retarded, others will voluntarily withdraw, and still others may be referred to other clinics. This latter consideration is especially true for the mentally retarded who initially seek help in an OPC and who may then be referred to an MR clinic. With respect to incomplete services, it is worthwhile noting that although about one-fourth of the clients of MR clinics were terminated in 1967, the great majority of these terminations were because the persons involved were not retarded and were voluntarily withdrawn.[94]

EMPLOYMENT PROGRAMS

State-federal vocational rehabilitation program: State vocational rehabilitation (hereinafter referred to as VR) agencies offer a range of services to assist the disabled to obtain or retain productive employ-

[92] Bernard Ferber and I. Jay Brightman, "Cost Determination in Mental Retardation Diagnostic Clinics," *American Journal of Mental Deficiency* (January 1962): 541.

[93] In Chapter VI a method of estimating the cost of a full course of clinical services will be developed.

[94] If there were a constant caseload, and if wages were constant, and if all retardates received a full course of treatment, then the average cost per termination (terminations would be about 8% of the total caseload annually) would be equal to the total expenditure over time for clinical care for a retarded child.

ment, or locate more suitable employment. The initial steps are always diagnosis, evaluation, and counseling to help clients select a suitable vocational goal and to outline the services needed to attain it. Any reasonable vocational goal may be selected, including homemaking and sheltered employment. The major services provided are physical restoration and vocational training. If necessary, an allowance for maintenance and transportation is provided and needed equipment and occupational licenses are purchased. After job placement and a short follow-up, the cases are usually closed.[95]

Counseling, diagnosis, and job placement are provided without charge. Since 1965 the states have the option to provide the other services without charge, or to use a means test to ascertain whether part of all of the cost should be borne by the client.

The number of retarded persons who are rehabilitated through the VR program has been rising rapidly in recent years. In 1968 mental retardation was the major disabling condition of almost 11% of all rehabilitants, or about 22,000 persons. During 1970, this number rose to over 30,000, and encompassed almost 12% of all rehabilitants.[96]

Over 6,000 more retarded clients were closed out as not rehabilitated in 1968.[97] Not all of these were unemployable. In 1967 almost half of the mentally retarded who were closed out as not rehabilitated declined further services or could not be located or contacted.[98] It can be presumed that most located employment. In addition, a number of clients who report other disabling conditions are also retarded. In 1963 it was reported that mental retardation was a secondary disability of 1% of all rehabilitants, but this is probably a substantial underestimate.[99]

Compared to other rehabilitants, retarded rehabilitants in 1969 were more likely to be under 20 years of age (67% as compared to 18%), male (63% as compared to 55%), never married (91% as compared to

---

[95] At the federal level the rehabilitation program is administered by the Rehabilitation Services Administration, SRS, USDHEW.

[96] USDHEW, SRS, RSA, *Characteristics and Trends of Clients Rehabilitated in Fiscal Years 1966-1970*, p. 18. This estimate assumes that the proportion of retarded rehabilitants among those for whom no diagnosis was reported was the same as among rehabilitants for whom a diagnosis was reported.

[97] USDHEW, SRS, RSA, *Major Disabling Condition of Rehabilitated and Not Rehabilitated Clients of State Vocational Rehabilitation Agencies—Fiscal Year 1968*, p. 3.

[98] USDHEW, SRS, RSA, *Reasons for Unsuccessful Closures among Selected Groups of Clients, Fiscal Year 1967*, September 1968.

[99] USDHEW, SRS, RSA, *The Rehabilitated Mentally Retarded*, April 1964. Rehabilitation counselors would have no incentive to report additional disabilities for clients whose eligibility for rehabilitation has been established and would be understandably reluctant to label clients as retarded.

35%), referred to rehabilitation by educational institutions (55% as compared to 10%),[100] and to have no dependents (92% as compared to 54%). The last three of these characteristics are explained by the comparative youthfulness of retarded rehabilitants. About 1 in 5 of rehabilitants in both groups were nonwhite. About three-fifths of these rehabilitants were mildly retarded. Slightly less than one-third were moderately retarded, and a little less than one-twelfth were severely retarded.

In 1968 the average cost of case services for successfully rehabilitated retarded clients with cost was $599, as compared to $611 for all rehabilitants.[101] In 1970 these figures had risen to $709 and $713. These figures, however, do not take account of the cost of counseling, placement, program administration, and services provided to unsuccessful clients (an unavoidable cost of operating the program).

Total expenditures by state VR agencies divided by the number of rehabilitants was $1,899 in 1968 and $2,181 in 1970.[102] The much higher figures would take account of all omitted costs to the rehabilitation program (*except* administration of the federal program), if the program had a constant number of clients. Although the program is, in fact, expanding rapidly, the net effect is small. (In an expanding program, expenditures on clients whose cases will be closed in future years are greater than expenditures on the current year's rehabilitants which were incurred in previous years.)

This is the average for all rehabilitants. Although the amount spent on case services for the retarded is slightly below average, the retarded usually require considerably greater amounts of counseling time than other clients. This is not a negligible consideration. Almost 30% of rehabilitation funds are used for counseling and placement.[103] If we assume the retarded require twice the counseling time of other rehabilitants, then actual cost per rehabilitated mentally retarded client would have been $2,456 in 1968 and $2,830 in 1970 (after making a slight downward adjustment for differences in the costs of case services).[104]

[100] USDHEW, SRS, RSA, *A Profile of Mentally Retarded Clients Rehabilitated during Fiscal Year 1969*, September 1971.

[101] USDHEW, SRS, RSA, *Characteristics and Trends of Clients Rehabilitated in Fiscal Years 1968-1970*, p. 11, and unpublished data. About 8% of rehabilitants are served without any expenditures for case service costs.

[102] USDHEW, SRS, RSA, *State Vocational Rehabilitation Agency Program Data 1968 and 1970*. This includes basic support (section 2), innovation grants (section 3), and social security trust funds used for vocational rehabilitation.

[103] Ibid.

[104] Even this figure understates the value of all resources expended on the rehabilitation of the retarded, since it does not include services provided by other agencies or paid for by the families of the retarded.

Sheltered workshops and work activity centers: A sheltered workshop can be defined as a work-oriented facility with a controlled environment. In effect, the job is engineered to fit the capabilities of the worker, while in unsheltered employment the worker is trained to fulfill the specifications of the job.

Sheltered workshops serve two roles. They are rehabilitation facilities that prepare workers for unsheltered employment through vocational training, molding of attitudes, development of physical capabilities, and assistance in obtaining suitable employment. And they are residual employers of the severely handicapped for whom employment in competitive situations cannot be envisioned in the near future.[105]

Work activity centers are "centers planned and designed exclusively to provide therapeutic activities for handicapped clients whose physical or mental impairment is so severe as to make their productive capacity inconsequential."

In 1966 the Fair Labor Standards Act was amended to require sheltered workshops to pay handicapped clients not less than 50% of the prevailing minimum wage. Exceptions were made in the cases of: (1) clients who are in training or evaluation programs; and (2) clients who are so severely disabled that their productivity cannot justify a payment of 50% of the minimum wage. Clients with severe disabilities may not be paid less than 25% of the statuatory minimum, and the actual rate must be related to productivity. For work activity centers, however, there is no minimum wage requirement.

In practice, the distinction between sheltered workshops and work activities centers is blurred and investigators frequently do not distinguish between them.

The most reliable data regarding sheltered workshops has been gathered under the auspices of the Regional Rehabilitation Research Institute at Cornell University. Much of the information was summarized in a paper prepared by William H. Button.[106]

Button presented two bases for estimating the number of sheltered workshops in the United States in 1968. In that year, 1,255 sheltered workshops (including work activities centers) were exempted from pay-

---

[105] One hesitates to describe workshops providing the latter service as terminal employers, since this connotes a finality which may be more aptly described as long-term.

[106] William H. Button, "Sheltered Workshops in the United States, an Institutional Overview," in *Rehabilitation, Sheltered Workshops, and the Disadvantaged.* Proceedings of a conference sponsored by Region II Rehabilitation Research Institute (Ithaca, New York: Cornell University, 1970), pp. 3–48.

ing the full federal minimum wage.[107] In addition, an estimated 50 sheltered workshops did not have such exemptions. Button felt that this overstated the number of sheltered workshops, since a single work-shop may have several physical locations—place of production, ware-house, retail outlets—and each location must maintain an exemption certificate.

A survey of rehabilitation facilities submitted to the Rehabilitation Services Administration by each state indicated that there were 1,127 sheltered workshops in 1968. Button felt that this was an understate-ment since certain states reported only those sheltered workshops with which the state rehabilitation agency had service-referral agreements. He concluded that the best estimate of the number of sheltered work-shops was 1,200. About half could be further subclassified as work activity centers.

To estimate the number of persons served, Button relied on a sub-stantial sample of 196 workshops in operation in 8 states.[108] During 1966 and 1967, the clientele of these workshops averaged 14,000 per day. Extrapolating from these data, he estimated that the average daily attendance in 1968 in all workshops in the United States was 86,000 of whom 30,000 were in long-term status (24 months or longer). Most of the remainder were trainees. He estimated that approximately 190,000 persons were served annually (clients at the beginning of the year and new admissions). Most workshop clients remain in workshops for less than a year.

Information on the primary disabilities of about half of the clients of the 196 workshops indicated that 30% were mentally retarded. This was the largest single diagnostic category and was about twice as high as the second highest—mental illness. Extrapolating from this data would indicate that about 26,000 mentally retarded persons were served in workshops on an average day in 1968 and about 57,000 were served during the course of the year. The actual number is, of course, higher, since some clients with primary disabilities other than mental retarda-tion were also retarded.

On the basis of data supplied to the Department of Labor by work-shops applying for exemption from the federal minimum wage, it is estimated that the number of clients served by workshops increased by 32% between 1968 and 1970. Assuming the same rate of increase ap-

[107] Based on data available from the Wages, Hours and Public Contracts Division of the U.S. Department of Labor.

[108] New York, New Jersey, Pennsylvania, Tennessee, Florida, Colorado, Ohio, and Texas.

plied to retarded clients, the number of retardates served in sheltered workshops would have risen to about 34,000.[109]

No information on the demographic characteristics of the mentally retarded in workshops was available. In 73 workshops serving nearly 4,000 clients (*all disabilities*), 79% were white and 54% were male. Information from the 196-workshop sample indicated that 36% of *all* clients were 14 to 25 years old, 18% were 26 to 35 years old, and that the percentage of clients decreased among older age groups, falling to 11% in the 56 to 65 age interval. It is probable that the retarded are younger than other clients. Of 360 retarded persons in sheltered workshops in California in 1961, only 2 were over 45 years of age, while 46% were under 20.[110]

To estimate the cost of operating sheltered workshops, Button again relied on his sample of 196 workshops. Extrapolating to a national basis, total operating costs in 1968 (assuming total income equals total cost) were estimated at $317 million, of which $251 million (79%) was business income, $25 million (8%) was from referral sources (mostly state VR agencies), $25 million (8%) was from community sources, and $17 million (5%) was from all other sources (client fees, federal grants, etc.).

It is apparent that workshop activities themselves support the greater part of their costs of operations. The net social cost, if such a term may be used, is only of the order of $67 million (total operating costs minus business income). This amounts to $763 per client in average daily attendance. We will assume that these same figures are also applicable to the retarded. It will also be assumed that the net social cost per client increased at the same rate as public institution costs per client between 1968 and 1970 (to $1,020).

If workshops were exclusively concerned with providing long-term employment, this would be a transfer cost and not a net social cost. However, since two-thirds of the clients are in training programs, and since most clients are paid on the basis of actual productivity, it seems more correct to regard the $67 million as a training cost. If anything, workshop clients subsidize the training operation by being paid less than would be warranted on productivity grounds, so that the net social cost should be higher. This amounts to a hidden tax on workshop clients.

---

[109] Based on data from the Division of Special Minimum Wages, Branch of Handicapped Worker Problems, U.S. Department of Labor.

[110] Nathan Nelson, *Workshops for the Mentally Retarded in California* (Sacramento, California: State Department of Education, Vocational Rehabilitation Service, 1962), p. 16.

A 1964 survey of 302 sheltered workshops found that volunteers contributed 26,712 hours of work per month.[111] Extrapolating these hours of work to 1,200 workshops in 1968, and valuing each of these hours at $1.50 (as in the case of public institutions) we estimate that the total value of volunteer work to workshops was $1,900,000, of which 30% is allocated to services provided to the retarded. In 1970 this estimate is increased to $2,800,000 to reflect increases in average hourly earnings of workers and the increase in the workshop population.

In sum, almost $75 million was expended on employment programs for the retarded in 1968 and $125 million in 1970. In the last chapter it will be shown that these programs need to be greatly expanded.

Other training programs: In 1970 federal outlays on manpower programs totaled slightly over $2.5 billion, the bulk of which was expended by the Department of Health, Education, and Welfare and the Department of Labor.[112] Subtracting the expenditures of the Rehabilitation Services Administration leaves over $2.1 billion, most of which has relevance, to a greater or lesser degree, for the mentally retarded. Although there is no basis on which to estimate the number of retardates served by these programs, a brief discussion of them is worthwhile.

The most important, as far as the retarded are concerned, are the training programs administered by the Department of Labor (several of which are partly funded by DHEW). These programs (On-the-Job Training, Institutional Training, Job Corps, New Careers, Operation Mainstream, Neighborhood Youth Centers, etc.) served over 1 million persons and obligated slightly over $1.9 billion in 1970.[113]

The average reading level of 33,000 persons enrolled in Job Corps during June 1968 was 5.2 years, and the average mathematics level was 5.3 years. (Almost 100,000 persons were enrolled in the program during the course of the year.) In short, over half could perform no better on reading and mathematics tests than a mildly retarded individual. In fact, 29% read at a third-grade level or less, and 24% could do no better in mathematics.[114] It can be presumed that many of these individuals were, in fact, retarded.

Other manpower programs have not reported comparable data on mathematics and reading achievement. However, of 6,400 persons en-

---

[111] Rich and Gilmore, "Volunteer Work with the Retarded," p. 231.

[112] *Special Analyses, Budget of the United States, Fiscal Year 1971* (Washington: USGPO, 1972), p. 134.

[113] Ibid., p. 148; and U.S. Department of Labor, *Manpower Report of the President*, March 1972, p. 261.

[114] *Manpower Report of the President*, p. 194. *Statistics on Manpower*, p. 101.

rolled in Operation Mainstream (September 1967 to August 1968), 29% had completed 6 years or less of school (presumed to be the upper limit to what the mildly retarded may attain), compared to only 7% among Job Corps enrollees. Of 138,000 *out-of-school* youth enrolled in Neighborhood Youth Center projects (September 1967 to August 1968), the median educational attainment was 8.9 years, compared to 9.0 in the Job Corps and 8.6 in Operation Mainstream.

The academic levels of enrollees in other manpower programs were considerably higher. Only 3.8% of the enrollees in the New Careers program, which served about 10,000 persons in 1968, reported a sixth-grade education or less; their median level of education was 11.4 years. Among 48,400 *in-school* youths enrolled in Neighborhood Youth Center projects (September 1967 to August 1968), the median years of school completed was 9.4, which hopefully would increase substantially before the enrollees terminated their education. Among 125,000 trainees in on-the-job training during 1968, median years of education was 12.0.[115] It should be noted that the Department of Labor has entered into a number of agreements with private firms, the National Association for Retarded Children, and state associations for retarded children for the express purpose of providing on-the-job training for the retarded. However, this would amount to only 1 or 2% of the total number of on-the-job trainees. It can be concluded that the Department of Labor's programs provide vocational training to a substantial number of retardates, although most are not specifically identified as such.

In 1968, 456,000 students were enrolled in adult basic education programs and in 1970, 3.7 million students were enrolled in post-secondary school and adult vocational education programs. Although many were undoubtedly retarded, there is no way of estimating their number.[116]

INCOME MAINTENANCE

In 1968 the Social Security Administration reported that 55% of the adults who were allowed disability benefits because of "childhood disability" had a primary diagnosis of mental deficiency. This undoubtedly understates the true percentage who were retarded, since a sub-

---

[115] See *Statistics on Manpower*, pp. 86–101, for these quoted statistics or the numbers from which they were derived.

[116] Adult basic educational programs are designed to correct the educational limitations of persons 16 years of age or over with less than an eighth-grade education. USDHEW, OE, National Center for Educational Statistics, *Adult Basic Education Program Statistics*, June 1969, p. 1.

stantial proportion of those with other primary diagnoses were also retarded. Conservatively, we will assume that 65% of all persons receiving "childhood disability" benefits were retarded. On this basis there were in fiscal year 1968 an estimated 158,000 adult mentally retarded beneficiaries under this program who received $118 million during the course of the year, or about $742 per person (Table 20). In 1970 the comparable figures were 176,000, $154 million, and $878 per person. About one-fourth of the beneficiaries were over age 45 and another one-fourth were between 35 and 45.[117]

Although there are no estimates of the proportion of "childhood disability" beneficiaries who are retarded under the railroad retirement, Civil Service retirement, or Veteran's Administration programs, one would expect that the experience of these programs would be comparable to that of the Social Security Administration—an observation that has been affirmed by persons involved in this program in the three agencies. On that basis, the three programs combined served about 26,000 retarded "childhood disability" beneficiaries in 1968, and aggregate payments were $16.5 million. In 1970 these estimates rose to 27,000 beneficiaries with aggregate payments of $20.4 million.[118]

A 1962 study of 2% of the national caseload of APTD recipients reported that almost 15% had a primary diagnosis of mental deficiency.[119] Considering both primary and secondary diagnoses, it was estimated that almost 18% were mentally retarded.[120] Data from an as yet unpublished survey in 1970 indicated that 19.3% of adults on APTD had a primary or secondary diagnosis of mental retardation. Assuming that the correct percentage was 19%, there would have been about 133,000 retarded persons receiving APTD in 1968 and annual payments would have been approximately $125 million (19% times total disbursements). In 1970 the comparable figures rose to 178,000 and $185 million.

[117] Based on unpublished social security data. See also Phoebe H. Goff, "Childhood Disability Beneficiaries, 1957–64: Characteristics and Geographic Distribution," *Social Security Bulletin* (February 1967): 14–23. USDHEW, Social Security Administration, *Social Security Disability Statistics, 1965*, December 1967. Adults are entitled to a social security "childhood disability" benefit if they become disabled before age 18 and if one of their parents was an insured worker who died, retired, or became disabled.

[118] This assumes that the average benefit paid to mentally retarded "childhood disability" beneficiaries was the same as for all "childhood disability" beneficiaries.

[119] USDHEW, Welfare Administration, Bureau of Family Services, *1962 Study of APTD Recipients: National Cross-Tabulation*, January, 1967, Table 21.

[120] USDHEW, SRS, *Federally Aided Public Assistance Programs: Program Facts*, April 1968.

Table 20. Income maintenance payments to the mentally retarded, 1968 and 1970

Type of program	Percentage of program beneficiaries who are retarded	Number of retardates served		Average payment		Total cost	
		1968	1970	1968	1970	1968	1970
"Childhood Disability Beneficiaries"							
Social Security	65%	158,000	176,000	$ 742	$ 878	$118,000,000	$154,000,000
Railroad Retirement	65	4,700	5,200	940	1,089	4,400,000	5,700,000
Civil Service Administration	65	1,600	1,900	624	976	1,000,000	1,800,000
Veterans Administration	65	19,500	20,100	569	640	11,100,000	12,900,000
Public assistance							
Aid to the permanently and totally disabled	19	133,400	177,700	934	1,043	124,600,000	185,300,000
Aid to the blind	5	4,100	4,100	1,084	1,204	4,400,000	4,900,000
Total						$263,500,000	$364,600,000

A 1962 study of persons receiving Aid to the Blind found that 5% were retarded.[121] This figure appears low in view of our earlier conclusion that about one in four blind children is retarded. However, persons blinded after childhood are far less likely to be retarded. In addition, a substantial proportion of blind and retarded adults are presumably institutionalized, since the barriers to community adjustment are formidable. Assuming that this percentage is also valid for 1968 and 1970, the total number of retarded persons receiving this category of public assistance would be a little over 4,000 in both years and aggregate payments would have been about $4.4 million in 1968 and $4.9 million in 1970.

One problem with these data is that some persons receive payments from both public assistance and social security and therefore would be counted twice in our figures. In 1962, for example, about 14% of the persons receiving APTD also received social security benefits.[122] If this were the proportion of mentally retarded public assistance recipients receiving "childhood disability" benefits under one of the three programs, the net number of mentally retarded adults receiving income maintenance as "childhood disability" beneficiaries or through public assistance under the APTD or AB programs would be of the order of 360,000 persons in 1970. The Social Security and APTD programs were by far the most important income maintenance programs for the mentally retarded, accounting for about 98% of total beneficiaries. The amounts paid were appallingly low, ranging from less than $900 per year from Social Security to a little over $1,200 per year under the AB program in 1970. Total payments were about $260 million in 1968 and $365 million in 1970.

These estimates do not include income maintenance payments made to retarded persons receiving adult disability, retirement or survivors' benefits from the Social Security program or payments to retardates from Aid to Families with Dependent Children, Old Age Assistance, or General Assistance programs. It has been estimated that there are 133,000 AFDC children alone who are mentally retarded.[123]

The above groups were omitted from the estimates because the aged, the young, and those who become physically disabled as adults, would qualify for the benefits they receive *irrespective* of the fact that they are retarded. Our concern is with those payments that are made because a person is incapable of self-support *due* to retardation.

[121] Ibid.

[122] *1962 Study of APTD Recipients*, Table 60.

[123] *Mental Retardation Activities of the Department of Health, Education, and Welfare*, p. 45.

It is probably true, however, that the difficulties of caring for retarded children prevent some AFDC mothers or widows receiving social security benefits from seeking employment. Moreover, some of these mothers may themselves be retarded, which may contribute to their dependency. In addition, retardation may cause some persons to retire early. Finally, retardation exacerbates the effect of physical disability. To the extent that these situations occur, income maintenance payments under retirement, adult disability, and dependent children's programs should be considered a consequence of mental retardation. Our estimate of total transfer payments is, therefore, conservative.

Another omission from these estimates is vendor payments for medical care provided to retardates under public assistance. No satisfactory way of estimating these payments could be developed.

OTHER EXPENDITURES

Almost all of the federal effort in research, training, and construction relevant to programs for the retarded is carried on by the various constituent parts of the U.S. Department of Health, Education, and Welfare (hereafter referred to as DHEW). The Secretary's Committee on Mental Retardation (hereafter referred to as SCMR) has, for a number of years, maintained an inventory of DHEW programs that are concerned with mental retardation. Unless otherwise noted, all data are from this source.

Construction: Until the passage of the Mental Retardation Facilities and Community Mental Health Centers Construction Act in 1963 (PL 88–164), the major source of federal funds for mental retardation facilities was the Public Health Service through the Medical Facilities and Construction Act (Hill-Burton). These expenditures, usually used for additions to public institutions, neared the $5 million level at their peak in 1962. With the passage of PL 88–164 and the granting of construction authority to other agencies, expenditures under the Hill-Burton Act for mental retardation facilities declined rapidly, to $785,000 in 1968, and were phased out in 1970.

PL 88–164 authorized federal funds for the construction of three types of facilities for the retarded: mental retardation research centers, university-affiliated facilities (UAFs), and community facilities stressing comprehensive services. The three types of facilities were for research, training of personnel, and services, respectively. As of December 1970, 12 research centers, 19 UAFs, and 362 community facilities had been approved and funded. Their total cost was $318 million, of which 45%

was federal funds. Almost two-thirds was used for community facilities. Although these facilities are funded separately, they are often joined and operated as one facility.

Another relevant construction program was authorized by the Vocational Rehabilitation Amendments of 1965, which authorized funds for the construction of rehabilitation facilities and sheltered workshops. Most of these projects are multidisability in nature, although some workshops have been constructed specifically for the retarded.

In 1968 federal obligations of approximately $14.8 million were incurred for community facilities, and $2.7 million for vocational rehabilitation facilities specifically for the retarded. In 1970 the comparable figures were $13.5 million and $4.0 million. No obligations were made for construction of UAF's or mental retardation research centers during these two years.[124] The total costs of these facilities was estimated by assuming that the federal share of the costs of community facilities was 36% (the actual federal share for such projects approved through December 1970) and that it was 50% for Hill-Burton projects. The federal share of vocational rehabilitation projects was assumed to be 50% in the case of new construction and 20% in the case of improving existing facilities (about 75% of the funds were used for the latter purpose).

In 1968 an estimated $47 million was obligated, although not necessarily spent in that year, by all levels of government and private non-profit agencies for the construction of the types of mental retardation facilities that have been described. In 1970 this figure actually declined to $41 million. About two-fifths of these totals was provided from federal funds.

It was not possible to identify all construction expenditures relevant to mental retardation. Among the more important omissions are educational classrooms, mental retardation clinics, and multi-disability facilities. The first two are primarily funded by state and local governments, and there is no readily accessible information on their scope. In the last case, it is difficult to ascertain how many retardates are served in these facilities. It is worth noting that almost $25 million was expended for the establishment of rehabilitation facilities and workshops in 1969.

Training. The federal government sponsors several types of training programs in the field of mental retardation. Fellowships and traineeships may be directly awarded to students, usually on a graduate level, but in some cases to college seniors, and funds may be granted to

---

[124] The Research Centers Construction Program was completed in 1968.

Table 21. Estimated construction costs of selected mental retardation facilities, 1968 and 1970

Type of facility	Federal share		State, local, or private nonprofit agency share		Total cost	
	1968	1970	1968	1970	1968	1970
Hill-Burton projects	$ 785,000	$ -0-	$ 785,000	$ -0-	$ 1,570,000	$ -0-
Community facilities	14,808,000	13,531,000	26,325,000	24,055,000	41,133,000	37,586,000
Vocational rehabilitation projects	2,692,000	4,023,000	1,147,000	848,000	3,839,000	3,871,000
Total	$18,285,000	$17,554,000	$28,257,000	$24,903,000	$46,542,000	$41,457,000

educational institutions to set up training courses, including paying staff salaries.[125]

SCMR estimated that DHEW expended almost $39 million for training purposes in 1968 and $42 million in 1970. However these totals include $10 million in grants from the National Institute of Neurological Diseases and Strokes (NINDS) in 1968 ($9 million in 1970), part of which was for training relevant to, but not specifically concerned with, mental retardation. Federal expenditures for training specifically concerned with mental retardation would be of the order of $35 million and $38 million.

During the fall of 1968 there were 39,458 students preparing to be special education teachers of the mentally retarded. Of these, 27,444 were undergraduates and 12,014 were graduate students. Approximately 85% of the former and 17% of the latter were full-time students.[126] Altogether there were about 25,400 full-time and 14,000 part-time students.

These data illustrate the enormous growth of interest in special education programs for the retarded. In 1962 only 6,149 students were preparing for this specialty, and in 1954 the number was only 805.

Among the full-time graduate students, the primary sources of support were: federal scholarships 48%; State, local, or private scholarships 14%; research or teaching assistantships 17%; own resources 22%. From a social standpoint, the cost of training these students is equal to the value of educational resources they utilize and the earnings they forgo. Fellowships and traineeships are means by which other parties share in these costs, but are not, in and of themselves, a measure of the costs of training.

To estimate the social costs of training these students in 1968 we assume: (1) that the value of educational resources used for full-time students was $2,500 per year (staff salary, plant operation, materials, rental value of classrooms),[127] and for part-time students it was $1,000

---

[125] As used here, training refers to the training of individuals to provide care to the retarded and not the training of the retarded themselves.

[126] Herman Louis Saettler, "Students in Training Programs in the Education of the Handicapped," doctoral thesis submitted to the Graduate College of the University of Illinois, 1969. The large number of part-time graduate students consists, for most part, of teachers working for advanced degrees.

[127] Total current expenditures per student enrolled are several hundred dollars higher. If we allowed for the part-time status of many students and the fair rental value of buildings, the total value of resources expended per full-time student would be considerably higher, probably around $1,000 more. A substantial portion of this cost, however, is used for research purposes and I am reluctant to attribute the full amount of resources expended by higher education institutions to instructional costs.

per year; (2) that the forgone earnings of a full-time graduate student were $5,000 per year, and of full-time undergraduates $3,000 per year; and (3) that part-time students have no forgone earnings. These figures are speculative. The labor market entry wage for college graduates was around $7,500 per year, and for high school graduates it was probably around $4,500. However, many students work part-time while attending school, which would mean that actual forgone earnings were less than these amounts. On these assumptions, the social cost of training special education teachers for the retarded was $158 million for the 1968–69 school year.

The number of students on federal fellowships was only about 1,000. Thus, most of the federal training effort is aimed at establishing programs, in-service training, or short training courses that will enable persons to switch into mental retardation from other fields, and was not supporting students training to become special education teachers of the retarded.

It is probably sufficient to subtract $10 million from federal training expenditures to adjust for the federal share of the training of special education teachers. Thus, we estimate that about $183 million was expended in 1968 to train people to work with the retarded ($158 million plus $25 million).

Training costs in 1970 were estimated by assuming that: (1) the number of students preparing to be special education teachers of the retarded increased in the same proportion as the enrollment of all college students between 1968 and 1970 (14%); (2) forgone earnings increased in the same proportion as changes in the average hourly earnings of workers on private payrolls; and (3) educational costs increased at the same rate as average expenditures per student in secondary and elementary education. On this basis, estimated training costs in 1970 were $235 million.

These estimates do not include the training of people in areas that are not specific to mental retardation, but who will be involved with the mentally retarded (social workers, psychiatrists, special education teachers for the physically handicapped, etc.). Nor do they include nonfederal expenditures on short-term training courses.

Research. SCMR reported that $25 million of USDHEW funds were expended for research in mental retardation in 1968 and $31 million in 1970. As in the case of training, NINDS included expenditures that were related to, but not specifically concerned with, mental retardation. However, I prefer not to adjust the estimate downward. Although insights into the nature, causes, and possible solutions to the problem of mental retardation may be only one of the goals of a research project, or even incidental to the project, these insights might well be sufficient to justify the project.

The National Science Foundation estimated that in 1968 60% of all funds used for research and development *in all fields* ($25 billion) was supplied by the federal government, 36% was supplied by industry, 3% by colleges and universities, and 1% by other nonprofit organizations.[128] One suspects that the federal share is overstated. Assuming the actual federal share to be 50%, and assuming that this is also applicable to mental retardation, total research expenditures in mental retardation would have been of the order of $50 million in 1968 and $62 million in 1970.

Agency operating expenditures. An itemization of the resources used for the care of the retarded should include administrative expenses that are not included in program data (e.g., costs of administering grant programs, public information services, consultations, conferences, etc.)

SCMR reported that the combined budgets of the President's Committee on Mental Retardation (PCMR) and of SCMR itself were $705,000 in 1968 and $691,000 in 1970. A highly speculative estimate of other administrative expenses incurred on behalf of the retarded in other DHEW agencies was derived by multiplying the total *administrative* expenses of the Office of Education, Social Security, and the Social and Rehabilitation Service times the proportion of their *total* budget that was used for mental retardation.[129] In 1970 the amounts were $1.1 million, $3.9 million, and $1.1 million respectively. Administrative costs in the Health Services and Mental Health Administration, the National Institute of Child and Human Development, and the National Institute of Neurological Disease and Strokes were estimated at $.3 million.[130]

It can be assumed that the administrative costs incurred by the federal government for the APTD and AB programs are at least as high per beneficiary as those of "childhood disability" beneficiaries under Social Security, or $4 million. A similar imputation to "childhood disability"

---

[128] USDHEW, OE, *Digest of Educational Statistics*, 1968, p. 127.

[129] The data for these estimates were taken from the *Budget of the United States*, 1970 and 1972. The estimate for the Social Security trust fund was derived by multiplying administrative expenditures of the fund by the proportion of beneficiaries who were disabled in childhood.

[130] This was estimated by multiplying the ratio of total expenditures on the retarded in these three agencies to total expenditures in the Social and Rehabilitation Service times administration costs in the latter agency.

beneficiaries under the Railroad Retirement Act, Civil Service Retirement and the Veteran's Administration would increase federal administrative costs by $.6 million.

In total, the above programs spent $11.8 million in administrative costs on behalf of the retarded in 1970. This underestimates total administrative costs, since it does not include the cost of operating private nonprofit organizations and many state agencies concerned with mental retardation.

Comparable calculations for 1968 yielded an estimate of $7.1 million.

AGGREGATE COST OF CARE

Table 22 summarizes the costs of the various programs that have been described. Each of these programs has an effect on the well-being of the retarded, but as a measure of the value of all resources devoted to their well-being it is hopelessly inadequate. Such a total would include the value of all normal consumption expenditures (including the provision of public services, such as police protection) and would probably be in the $20 to $30 billion range.

A more useful cost concept is one limited to measuring the value of resources used to assist the retarded in their intellectual and social development—i.e., one that excludes consumption expenditures. Developmental expenditures are equivalent to the concept of investments in people described at the beginning of this chapter.

The developmental costs included in Table 22 were estimated by subtracting: (1) income maintenance payments; (2) agency operating expenses of income maintenance programs; and (3) 20% of the total expenditures on residential care. This surprisingly low adjustment for consumption expenditures in institutional care is based on the observation that the quality of life among institutionalized retardates is not high. The average per capita food expenditure among institutionalized retardates was less than $300 per year in 1961; the median clothing allowance was $29 a year per person.[131]

The programs reported in Table 22 expended an estimated $3.116 billion for developmental purposes in 1968 and $4.029 billion in 1970. The definition of developmental costs can be further restricted by limiting it to costs incurred for the current provision of services. Research, training, construction, and associated agency operating expenditures are part of the costs of future services. This estimate is $2.835 billion in

[131] National Association for Retarded Children, *A Survey and Study of State Institutions for the Mentally Retarded in the United States*, 1963, pp. 29, 52.

Table 22.   Expenditures on selected programs serving the retarded

	1968	1970
Residential care	$1,284,400,000	$1,619,500,000
Special education	1,057,900,000	1,463,600,000
Regular academic education	648,000,000	748,600,000
Clinical program	26,000,000	54,400,000
Employment programs	75,000,000	124,800,000
Construction	46,500,000	41,500,000
Training of personnel	183,000,000	235,000,000
Research	50,000,000	62,000,000
Income maintenance	263,500,000	364,600,000
Agency operating expenses	7,100,000	11,800,000
Total	$3,641,400,000	$4,725,800,000

1968 and $3.689 billion in 1970. It should be noted that a portion of the research, training, and construction costs that were incurred in the past should be allocated to current developmental costs.[132] Only in the case of past construction costs have we made a *partial* allowance for any of these variables (through imputed rental values). It is sometimes suggested that current expenditures for these purposes be included in costs of current services as a proxy variable for the use of resources invested in these ways in previous years.

Whichever version of developmental costs is preferred, it is only a partial measure of actual developmental costs incurred for the retarded. Among the omissions are: (1) the services rendered by private physicians, psychologists, or psychiatrists; (2) guardianship, counseling, homemaking, protective services, day care, foster family care, adoptive services, and other services rendered by state and local agencies. For example, in 1973 it is estimated that 43,000 retarded children will receive services under the Child Welfare Services Program and 456,000 will receive services under the Social Services Program.[133] In some

[132] When training and construction costs are privately borne, prospective earnings must be sufficiently high to attract people into the profession and capital into these uses. This, presumably will enable trainees and investors to recoup their training costs. Current earnings then would automatically reflect these past training costs, and fees charged would reflect the use of capital (depreciation). Subsidized training and construction reduces the prospective earnings needed to attract trainees and capital and, therefore, an adjustment is needed to reflect the current use of the previous investments.

[133] USDHEW, Secretary's Committee on Mental Retardation, *Mental Retardation Activities of the Department of Health, Education, and Welfare*, March 1972, pp. 34–35. The Community Services Administration (SRS, USDHEW) is the federal agency charged with administering these programs, usually through public assistance agencies.

states the retarded are committed to guardianship for life.[134] Many mentally retarded children received medical services through the Crippled Childrens Program (HSMHA, USDHEW). In 1970 almost 500,000 crippled children were served through this program.[135] (3) The value of parental care, an especially important consideration in view of the forgone earnings of many mothers.

In one respect, these estimates of the costs of developmental services include too much. It is unlikely that 80% of residential care expenditures should be considered developmental, since a large portion of these funds are used for custodial purposes.

Even the concept is defective. Childhood development depends greatly upon so called normal consumption. The consequences of inadequate recreation, diet, etc. are readily observable among many retardates.

Another cost concept is social costs, often referred to as "excess costs." This refers to the value of resources that would be available for other uses if retardation did not exist. Two situations can be envisioned: one where the retarded suddenly vanish, and one where the retarded are all within the normal intellectual range. This section will consider the latter possibility. Some of the issues of the first situation will be considered in Chapter VI. "Excess costs" are measured by the difference between what is spent on the retarded and what would be spent on these individuals if they were in a normal intellectual range. "Excess cost" is a more complicated variable than may appear. It should be noted that the concept of excess cost excludes "normal" investments in people and includes abnormal consumption expenditures.

The following adjustments are made to estimate "excess costs" from Table 22:

1) Income maintenance payments and maintenance costs in institutions are subtracted, since these costs would be incurred in any event.[136] Unlike the case of developmental costs, agency operating costs of income maintenance programs are *not* subtracted, since they

---

[134] Maynard C. Reynolds and Clayton L. Stunkard, *A Comparative Study of Day Class vs. Institutionalized Educable Retardates*, Cooperative Research Project No. 192, University of Minnesota, Minneapolis, Minnesota, 1960, p. 24.

[135] USDHEW, SCMR, *Mental Retardation Activities of the U.S. Department of Health, Education, and Welfare*, March 1972, p. 20.

[136] Consumption levels would undoubtedly rise among many retardates if not retarded, especially those in institutions. This creates no conceptual problem, since it is simply a manifestation of one of the ways in which the freed resources would be used.

represent a use of resources that society would not incur if the beneficiaries of these programs were not retarded.

2) Even in the absence of retardation children must be sent to school, so only the above average expenditures on the education of the retarded represent "excess cost." Excess education costs for noninstitutionalized retardates *in school* can be estimated by multiplying the difference in costs between special education and regular education programs by the number of children in special education classes. This came to $502 million in 1968 and $720 million in 1970.

This, however, overstates excess education costs for all retardates, since retardates spend fewer years in school than nonretardates. About 90% of all nonretarded children, age 5 to 19, attend school. The average annual education cost for *all* of these children was $790 in 1968 and $931 in 1970. Among noninstitutionalized retardates in this age group, about 25% did not attend school, 40% attended regular classes, and 35% attended special education classes in 1968. The average annual education cost for all of these children (weighted for the proportion of children attending each type of class) was, therefore, $937. An identical calculation in 1970 (with slightly changed percentages) yielded an estimate of $1,173. "Excess educational costs," therefore, were only about $147 per school-age retardate in 1968 and $242 in 1970. Excess educational costs for all retardates, therefore, are estimated at about $270 million in 1968 and $450 million in 1970.

3) Institutional costs are further reduced by $85 million in 1968 and $102 million in 1970, since this amount would have to be expended on institutionalized school-age retardates if they attended normal classes in the community ($790 × 108,000 and $931 × 110,000).

4) All other costs in Table 22 are assumed to represent abnormal expenditures.

After making these adjustments, our estimate of social (excess) cost in 1968 is $1.599 billion, if we include research, training, and construction, and $1.319 billion if we do not. In 1970 the comparable figures were $2.173 billion and $1.835 billion.

Machlup has argued that current expenditures on construction, training, and research, as well as fair rental values of property being used

---

Although a large share of residential costs are for custodial care, these should not be regarded as consumption, since it clearly refers to the provision of a type of lodging that is *not* normal. Technically, the only adjustment in custodial costs that should be made is a reduction to reflect any reduction in the use of resources devoted to housing outside the institution as a result of people having been institutionalized. The remaining custodial costs are an additional use of resources that society would not otherwise bear.

(and, extending his argument, an apportionment of part of past training efforts) should be included in estimates of social cost. To apply Machlup's reasoning, both existing buildings and equipment and resources used to build new buildings would be available for other uses if mental retardation did not exist.[137] If current expenditures on construction, training, and research are included in excess costs, we measure the resources that would be available for other purposes during the year if retardation did not exist now or in the future. If these variables are excluded, we measure the excess costs chargeable only to persons currently receiving services. These estimates of excess costs suffer from the same omissions as our previous cost measures. In addition, they present the problem that they hypothesize an impossible situation and are of little consequence for policy purposes.

These observations on the costs of mental retardation are made:

1) No inventory of programs relevant to mental retardation can be complete. Because it is a developmental disorder, almost any program designed to protect or enhance childhood development is relevant.

2) Many of the omitted programs are crucial to the development and welfare of the retarded—e.g., recreational activities.

3) Each of the different cost concepts contain serious empirical and conceptual deficiencies. From a policy standpoint, the "laundry list" approach is probably the most useful, since it summarizes the costs of the major programs for the retarded that are subject to the influence of policymakers.

4) In recent years there has been a growing trend toward community facilities which provide comprehensive services to the retarded, including residential care. In our calculations, we listed these services separately, although in some cases they were provided by the same facility.

COSTS OF SERVING DIFFERENT GROUPS
AMONG THE RETARDED

The cost of serving the retarded varies sharply depending upon their level of retardation, physical and emotional handicaps, age, and a host of other variables.

Special Education. In 1968 the student-classroom ratio was 1.8 times greater for special education programs for the retarded then for regular academic students. Since almost nine out of ten retardates in special

---

[137] A similar statement can be made for training. Research does not fit into this statement since its use is not limited by physical constraints. See Fritz Machlup, *The Production and Distribution of Knowledge in the United States* (Princeton: Princeton University Press, 1962), pp. 98–100.

education programs attended programs for the educable retarded, we will assume that the student-classroom ratio for the educable retarded can be approximated by that of all types of special education classes in that year. The error, if any, will be small. We estimate, therefore, that in 1970 it cost $1,409 per year for classroom activities, $56 for excess transportation costs, $15 for extra services, and $456 for capital costs for each student in classes for educable mentally retarded, or $1,936 altogether. In contrast, it cost $1,003 ($783 operating cost and $220 capital cost) per student in regular academic programs.

Kirk reported that classes for severely retarded children generally vary from 5 to 12 children per teacher, and that classes which have over 8 or 9 children require the assistance of a matron or aide.[138]

Since special education classes for the educable retarded average about 15 students per class, the operating costs of classes with 5 students would be about 3 times the average, $4,225 per year per child. If $280 for excess transportation costs, $15 for extra services, and $1,370 for capital costs are added to this sum, the total annual cost per student would be almost $5,900 in 1970.

If a class had 10 students, however, the total annual cost per student would be about $3,500 (operating cost $2,115, capital cost $684, excess transportation costs $280, extra expenses $15, and about $400 for an aide). This is probably a more reasonable estimate for most programs for the trainable retarded. The higher estimate, however, may be reasonable for "day development" classes.

Based on these assumptions, the cost per student of classes for the educable retarded is 1.9 times the cost of regular classes, while the cost of classes for the trainable retarded is 3.5 and the cost of day development classes is 5.9 times that of regular classes.

Actual costs vary greatly among school districts for a variety of reasons, among which are whether classes are operated full-time or part-time, the actual number of students in the classroom, and the types of students. (Some classes have both trainable and educable retardates, as well as those with varying degrees of associated handicaps.)

How do these estimates compare with reported costs? After reviewing several published studies Kirk observed: "If a generalization is to be made, it could be said that a program would cost twice (for a minimum program) to six times as much for the severely retarded as it would for a child in the regular grades of a public school."[139]

---

[138] Samuel A. Kirk, *Public School Provisions for Severely Retarded Children*, Special Report to the Interdepartmental Health Resources Board (Albany, New York: 1957), p. 36.

[139] Kirk, *Public School Provisions*, p. 52.

The Special School District of St. Louis County reported that in 1968 per pupil costs in classes for the educable retarded were $1,206,[140] which is about what our estimates of *operating costs* of classes for the educable retarded would be if adjusted to the earlier year. Per pupil cost in classes for the trainable retarded were considerably less than expected.

In a survey of over 1,000 severely retarded or severely physically disabled children attending Development Centers for Handicapped Minors in California (fiscal year 1968–69), average expenditures of $3,793 per child per year were reported.[141] This is somewhat less than the anticipated cost (excluding capital cost) of operating day development classes, (especially since per pupil educational costs in California are about 10% above the national average). However, these development centers serve some trainable retarded children, which would lower expected costs.

A report from California for the 1960–61 school year indicated that the cost per student in classes for the educable retarded was 1.9 times that of regular students, and that the corresponding ratio for classes for the trainable retarded was 3.5.[142] In the 1969–70 school year a Pennsylvania report indicated that these ratios were 1.9 and 3.9.[143] These are very close to our estimates and would be even closer if all retarded students attended class full-time and if transportation and capital costs could be adequately adjusted for.

In a sample of twenty-two school districts in five states, it was reported that the ratio of the per pupil costs for the educable mentally retarded to the per pupil costs of students in regular education was 1.9, which is identical to our estimate. In the case of the trainable retarded, however, the ratio was only 2.2, which is far below our estimate. Unfortunately, data were not presented that would make a detailed evaluation of this finding possible.[144]

Residential care. An assessment of costs among the institutionalized retarded is complicated by the fact that a large proportion are severely

[140] Report of Oral W. Spurgeon, superintendent.

[141] Report from the State of California, *Developmental Centers for Handicapped Minors* (no date).

[142] Study Commission on Mental Retardation, *Report of Survey by Committee on Existing Resources, Functions, and Coverage*, 1964, p. 16.

[143] Bureau of Special Education, Pennsylvania Department of Education, *Special Education Programs for Exceptional Children*, 1970, p. 7.

[144] Richard A. Rossmiller, James A. Hale, and Walter I. Garms, *Educational Programs for Exceptional Children* (Madison, Wisconsin: The University of Wisconsin, 1970), pp. 67 and 71.

physically or emotionally handicapped. Their educational needs will be more complex, and differences in cost among retardates of varying levels of intellectual deficiency will be less pronounced as compared to their counterparts in the community. I am not aware of any studies which have specifically ascertained the costs of serving different demographic groupings of institutionalized retardates.

The following information was collected on 107 public institutions with an average daily resident population of 500 or more in 1968:[145]

1. Average daily resident population.

2. Average annual per capita cost.

3. Resident to staff ratio.

4. Percentage of resident population under age 20.

5. Percentage of resident population with an IQ of 35 or less (profoundly and severely retarded).

6. Percentage of resident population with an IQ between 35 and 50 (moderately retarded).

7. Percentage of staff that are full-time professionals.

8. Average annual earnings of staff in 1965 by state (the last year in which such information was collected). Individual institution data was not available.

9. Whether the facility was located in a Standard Metropolitan Statistical Area (SMSA).

Analysis of scatter diagrams and the results of multiple regressions indicated that the relationships between these variables were essentially nonlinear. Therefore, the succeeding correlations and regressions are based on the logs of these variables.

The number of residents per staff member decreased as the percentage of profoundly and severely retarded residents in an institution increased ($r = -.24$) and the percentage of residents under age 20 increased ($r = -.56$). As a consequence, average per patient costs (which are largely determined by the number of staff employed) were higher in institutions with higher percentages of these demographic groupings ($r = .23$ and $.51$ respectively). These relationships were reversed among the moderately retarded, evidently because of their greater capability for self-care and possibly because they do some of the work of the institution. These results were not entirely expected, since it was felt that institutions might emphasize developmental services to the moder-

---

[145] Items 1, 2, 3, 8, and 9 were based on NIMH data. Items 4, 5, 6, and 7 were abstracted from AAMD *Directory of Residential Facilities for the Mentally Retarded*. In a few cases facilities were contacted by telephone and asked to supply missing information.

ately retarded because of their greater capability of benefiting from these services.

Log linear regressions have the property that the coefficients of the independent variables represent the percentage increase in the dependent variable that would be expected from a 1% increase in the independent variable.

The log linear regression of average annual per capita cost (dependent variable), with the percentage of residents under 20 and the percentage of profoundly and severely retarded residents, indicated that a 1% increase in the percentage of residents under 20 was associated with a 0.26% increase in average cost, and a 1% increase in the percentage of profoundly and severely retarded residents was associated with a 0.15% increase. The coefficient for the profoundly and severely retarded increased to 0.20% when the percentage of staff that held professional status was added to the equation. This change reflects the fact that the profoundly and severely retarded receive slightly less professional time than the moderately retarded.[146]

Adding average wages and salaries (statewide) to the equation decreased this coefficient to 0.16%. Apparently, wages are lower in states serving high percentages of the profoundly and severely retarded, possibly because of greater numbers of nonprofessional staff.

Adding the dummy variable for SMSAs did not affect the coefficient for the percentage of profoundly and severely retarded, but adding the institution-size variable (average daily resident population) reduced it to 0.12%. Although the correlation between the percentage of profoundly and severely retarded and institution size was negligible (0.02), both of these variables were strongly correlated with the resident-to-staff ratio, so that institution size, in effect, served as a proxy for the latter variable. Throughout these equations the coefficient for the percentage under 20 remained remarkably constant and relatively large; in the last equation it was 0.27%.

The cost differences implied by these regressions are considerable. It was calculated that, all other things equal, increasing the percentage of the resident population under twenty by ten percentage points would have increased average per capita costs by about $210 per year, which implies a cost difference between adult and child residents of almost

---

[146] The higher the percentage of profoundly and severely retarded, the lower the percentage of full-time professional staff members. The percentage of profoundly and severely retarded served as a proxy for the second variable, which tended to pull down the coefficient. When the percentage of full-time professionals among the staff was explicitly added to the equation, the coefficient for the severely and profoundly retarded rose.

$2,100. This indicates average costs among adults of about $2,300 and average costs among children of about $4,400 in 1968.[147]

Similarly, when an increase of ten percentage points in the proportion of the resident population that is profoundly and severely retarded was assumed, average costs increased $42 to $93, depending upon the variables that were controlled. This implies a cost difference of between $400 and $900 between profoundly and severely retarded institution clients and those with higher IQs.

The higher figure is probably the more relevant, since the lower figure assumes that the resident-to-staff ratio is independent of the level of retardation, when, in fact, the more severely retarded require more staff, although not necessarily at a professional level. Because of this latter qualification, the relevant coefficient should perhaps be 0.15 rather than the 0.20 that was used to compute the higher estimate. In any event, it can be assumed that the cost difference between institutionalized retardates under 20 and over 20 is considerably greater than any of these estimates, when the younger retardates are placed in special education programs. Our estimates reflect the fact that only about half of school-age retardates in public institutions are in special education programs. These observations are readily explainable in terms of the greater care needed by the severely and profoundly retarded, the developmental needs of youthful retardates, and frequent neglect of adult retardates.

The variable for the percentage of moderately retarded has not been included in these regressions because it is highly correlated with the percentage of profoundly and severely retarded ($r = .63$). Throughout these equations the coefficient for the percentage under 20 has remained highly significant statistically. The t tests ranged between 5.8 and 7.9. The t tests for the coefficient of the percentage of profoundly and severely retarded were much lower, ranging from 1.7 to 2.5.

VARIATIONS AMONG STATES

The variation in the provision of mental retardation services by state is remarkable (Table 23). In 1968 the number institutionalized per 100,000 population (hereafter referred to as the "rate") ranged from zero to 151; in 1966 in special education this rate ranged from 12 to

---

[147] The difference may be even greater. If we calculated average costs by inserting assumed values of 100% and 0% for children in the regression equation, the estimated annual costs would have been only $1,300 for adults and $4,300 for children. However, estimates based on assumed extreme situations are highly unreliable.

Table 23. Selected state data

State	Pub. inst., rate/100,000 pop., 1968	Pub. ment. hosp. Rate/100,000 pop. of MR resident patients, 1968	Priv. inst. & priv. ment. hosp. rate/100,000 pop. MR res. patients 1967	Spec. ed. classes for MR in local pub. schools, rate/100,000 pop., 1966	Daily exp./res. patient in pub. inst., 1968	Resident-to-staff ratio in pub. inst., 1968
Alabama	67.4	28.2	3.6	31.0	5.04	3.1
Alaska	40.1	14.5	0	86.0	32.51	1.0
Arizona	60.4	8.3	16.6	239.9	6.52	2.0
Arkansas	43.3	19.9	1.9	105.3	11.84	1.1
California	71.1	2.5	17.9	327.9	13.79	2.0
Colorado	122.9	2.4	3.6	245.4	9.97	1.6
Connecticut	139.9	9.8	9.9	205.7	10.93	2.0
Delaware	112.0	12.4	15.8	264.5	9.29	1.6
D.C.	166.4	14.1	7.0	1122.7	7.72	3.4
Florida	91.8	15.1	7.9	192.5	11.26	1.2
Georgia	41.1	43.0	1.9	160.0	12.47	1.4
Hawaii	109.3	1.8	0	283.5	9.97	2.2
Idaho	99.3	12.1	0	143.8	8.12	2.0
Illinois	83.8	13.8	23.0	134.0	11.45	1.7
Indiana	75.9	14.9	.9	154.5	10.51	1.6
Iowa	60.7	2.5	26.2	294.1	12.19	1.2
Kansas	87.1	4.3	9.4	125.2	13.46	1.2
Kentucky	34.4	21.7	6.6	140.6	9.94	1.6
Louisiana	75.7	21.6	15.7	112.3	10.89	1.3
Maine	94.3	22.6	14.1	88.1	10.61	1.7
Maryland	84.5	15.2	9.1	646.2	9.35	2.1
Massachusetts	147.3	21.0	11.0	225.7	9.35	2.4
Michigan	149.5	8.8	5.9	350.8	10.66	2.0
Minnesota	142.6	7.7	30.8	230.2	9.14	2.0
Mississippi	58.3	54.1	.9	52.3	3.79	2.9

State	Column 1	Column 2	Column 3	Column 4	Column 5	Column 6
Missouri	57.5	23.0	11.8	416.0	8.99	1.6
Montana	125.4	23.8	0	99.3	8.40	2.9
Nebraska	147.5	11.8	24.3	96.0	4.70	3.0
Nevada	—	35.6	3.2	390.5	—	—
New Hampshire	150.4	34.6	4.4	89.8	7.02	2.3
New Jersey	95.6	19.9	9.0	249.9	9.00	1.9
New Mexico	77.1	12.6	8.4	214.9	12.09	1.2
New York	152.3	19.6	5.8	256.3	8.72	2.1
North Carolina	93.3	17.9	5.7	250.5	8.79	1.8
North Dakota	252.0	13.7	1.1	95.3	6.31	2.2
Ohio	90.7	11.3	7.5	252.2	7.11	2.7
Oklahoma	92.5	13.8	22.2	150.1	10.45	1.5
Oregon	152.0	3.7	8.6	235.4	9.01	2.3
Pennsylvania	98.8	25.5	36.7	459.3	9.35	2.0
Rhode Island	97.3	23.7	14.0	211.6	14.10	1.7
South Carolina	127.9	30.6	0	132.7	2.46	2.8
South Dakota	187.3	3.3	0.8	121.5	6.40	2.6
Tennessee	57.8	17.2	3.0	275.7	8.35	1.6
Texas	96.1	13.4	18.8	215.8	6.79	2.2
Utah	77.4	1.2	22.1	225.3	6.83	2.3
Vermont	155.5	33.4	8.9	12.4	7.90	2.4
Virginia	80.9	33.6	6.5	160.0	5.97	2.6
Washington	111.3	5.6	1.9	340.1	10.79	2.1
West Virginia	26.0	63.3	0	97.7	10.97	1.2
Wisconsin	86.5	44.3	3.1	284.9	15.58	1.3
Wyoming	203.4	5.3	0	147.6	7.92	2.0

Sources: Column 1, USDHEW, NIMH, *State Trends in First Admissions and Resident Patients, Public Institutions for the Mentally Retarded—1964–1968*, March 1970.

Column 2, USDHEW, NIMH, *Patients in State and County Mental Hospitals, 1967*, Series 1, No. 2.

Column 3, see pp. 76–77 of this chapter.

Column 4, R. Mackie, *Special Education in the United States* (New York: Teachers College Press, 1969).

Columns 5–6, USDHEW, NIMH, *Provisional Patient Movement and Administrative Data*, 1968.

over 1,100. Staffing patterns and average daily expenditures in public institutions also showed sharp variation. Since one service may be an alternative to another, we would expect to find some systematic relationship among these variables.

As expected, states with high rates in public institutions had lower rates for the retarded in public mental hospitals ($r = -.35$). It was less expected to find that there was no significant relationship between the rates of persons in public institutions and the rates in private residential care ($r = -.07$), or the rates in special education classes ($r = .09$). The first of these unexpected relationships is not particularly important, since private institutions serve relatively few people and often accept out-of-state clients. The correlation in the second case was even in an unexpected direction. Possibly the sharp differences among states do not reflect differences in the mix of mental retardation services as much as differences in the degree of concern for the needs of the retarded.[148]

There was no relationship between average daily expenditure and the rate in public institutions ($r = -.01$), but a strong positive relationship between this rate and the resident-to-staff ratio ($r = .48$). Average daily expenditures were greatly affected by differences in wage rates among institutions and are not necessarily indicative of differences in quality of care. However, the resident-to-staff ratio may be used as a rough proxy for quality of care, and a low staffing pattern was clearly associated with relatively large institutional populations, possibly because services were not available to assist the retarded to return to the community.[149]

This last observation is important. It suggests that states which appear to be manifesting the greatest concern for the retarded may, in fact, be victims of their own neglect of the retarded. Low quality of care apparently prevents the release of many institutionalized retardates, causing a build-up of the institutional population. This is perhaps too strong a statement in view of the long waiting lists for institutional

[148] These correlation coefficients include the District of Columbia but exclude Nevada, since it did not have a public institution for the mentally retarded in 1968. The use of years before 1968 to show the extent of private residential care and special education by state is necessitated by the fact that these are the latest years for which reliable data by states on these variables are available.

[149] Indices of total residential care by state were obtained by summing the rates for public institutions, private residential facilities, and the retarded in public mental hospitals. The correlation coefficient between the index of total residential care and the resident-to-staff ratios, average daily expenditures in public institutions, and the rate of persons in special education programs by state was almost identical to those obtained between these variables and the rates for public institutions reported above.

placement in most states and the widely varying admittance practices, variables which we could not adjust for in the regression (e.g., states may maintain high staffing ratios by restricting admissions). Nevertheless, it is of interest to note that of the 22 states where the resident-to-staff ratio was below the national average in 1968 (indicating fewer residents per staff person and higher quality care) the percentage of the state's population in public institutions was also below the national average in 20. But of 28 states where the resident-to-staff ratio was above the national average (indicating less adequate care), the percentage of the state's population in public institutions was above the national average in 18. In the remaining 10 states in the latter group, the percentage of retardates in special education classes also tended to be below average, and it is probable that these states contain large numbers of retardates who are not receiving any form of special care.

The situation had changed little by 1970. Of 21 states where the staff-to-resident ratio was above average, 18 had less than the average proportion of their state population in these institutions. And of 29 states where staffing was below average, the percentage of the states population in the institutions was above average in 18.

DISTRIBUTION OF PROGRAM COSTS

Programs for the mentally retarded are funded by a combination of patient fees (part of which are paid by private insurance), private philanthropy, state and local governments, and a wide variety of federal agencies. In most cases, only broad statements can be made about the relative importance of these sources of funding.

Public institutions. In 1968 New York State was reimbursed 6.1% of its operating expenditures in public institutions: 1% was obtained from patient fees; 1.2% from various types of insurance funds, including trifling amounts from workmen's compensation and industrial pensions; and 3.9% from federal funds. Of the federal funds about three-fifths was obtained from Social Security (presumably childhood disability payments).[150]

The Arkansas Legislative Counsel compiled fiscal information for 1968 on 43 public institutions which served 33% of the total number of mentally retarded in public institutions and expended 35% of total operating expenditures.[151] Slightly less than 10% of the expenditures of these facilities were reported as paid by non-state sources—4% by patient fees and 5.7% by other sources, most of them presumably federal.

---

[150] Unpublished data.

[151] Unpublished data supplied by Charles Acuff, acting commissioner, Arkansas Department of Mental Retardation.

Both surveys understate the federal contribution to public institutions. In 1968 the Office of Education funded almost $14 million to provide improved services to the mentally retarded in state-supported school systems.[152] Another $9 million was granted to public institutions through the mental retardation Hospital Improvement Program (HIP) and Hospital Inservice Training Program (HIST), and a minimum of $30 million (federal share only) was paid to these institutions through Medicaid. The latter figure is minimal, since it is based on payments to only six states (although it is believed that these states utilized the bulk of Medicaid funds for this purpose).[153] In all, almost 8% of the operating expenditures of public institutions were derived from these sources. If another 2.5% was recovered from the various trust funds, the federal contribution was about 10.5%.

By 1970 Medicaid payments to public institutions had risen to an estimated $90 million, HIP and HIST payments to $11 million, and the Office of Education payments to state-supported school systems had risen to about $21 million (not all of which was granted to public institutions). Roughly about 13% of the operating costs of state institutions was recovered from these sources. If we add 2.5% to represent the trust funds, the federal contribution can be estimated at 15.5% in 1970, a substantial increase over 1968.

Patient fees reported by New York also seem unduly low. The Arkansas survey (4%) is probably more representative of the U.S., although this figure may include some payments by private insurance companies or the federal trust funds. These figures suggest that the states recovered 15.7% of the operating expenditures of public institutions in 1968 and 20.7% in 1970 (federal, 10.5% in 1968 and 15.5% in 1970; patient fees, 4% in both years; private insurance companies, 1.2% in both years.)[154]

Other residential facilities. Since retardates in public mental hospitals are older and less severely retarded than those in public institutions, their parents are less likely to be financially responsible for their care, and they are less likely to be encompassed under the "childhood disability" provisions of the federal trust funds or Veteran's Administration. It is likely, therefore, that the states will recover a smaller proportion of the cost of the care of the retarded in public mental hospitals

---

[152] The allotment to New York from this source alone was 1.7% of the operating expenditures of public institutions in the state.

[153] New York was not one of the six states.

[154] One reason for the understatement of reimbursements in the Arkansas study is that these payments are sometimes made directly to the state and not the institution. Institution records on reimbursement are probably, therefore, incomplete.

than in public institutions (although the substantial contribution of Medicaid to public mental hospitals casts some doubt on this conclusion).

Although private institutions are primarily supported by private philanthropy and patient fees, state and local governments purchase care for some retardates from private facilities. In addition, a substantial part of the $2 million expended by the Office of Civilian Health and Medical Programs for the Uniformed Services (OCHAMPUS) on residential care for the retarded in 1968 went to this class of facility, as well as some Medicaid payments and trust fund payments. Undoubtedly, most of the expense of caring for the retarded in private mental hospitals and general hospitals is borne by parents and private insurance companies, which, coupled with the high cost of this type of facility, probably explains the high turnover rate. Residential treatment centers for the emotionally and mentally ill are usually privately operated with state and local governments, private insurance, and patients' fees supporting about 30% of program expenditures each, and private philanthrophy 10%.[155]

Education and clinics. About 92% of the noninstitutionalized retarded attending special education classes, and an even higher proportion of those attending regular academic classes, are in public schools. The federal contribution to all public education expenditures amounted to only 7.9% during the 1969–70 school year (8.8% during the 1967–68 school year).[156] SCMR reported that in 1968 the U.S. Office of Education expended $38 million in direct services to the retarded, of which $14 million went to state residential facilities. Federal support of public special education classes was, therefore, only about 3%. In 1970 Office of Education expenditures on the retarded were estimated at $63 million, of which somewhat over $40 million went to community educational facilities. Federal support of public special education classes apparently, therefore, rose to about 4% in 1970.

Although one would expect the largest part of private day special education classes to be financed from private sources, a substantial number of public school districts purchase care from private schools.

Clinical facilities are primarily state-supported, probably of the order of 70% of expenditures, with the rest being equally divided among the federal government, patient fees, and private philanthropy.[157]

[155] Ronald W. Conley, Margaret Conwell, and Shirley G. Willner, *The Cost of Mental Illness*, 1968, Statistical Note 30, Survey and Reports Section, Biometry Branch, Office of Program Planning and Evaluation, NIMH, p. 7.

[156] Simon and Grant, *Digest of Educational Statistics*, 1971, p. 5.

[157] Conley, Conwell, and Willner, "The Cost of Mental Illness," p. 7.

Vocational training. The federal government matched state expenditures on vocational rehabilitation at the rate of 3 to 1 in 1968 and 4 to 1 in 1970.

About one-fifth of workshop costs are financed out of funds not obtained from business operations. Of this, a tiny portion, 1%, is obtained from patient fees; 38% from sources such as fund drives, parent organizations, and bequests; 33% from fees paid by referring agencies; and 29% from grants.[158] The referring agencies are usually vocational rehabilitation agencies and grants are derived primarily from the Rehabilitation Services Administration. Thus, about 53% of the nonbusiness income of workshops is derived from the federal government (three-quarters of 33% and 29%) and 8% from state governments.

Estimated cost distribution. An estimate of the cost of mental retardations programs is presented in Table 24. This estimate is limited to the operating expenditures of residential care programs and community programs providing developmental services—i.e., it does not include our estimates of fair rental values, patient and volunteer help, research, training, and construction expenditures, income maintenance programs, or agency operating expenditures.[159]

Table 24.   Estimated sources of funds for mental retardation programs providing direct services, 1968 and 1970 (in 000,000's)

	Total	Federal	State & local	Client fees	Insurance & philanthropy
			1968		
Residential care	$1,004	$110	$ 768	$ 89	$37
Community care	1,391	121	1,207	44	19
Total	$2,395	$231	$1,975	$133	$56
% Distribution	100.0%	9.6%	82.5%	5.6%	2.3%
			1970		
Residential care	$1,307	$196	$ 937	$123	$51
Community care	1,868	192	1,580	64	32
Total	$3,175	$388	$2,517	$187	$83
% Distribution	100.0%	12.2%	79.3%	5.9%	2.6%

[158] John R. Kimberly, *The Financial Structure of Sheltered Workshops* (Ithaca, N.Y.: Region II Rehabilitation Research Institute, New York State School of Industrial and Labor Relations, Cornell University, June, 1968), p. 6. The data are based on a sample of 123 workshops in New York, New Jersey, and Pennsylvania, collected in December 1966 and January 1967.

[159] A few facilities are included for whom the sources of funding were not discussed because they were obvious—e.g., state and federal prisons.

In some cases speculative assumptions about the importance of various sources of funds were made. Fortunately, our information on the major programs is reasonably good, and, in the aggregate, these estimates should be reasonably accurate. Since there is little purpose to be served in implying greater precision in the estimates for individual programs than exists, a distinction was made only between community care programs and residential care programs.

It is apparent that programs in mental retardation are overwhelmingly a state and local responsibility and will continue to be so in the future. Although the federal share increased significantly between 1968 and 1970 and, because of the influence of Medicaid, will continue to increase, it is unlikely that the federal share will exceed 20% in the foreseeable future.

The small proportion of funds derived from client fees must be interpreted cautiously, since we have not taken account of services rendered by private psychiatrists, psychologists, and physicians. Moreover, the distribution of fees among clients is extremely uneven. Families who place children in private residential or educational facilities may face staggering burdens and are unlikely to be impressed by the contribution of state and local government to the care of the retarded.

This estimate of federal funding of direct services to the retarded is considerably higher than the SCMR estimate for HEW for 1968 or 1970. One reason is that unlike the SCMR estimate we estimated the federal share of the cost of serving the retarded in facilities not primarily operated for the retarded (e.g., mental hospitals). In addition, we included trust fund disbursements to institutionalized "childhood disability" annuitants and outlays by OCHAMPUS.

If to the $231 million estimate for the federal government, we add $82 million for federal expenditures on research, construction, and training activities directly relevant to mental retardation in 1968 (SCMR estimate), another $12 million for agency operating expenses (including the costs of operating PCMR and SCMR), then total federal expenditures on programs (other than income maintenance) for the retarded came to $321 million in 1968. In 1970 this estimate had risen to $492 million.

SUMMARY

1. Programs for the mentally retarded have varying goals and serve a wide range of functions: developmental, supportive, protective, rehabilitative, and modification of the work or social milieu.

2. Approximately 275,000 mentally retarded individuals were institutionalized during 1968 and 1970. The average cost per patient was

about $6,000 per year in 1970, having increased about 30% since 1968.

3. The reasons for institutionalization are usually the difficulty of providing adequate care in the home; illegal, immoral, or otherwise undesirable behavior; and a lack of living arrangements in the community. The severely retarded and male retardates are more likely to be institutionalized than the mildly retarded and female retardates.

4. In 1970 almost 690,000 retarded children attended public or private special education classes in the community and about 740,000 attended regular academic classes. Another 450,000 retardates, age 5 to 19, were not in school. Since 1968 the proportion of school-age retardates in special education programs has increased slightly and the proportion who are not in school has decreased slightly. The per student cost of special education was almost twice that of regular academic classes.

5. Almost 180,000 retardates received clinical services in 1970.

6. Another 65,000 adult retardates were rehabilitated or in sheltered workshops. Most of those in the latter type of facility were being prepared for work in competitive situations.

7. About $365 million was disbursed to 360 thousand retarded individuals by income maintenance programs, primarily "childhood disability beneficiaries" under Social Security and APTD in 1970.

8. Over $3.6 billion was expended under the programs described in this chapter in 1968. In 1970 this figure rose to $4.7 billion. Slightly over $3 billion could be ascribed to developmental purposes in 1968 and $4 billion in 1970. The "excess costs" of these programs were $1.6 billion in 1968 (if we include research, training, and construction expenditures) and $2.2 billion in 1970.

9. Classes for the educable retarded cost about 1.9 times as much as regular academic classes; classes for the trainable retarded about 3.5 times as much, and day development classes 5.9 times as much.

10. Variation among states in the provision of services to the retarded is wide. There is a suggestion that the states which provide the most extensive care in residential facilities have the smallest proportion of their population institutionalized.

11. State and local governments funded over four-fifths of the operating costs of the programs discussed in this chapter.

V

The Effects of
Mental Retardation

The resources used for the development and care of the retarded are only one aspect of this condition. The other aspect, and by far the more important in terms of social welfare, is the effects of mental retardation.

TYPES OF EFFECTS

The adverse effects of mental retardation are many. In general, an adverse effect is one that causes a person's mental or physical well-being to be below what it would have been had the person been of normal intelligence. A brief summary of the major ways in which mental retardation affects social welfare will help place this chapter in better perspective.

A. **Reduction in productive capacity**. Loss of productive capacity measures the reduction in the standard of living that occurs because of mental retardation. It has three components.

1. *Reduced production of goods and services that enter into measures of gross national product.* This occurs because some retardates are unemployed (seeking, but unable to find work), have withdrawn or never entered the labor market (not seeking work), are employed in unskilled jobs with below average productivity, or tend to be less efficient in the performance of their jobs. In addition, there are ripple effects. Lower earnings reduce capital accumulation. Less capable workers may require the use of a less advanced technology which af-

fects all workers. The mother of a retarded child may forgo work in order to care for her child.

2. *Reduced value of homemaking services and other unpaid work.* Homemaking services must be divided into three components: (1) the physical task of organizing, decorating, and maintaining a living residence; (2) child care; and (3) the managerial task of coordinating and performing these tasks within a given budget. Other unpaid work refers to the many productive activities adults carry on that are not remunerated or normally considered homemaking—lawn maintenance, painting, charitable activities.

Although not reflected in gross national product, these activities are as much a part of the nation's well-being as the production of automobiles and refrigerators.

3. *Reduced value of use of leisure time.* People allocate time to travel, health care, watching television, spectator sports, etc., as well as to work and to homemaking services and child care. Since the ultimate goal of any of these uses of time is increased well-being, they should all, including the various uses of leisure time, be considered as a use of productive capacity (people's time). Leisure is as important a consumption goal as any of the commodities purchased in the market. Mental retardation will reduce a person's ability to enjoy leisure time in the same way that it reduces a person's ability to earn in paid employment.

Although it is conceptually confusing to include the use of leisure time (normally regarded as consumption) as a category of productive capacity, this difficulty can be resolved if leisure time activities are regarded as production that is simultaneous with consumption.

B. Illegal behavior, undesirable behavior, and accidents. Any distinction between these three categories is tenuous. Accidents and illegal behavior are, by definition, undesirable. Illegal behavior refers to thefts, assaults, homicides, etc. Undesirable behavior refers to such things as alcoholism, promiscuity, excessive gambling, etc. (which may also be illegal in some areas). Undesirable behavior and accidents may be distinguished by regarding the former as intentional and the latter as unintentional.

C. Psychic effects. This broad term refers to the moods, feelings, perceptions, and attitudes of people, and the pain they sometimes suffer. The problems of the retarded often cause frustration, insecurity, and bitterness among themselves and their families, regardless of whether they suffer material losses. Many retardates die prematurely. Although conceptually confusing to assign a psychic loss to the deceased, society generally assumes that life has an intangible value that merits prolongation under almost any circumstances.

D. Other effects. A complete list of the ways in which mental retardation may adversely affect well-being would require many pages. Some of the more important of these other effects are:

1. decreased social acceptability;
2. dependence on others for basic needs (dressing, eating, toileting, transportation, etc.);
3. unwise decisions as to how they spend their money;
4. possible disruption of family relationships;
5. poor intellectual development of the children of the retarded;
6. rejection from military service.

These effects are not independent of each other. Many adverse psychic effects would be ameliorated if the retarded were provided with an adequate and secure standard of living and assisted to greater independence in providing for their daily needs. Similarly, illegal and undesirable activities would decrease and their children's intellectual development would improve. Nevertheless, these are conceptually distinct effects and should be distinguished.

The effects of mental retardation are often conflicting. Although remunerated employment decreases as a result of retardation, this overstates the number of persons economically idle because of this condition. Some of the retarded who would have been in the labor force will instead become full-time homemakers, and many may increase their unpaid efforts at home.

It is conceivable that among some groups retardation could cause the provision of homemaking services to be greater than among the nonretarded, if the number of women prevented from keeping house is more than offset by women turning to homemaking as an alternative to paid work (a realistic possibility among mildly retarded females). Such a finding, if made, must be interpreted cautiously. It would not mean that there should be no concern about loss of homemaking services among this group (since some are unable to keep house), but rather that the norms applicable to the general population would not be applicable here.

The seriousness of these effects will vary immensely among retardates and will depend upon many factors other than the degree of retardation.

MEASUREMENT CONSIDERATIONS

From a measurement standpoint, the effects of mental retardation can be grouped into three categories:

1. those which are tangible and potentially have a market-determined value—e.g., loss of earnings, some unpaid work;

2. those which are tangible but do not have a market-determined value—e.g., homemaker's services;

3. those which are intangible and which obviously do not have a market determined value—psychic benefits, increased ability to care for personal needs.

Any defined effect of mental retardation is potentially measurable. This does not mean that it is always worth the effort, or that the present state of knowledge is such that it could be done quickly or easily. But the point must be underscored that if an effect is definable it can be made measurable.

Empirical analysis has three goals: completeness, accuracy, and comparability among the different variables. As we have observed, lack of data precludes completeness in our analyses or achievement of great accuracy in most of our measurements. Comparability is possible only for effects that have a market-determined value, such as loss of earnings, or that can be given a market value, such as homemaking and other unpaid work.

In cases of intangible effects, direct measurement is difficult. Usually, one measures observable tangible effects that are presumed to be related to the intangible effects and are themselves often of great importance. As examples, the academic skills of the retarded, ability to handle various aspects of self-care, job-retention rates, absenteeism, etc.

Although considerable accuracy is possible in the measurement of these variables, it must be stressed that for all practical purposes there is no comparability among them. There is no way of combining these indices to derive any meaningful total. Later in this chapter, various approaches to placing a monetary value on the services of homemakers will be discussed. Although comparability is thereby achieved, accuracy becomes questionable.

The effect of retardation on earnings can be measured with considerable accuracy. Moreover, this loss can be considered a reasonably good indication of the reduction in gross national production due to mental retardation.

This is because earnings, in theory, measure the value of what additional workers would add to total production—i.e., the value of the marginal product. Workers would not normally be paid more than they add to a firm's output, and if they were paid less, employers would hire additional workers, until the combined pressures of bidding-up wages (to attract more workers) and declining marginal productivity brought earnings and marginal product into equality.

Of course, earnings will not equal the marginal product of workers in all cases. In a technologically dynamic economy, marginal products frequently change, and wages are drifting toward equality with this variable. In addition, distortions occur because of monopolistic firms, union pressures, the difficulties of entering particular lines of work, the difficulties of measuring marginal products, complementarity of jobs,[1] and many other factors, such as seniority, altruism, favoritism, "featherbedding," etc.

LOSS OF EARNINGS AMONG INSTITUTIONALIZED RETARDATES

The major focus of this chapter will be on the extent of and reasons for reduced employment and earnings among the retarded. This is not because other effects of retardation are not of equal, and perhaps superior, importance. Rather, it is because we have little firm data on these other effects. We will first estimate the loss of earnings among institutionalized retardates and then turn to the more complicated task of assessing the vocational performance of noninstitutionalized retardates.

The procedure for estimating earnings and employment loss among the retarded is to ascertain by how much these variables would increase if their vocational achievement was comparable to that of the general population. In short, we are measuring the extent to which earnings and employment are *below average* among the retarded.

In the case of institutionalized retardates, this requires three types of information: a demographic distribution of the institutionalized retardates and the average employment rates and earning levels among the general population according to the same demographic grouping.

Age and Sex of Institutionalized Retardates. Table 25 presents estimates of the age and sex of institutionalized retardates in 1968 and 1970. This includes estimates from the previous chapter for residents in all facilities, with the exception of general hospitals, where the shortness of the length of stay made the number of retardates placed in these facilities negligible at any point in time.

As would be expected, the data were not conveniently available in this form. The following procedure was employed to develop this table. Information on the age and sex of about 95% of the retarded residents of public mental hospitals was available from NIMH for both years. It was assumed that all retarded residents had the same age and sex distribution as those reporting.

---

[1] Complementarity occurs when one job requires the performance of another job. If it takes three workers to operate a machine, the absence of any one will cause the productivity of the others to fall drastically. Wages then become a measure of bargaining strength rather than the marginal product. The mentally retarded are at an obvious disadvantage.

Table 25.   The mentally retarded in facilities providing residential care, by age and sex, 1968 and 1970

Age	1968		1970	
	Male	Female	Male	Female
Under 15	40,619	29,549	45,534	33,115
15–17	15,645	10,867	14,696	10,209
18–19	9,706	6,778	9,162	6,307
20–24	20,448	13,252	19,323	12,301
25–34	25,382	16,524	24,282	15,571
35–44	19,078	13,998	17,298	12,524
45–54	14,248	12,000	12,929	10,745
55–64	8,732	7,152	8,030	6,419
65+	4,566	6,308	4,354	6,000
Total	158,424	116,428	155,608	113,191

Information on the age and sex of about 80% of the residents of public institutions was available from NIMH for 1968. In 1970 no information was available on the sex distribution of residents and the age distribution employed only a few broad age spans (under 15, 15–24, 25–34, 35+). It was assumed that the sex distribution of residents in 1970 was the same within each of these broad age groupings as in 1968. Then, it was assumed that within these broad age groups the relative distribution of residents among the more detailed age groupings remained constant.

The age and sex distribution for retarded residents of private institutions and private mental hospitals was based on data for 6,243 residents of private institutions in 1967, the most recent data available.[2] The only information on the age and sex of prisoners in federal and state prisons dates back to the 1960 census.[3] It was assumed that this distribution was representative of retarded prisoners in 1968 and 1970 (females constituted less than 4% of the prison population).

A detailed age and sex breakdown of retardates was required because employment rates and earnings differ among age groups and between sexes, and because the age and sex distribution of the institutional

[2] NIMH used an open-end 55-and-over age grouping for public and private institutions. This grouping was subdivided into a 55-to-64 and 65-and-over age classification by assuming that the percentage distribution in these age groups was the same as their age and sex counterparts in public mental hospitals. Using information on 6,000 residents in private institutions to estimate the age and sex of 25,000 residents in all private institutions appears questionable, but since only one-third of these residents are over 20, any bias in our measure of lost earnings will be small.

[3] Department of Commerce, Bureau of the Census, *U.S. Census of Population: 1960*, Series PC(2)–8A.

population is not representative of the population. For example, the excess of males in institutions means that the average loss of workers and reduction in earnings will be greater than would be true if the sexes were distributed equally.

Employment rates and earnings differ by race as well as age and sex. In principle, our estimates should also be adjusted for this variable.

The only information on the racial composition of different age and sex groups among residents of institutions dates back to the 1960 census, where this information was published for different types of residential facilities.[4]

Surprisingly, despite the high prevalence of retardation among nonwhites, the percentage of nonwhites in public institutions was about half of the percentage of nonwhites in the U.S. population. Perhaps nonwhites are better able to accept the mentally retarded in their families, or nonwhites may be less likely to know of the availability of institutional care. Possibly, public and private agencies were less concerned with the problems caused by mental retardation in nonwhite families than in white families.

On the other hand, the proportion of nonwhites in public mental hospitals exceeded their proportion in the population, which was probably also true for retarded nonwhites in these hospitals. Evidently, retarded nonwhites are less likely than retarded whites to be institutionalized, but as they become older they are more likely to be placed in mental hospitals (or to be imprisoned). In public institutions the percentage of nonwhites among residents under 20 was about twice the percentage among residents over 20 which suggests that this pattern is being altered. In view of this possibly changing percentage of nonwhites among the institutional population, it did not appear wise to attempt to estimate the racial composition of the institutionalized retarded in 1968 and 1970 on the basis of 1960 data. It is doubtful if failure to adjust for race differences will significantly affect our results, since the racial composition of the institutionalized population does not appear to radically differ from that of the U.S. population.

Employment rates. Civilian labor force participation rates (LFPR) and unemployment rates by age and sex for 1967 were available from the 1968 *Manpower Report of the President.*[5] Employment rates for

---

[4] Ibid.

[5] U.S. Department of Labor, *Manpower Report of the President,* April 1968, pp. 225, 237. The LFPR includes the percentage who at a point in time are employed and unemployed. Persons are counted as unemployed if they are currently available for work and had engaged in some specific job-seeking activity within the past four week period.

each demographic group were calculated by multiplying the LFPR times the percent of the LFPR that is employed (100% minus the unemployment rate, see Table 26). Unemployment rates in 1967 were chosen to measure employment loss in 1968 and 1970, rather than the actual rates existing in those years. Under normal conditions, employment rates are highly stable over time. However, they do vary with the level of unemployment. Nineteen sixty-seven, with an unemployment rate of 3.8%, is probably a more representative year than 1968, when unemployment fell to its lowest point since World War II, or 1970 when unemployment reached 4.9% and was rapidly rising.

Table 26.   Percentage employed by age and sex, United States, 1967

Age	Male	Female
18–19	54.9	42.4
20–24	78.7	49.3
25–34	95.4	39.6
35–44	95.9	46.1
45–54	93.5	50.2
55–64	82.9	41.2
65+	43.4	17.4

Table 27 shows the extent to which employment would increase if the institutionalized retarded above age 18 had the same employment rates as the general population. It was calculated by multiplying the employment rates for each demographic grouping times the number of institutionalized retardates with these characteristics. Technically, this slightly understates the true loss of employment, since a small percentage of youths below age 18 are employed, usually on part-time and low-paying jobs. Limiting our analysis to persons 18 years old and over

Table 27.   Employment loss among mentally retarded persons in residential facilities, United States, 1968 and 1970

Age	1968		1970	
	Male	Female	Male	Female
18–19	5,300	2,900	5,000	2,700
20–24	16,100	6,500	15,200	6,100
25–34	24,200	6,500	23,200	6,200
35–44	18,300	6,500	16,600	5,800
45–54	13,300	6,000	12,100	5,400
55–64	7,200	3,000	6,700	2,600
65+	2,000	1,100	1,900	1,000
Total	86,400	32,500	80,700	29,800

will not significantly affect our conclusions and will be more consistent with our subsequent work in this and the next chapter.

In 1968 the estimated employment loss among the institutional population was slightly less than 120,000 persons. In 1970 this decreased to less than 110,000, partly because of a reduction in the number of institutionalized retardates and partly because the proportion of retardates under age 18 in institutions has grown.

These estimates represent average employment loss at a point in time (both full-time and part-time). Because some people work intermittently, the number employed during the course of a year, if not institutionalized, would be somewhat greater.

Earnings. Amazingly little information on earnings is available in the demographic detail needed for our estimates. A special survey conducted in May 1967 for the Department of Labor by the Bureau of the Census ascertained the usual wage and salary earnings of the employed labor force during the week preceding the interview by age, sex, and race.[6] The problems with this data were that it provided median earnings figures only, did not include self-employment earnings, and did not adjust for the zero earnings of unpaid family workers.

A separate survey by the Census Bureau reported mean and median total money income of persons by age, sex, and race for 1967.[7]

It was decided to use the first source of data. One reason is that the census data on income included rents, corporate dividends, and interest paid to individuals. Income from these sources represents the contribution of capital to output, not the efforts of the recipient. Another problem with the census survey was that it included the earnings of people over the full year prior to the survey. Our estimates of labor force loss, on the other hand, refer to an average one-week period. In consequence, the census survey would include a greater proportion of intermittent workers, depressing estimates of median and mean earnings. These biases are conflicting. The first (the inclusion of unearned income) would cause an overstatement, and the second (the inclusion of an excessive proportion of intermittent workers) would cause an

[6] People on vacation, or sick leave, or who were on strike or laid off because of bad weather were counted as having their usual weekly earnings. With the exception of the latter two categories, which were small, this procedure is appropriate, since paid leave is a form of *deferred* compensation designed to even out income during the course of a year.

[7] U.S. Department of Commerce, Bureau of the Census, *Current Population Reports, Income in 1967 of Persons in the United States*, series P-60, No. 60, June 30, 1969, pp. 25–26. The Census Bureau also publishes data on earnings by sex and race, but not by the crucial variable of age.

understatement of the average contribution to output of a worker during a point in time.

A major drawback to using the Department of Labor survey is that only median earnings are available. Median earnings are usually considerably below average earnings because the income distribution of the population is sharply skewed to the right; i.e., there are many more low-salaried workers than high-salaried workers. It is average earnings, however, that are needed to estimate the loss of earnings among the institutionalized retarded. The distributions in which a wide divergence has been noted between mean and median income in the past have been distributions of annual income. These distributions include a large proportion of (a) intermittent (less than full year) workers; and (b) nonworkers receiving interest, rent, or dividend income, factors which may contribute heavily to the number of low income recipients in distributions of income. It was assumed that the Department of Labor data, which excluded nonearned income and was restricted to a one-week period preceding the interview, would greatly reduce these problems and that median earnings could, therefore, be used to approximate average earnings.

Median weekly earnings by age, sex, and race were calculated from the Department of Labor data. These median weekly earnings were then converted to an annual basis by multiplying each by 52.[8] These median wage and salary earnings were next adjusted to allow for the effect of unpaid family workers and the self-employed.[9] Surprisingly, the net effect of these adjustments was small and usually in a downward direction.

[8] The Department of Labor data was available in far greater detail that could be utilized for our purposes. The age intervals were five years after age 25 and one year below this age. Each age group was divided into four groups. There were three categories of part-time workers (less than 35 hours per week): voluntary part-time; part-time for economic reasons, usually full-time; and part-time for economic reasons, usually part-time. The other category was full-time workers and those working part-time for noneconomic reasons (vacation, sick leave, etc.), but usually full-time. In addition, persons under 25 were further subdivided according to whether they were in school or not. The median earnings of these groups were combined into our larger categories by weighting each median earning figure by the ratio of the number of persons in that group to the total number of persons in the combined groups.

It is customary to multiply weekly earnings by 50 rather than 52 in order to estimate annual earnings, on the assumption that most people enjoy a two-week vacation annually. However, the procedure used here is the more appropriate, since paid vacations are a form of deferred compensation.

[9] Two sources of information were used: a distribution of unpaid family workers and the self-employed by age and sex for May 1967. U.S. Department of Labor, Bureau of Labor Statistics, *Employment and Earnings and Monthly Report on the Labor Force*, June 1967, p. 17); and a distribution of unpaid family workers and

The results of these calculations are presented in Table 28. The calculations are presented by race, as well as age and sex, since this information will be used later in the chapter.

Table 28.   Estimated annual earnings of employed workers, United States, 1967

| | Wage & salary workers | | | | All workers | | | |
Ages	White male	White female	Non-white male	Non-white female	White male	White female	Non-white male	Non-white female
15–17	$1,060	$ 853	$1,178	$1,048	$ 976	$ 822	$1,082	$ 981
18–19	2,665	2,584	2,436	1,976	2,577	2,559	2,374	1,958
20–24	5,042	3,750	4,016	3,113	4,996	3,716	3,979	3,081
25–34	6,818	3,799	5,011	3,082	6,832	3,657	4,995	3,008
35–44	7,413	3,768	5,009	2,844	7,472	3,581	5,003	2,738
45–54	7,172	3,817	4,654	2,557	7,230	3,579	4,641	2,405
55–64	6,336	3,633	4,031	2,188	6,355	3,439	3,989	2,065
65+	4,123	2,493	2,185	1,060	4,055	2,401	2,096	1,033

Since our estimates of earnings loss will be for 1968 and 1970, the earnings in Table 28 must be increased to reflect: (a) the change in price levels between 1967 and these two years; and (b) the change in worker productivity. This was done by multiplying estimated earnings in 1967 by the percentage change in average weekly earnings of workers on private payrolls. Between 1967 and 1968, these earnings increased

the self-employed and the earnings of the latter by race and sex for 1967 (U.S. Department of Commerce, Bureau of the Census, *Current Population Reports, Series P-60, N. 60,* June 30, 1969, pp. 44–46).

An age, race, and sex distribution of unpaid family workers and the self-employed was estimated by assuming that the proportion of these types of workers in each race and sex group was constant over all age groups. For example, if *a%* of white males were unpaid family workers (from the census data), it was assumed that this was the proportion of white males among unpaid family workers in each age and sex group (from the Department of Labor data). The next step was to calculate the percentages of wage and salary workers, self-employed, and unpaid family workers in each demographic group. Then the percentages of each class of worker in each demographic group were multiplied by a weight which reflected the earnings of that class of worker *vis-à-vis* the earnings of wage and salary workers. Wage and salary workers were given a weight of 100%, unpaid family workers a zero weight, and the self-employed a weight obtained by dividing the earnings of wage and salary workers by the earnings of the self-employed in each race and sex group. It was assumed that the relationship of the earnings of the self-employed to wage and salary workers was constant throughout all age groups in each race and sex grouping. These products were summed and the total multiplied by our previous estimate of the median annual earnings of wage and salary workers for each demographic group.

5.8% and between 1967 and 1970, 17.3%. These estimates are presented (Table 29) for all workers (including unpaid family workers, the self-employed, and wage and salary workers) by age and sex only.[10]

Table 29. Estimated annual earnings of employed workers, United States, 1968 and 1970

Age	1968		1970	
	Male	Female	Male	Female
18–19	$2,702	$2,651	$2,996	$2,940
20–24	5,159	3,855	5,721	4,274
25–34	7,016	3,754	7,779	4,163
35–44	7,648	3,659	8,481	4,057
45–54	7,405	3,644	8,211	4,041
55–64	6,511	3,496	7,220	3,877
65+	4,105	2,364	4,552	2,622

Earnings loss. We now have two matrices. One estimates how many of the institutionalized retarded would have been employed in 1968 and 1970 if they had the same employment rates as their age and sex counterparts in the general population. The other estimates what their average annual earnings would be if they had the same earnings rates. Multiplying one matrix times the other shows the total earnings loss among the institutionalized retarded (Table 30) that can be attributed to their retardation and other physical and psychiatric difficulties impeding their adjustment outside the institution.

Table 30. Earnings loss among the institutionalized retarded, 1968 and 1970

	1968	1970
Males	$561,137,000	$578,891,000
Females	115,831,000	127,662,000
Total	$676,968,000	$706,553,000

In 1968 this loss was over $675 million and in 1970 it rose to over $700 million. Most of the rise was due to price level changes. During this period, output per worker remained virtually constant.[11] This estimate of earnings loss may be a slight overstatement, because, as noted in Chapter IV, many of the institutionalized retarded work as patient

[10] U.S. Department of Labor, *Manpower Report of the President*, March, 1972, p. 217.
[11] Ibid., p. 274.

aides or in other capacities. In addition, a small number worked in the community.

LOSS OF EARNINGS AMONG NONINSTITUTIONALIZED RETARDATES

Almost 95% of the retarded are not in institutions. Our next task is to estimate the extent to which earnings are below average among this large group.

Ideally, this would be calculated in the same way as loss of earnings was estimated for the institutionalized retarded. After estimating the distribution of the noninstitutionalized retarded by age, sex, race, and degree of intellectual deficit, the employment loss would be calculated by comparing actual employment rates within each demographic group with their age, sex, and race counterparts in the general population. The earnings loss would be calculated by: (a) multiplying this employment loss by the average earnings of the population counterparts of each demographic group; and (b) multiplying the difference in earnings between the employed retarded and their population counterparts by the number of employed retarded.

Unlike the calculations for institutionalized retardates, degree of intellectual deficit is specified as a crucial variable. Among the institutional population, zero productivity could be assumed for all persons, regardless of intellectual deficit. Among the noninstitutionalized retarded, productivity will vary greatly by this variable.

Unfortunately, our knowledge of the demographic characteristics of the noninstitutionalized retarded is too limited to justify the sweeping generalizations that would be required for this ideal approach. Our procedure, therefore, will be to utilize one broad age group, 20 to 64 years of age, and adjust by sex and level of retardation only.

Working-age retardates in the community. In Chapter III we estimated that there were, in 1968, 2,855,000 adults, age 20 to 64, with IQs below 70 and 2,915,000 in 1970. In this chapter we estimated that there were almost 151,000 retardates in this age range (Table 26) in residential care in 1968 and 139,000 in 1970, leaving approximately 2,704,000 in the community in the earlier year and 2,776,000 in the later year. Assuming equal numbers of male and female retardates, there were about 1,339,000 noninstitutionalized adult male and 1,364,000 noninstitutionalized adult female retardates in 1968. Comparable data for 1970 are 1,377,000 and 1,399,000.

In Chapter III we estimated that 35% of the retarded in residential facilities had IQs of 50 or over, 40% were in the 25 to 49 IQ range, and 25% were in the 0 to 24 IQ range. Assuming these proportions also apply to retarded adults in residential care, there would be about 53,000 adult retardates in the upper-IQ range, 60,000 in the middle range, and 38,000 in the lowest-IQ range in 1968. In 1970 the comparable figures were 49,000, 55,000, and 35,000.

The percentages of adult retardates in residential care in each IQ range are slightly higher than our estimated percentages (Chapter III) of the total number of persons in these IQ ranges who are institutionalized. This is as expected, since, all other things being equal, retarded adults are more likely to be institutionalized than retarded children.

On the basis of the information shown in the table on page 83, we estimate that 60% of the upper-grade, 58% of the middle-grade, and 54% of the lowest-grade retardates in residential care are male. Assuming equal numbers of male and female retardates in each IQ range, this provides sufficient information to estimate the intellectual and sex distribution of noninstitutionalized adult retardates.[12]

Table 31. Estimated number of noninstitutionalized retardates, age 20–64, by IQ and sex, 1968 and 1970

IQ	Number in population		Number in institutions		Total in community	
	Male	Female	Male	Female	Male	Female
1968						
0–24	47,000	47,000	21,000	17,000	26,000	30,000
25–49	116,000	116,000	35,000	25,000	81,000	91,000
50–69	1,264,500	1,264,500	32,000	21,000	1,232,500	1,243,500
Total	1,427,500	1,427,500	88,000	63,000	1,339,500	1,364,500
1970						
0–24	48,000	48,000	19,000	16,000	29,000	32,000
25–49	118,500	118,500	32,000	23,000	86,000	96,000
50–69	1,291,000	1,291,000	29,000	20,000	1,262,000	1,271,000
Total	1,457,500	1,457,500	80,000	59,000	1,377,000	1,399,000

Follow-up studies. Tables 32 to 35 present selected information from follow-up studies of the adult retarded. As in the survey of epidemiological studies, each study will be identified by the author's last name or, in the case of coauthors, by the last name of the first listed

[12] In earlier chapters it was suggested that there may be a slight excess of females in the lower-IQ ranges and it was pointed out that a few institutionalized retardates have IQs above 70. Adjustments for these factors were not made because they would have been of minor and questionable significance.

author. References and brief descriptions of the studies are given at the end of Table 32.

There are many problems in interpreting the results of these studies. To begin with, sample sizes are relatively small. In addition, these studies differ substantially in the age, IQ, sex, and racial composition of the subjects. Although these are factors which substantially effect employment status, many studies failed to report results for separate demographic groups. Others do not distinguish subjects by level of IQ, although the *average* IQ is often around 70, and some alleged retardates in these studies have IQs in the 90s. Only one study adjusted for the effect of age—a variable which will be shown to be crucial. Some studies even failed to report separate results for males and females.

In addition, most studies dealt with the community adjustment of former residents in institutions for the retarded or former pupils in special education classes. Only a few included retardates who attended regular academic classes. In the first case, particularly, there is a strong adverse selection factor.

Although most follow-up studies have found poor employment records among the retarded, this is largely a consequence of the fact that they evaluated former special education students within a few years after their having left the school systems. Most teenagers have relatively poor employment histories and retarded teenagers are no exception.

Another problem with follow-up studies is that they use different criterion of vocational adjustment. Some count only retardates earning wages as gainfully employed; others include housewives.[13] One important study included retarded women, if their spouses were gainfully employed. Some studies are concerned only with whether the subjects are currently employed, others ask whether the subjects are usually employed, and still others ask whether retardates have ever been employed.

Several other points about these study summaries should be borne in mind:

a) Whenever possible, employment and unemployment rates were calculated only for nonstitutionalized retardates who were not attending school. Thus the rates of employment here will not always agree with those reported in the original studies, since some of these surveys based employment rates on all persons in the original sample, including

---

[13] In none of the studies were retarded women keeping house counted as unemployed. This is why the percentages employed and unemployed sometimes total 100% and sometimes do not.

Table 32.   Employment status of adults formerly in special education
            classes, selected follow-up studies

Name of study	Number in community	Year of evaluation	Place of study	Descrip. of special educ. class	Time lapse between eval. & previous contact (in years)
1. Channing study[a]	603	1923–24	Seven large U.S. cities		3–7
	178				
	28				
	148				
	229				
	150				
	20				
	54				
	70				
	29				
2. McKeon study[b]	190	1943	Worchester, Massachusetts	Educable	1–11
3. McIntosh study[c]	707	1947	Toronto, Canada	Jarvis school for boys	1–11
	52				
4. Delp study[d]	41	1951	St. Paul, Minnesota	Trainable	1–14
5. Mullen study[e]		1951	Chicago, Illinois	Ungraded	1–5
	116				
	73				
6. Phelps study[f]		1952	Ohio		2–4
	105				
	58				
7. Bobroff study[g]		1953	Detroit, Michigan		12
	95				
	29				
8. Collman study[h]		1954–55	London, England		2–3
Normal group	49				
	57				
Dull group	101				
	99				
Educationally subnormal group	139				
	84				
	33				
	53				
	37				
	14				
	8				
	24				
	36				
	13				

Age	Sex	IQ	Race	Unemployed (%)	Employed at time of interview (%)	Never employed (%)	Unemployed 20% of time or more (%)
17–24	Males	Med. 64		28.9	71.7	2.0	
17–24	Females	Med. 62		30.3	69.7	16.5	
	Males	Less than 50					61
		50–59					54
		60–69					54
		70 or more					63
	Females	Less than 50					80
		50–59					54
		60–69					53
		70 or more					52
16–27	Males	52–83		0	99.5		
16–30 Med. 21	Males	40–100 Med. 73 below 60		3.1 13.5			
9–32 Med. 22	Both	Med. 36– (all but 3 below 50)			24.4		
16–40 Med. 19		Med. 68					
	Males			12.9	87.1		
	Females			21.9	60.3		
Med. 21.7	Males Females	Med. 60.6		10.5	67.5		
28–30	Males	40–99 (Mean approx. 70)		7.4	92.6	n/a	
	Females			n/a	41.4	21	
Not given evidently late	Males Females	90–109 90–109			} 99		
teen's and early 20's	Males Females	70–89 70–89			} 97		
	Males Females	Med. 63 Med. 58			} 72	12.1	
	Males	70 or over			57.6		
		60–69			77.4		
		50–59			75.7		
		40–49			35.7		
	Females	70 or over			62.5		
		60–69			79.2		
		50–59			75.0		
		40–49			23.1		

Table 32.   (Continued)

Name of study	Number in community	Year of evaluation	Place of study	Descrip. of special educ. class	Time lapse between eval. & previous contact (in years)
9. Saenger study[i]	348	1956	New York City	Trainable	1–27
10. Ferguson study[j]	11 29 88 70 4	1957	Glasgow, Scotland		9
11. Dinger study[k]	19 122	1960	Altoona, Pennsylvania	Educable	1–18
12. Orzack study[l]	41 20	1965	Bridgeport, Connecticut	Educable classes in in high school	Evidently brief
13. McFall study[m]	50	1965	New Jersey	Educable	4–14
14. Mudd study[n]	546	1966	Massachusetts	Educable	4–5
15. Tobias study[o]	66 22 44 77 40 37 90 36 54 48 21 27 43 25 18 59 30 29	1966–67	New York City	Educable	3–7

Age	Sex	IQ	Race	Unemployed (%)	Employed at time of interview (%)	Never employed (%)	Unemployed 20% of time or more (%)
	58% were male	Below 55 on highest test					
17–40					27	64	
17–20					16	77	
21–25					29	61	
26–30					25	63	
31–35					31	55	
36–40					30	59	
25	Males						
		Below 50		45.5	54.5		
		50–59		37.9	62.1		
		60–69		8.0	92.0		
		70–79		1.4	98.6		
		80 and over		0	100.0		
18–36 Med. 24	Males	50–85 Mean 70		14.7	85.3		
15–33 Med. 27	Females	58–85 Mean 69		12.3	27.3		
Not given, evidently late teens	Males Females				51 35		
						26	
21–22	Males	50–79			82.9	6.6	
20's (Med. about 23)							
	Males	50–75	Negro		54.5	13.6	
		50–65	Negro		54.6	22.7	
		66–75	Negro		54.6	9.0	
		50–75	Puerto Rican		67.5	7.8	
		50–65	Puerto Rican		70.0	10.0	
		66–75	Puerto Rican		64.9	5.4	
		50–75	White		63.3	13.3	
		50–65	White		55.6	19.4	
		66–75	White		68.5	9.3	
	Females	50–75	Negro		33.3	33.3	
		50–65	Negro		33.3	33.3	
		66–75	Negro		33.3	33.3	
		50–75	Puerto Rican		30.2	30.2	
		50–65	Puerto Rican		36.0	28.0	
		66–75	Puerto Rican		22.2	33.4	
		50–75	White		30.5	37.5	
		50–65	White		20.0	46.7	
		66–75	White		41.4	27.6	

Table 32.   (Continued)

Name of study	Number in community	Year of evaluation	Place of study	Descrip. of special educ. class	Time lapse between eval. & previous contact (in years)
16. Grate study[p]	67	1967	Oregon		1–3
17. Sweeny study[q]	28 53	1967	Delaware	Work study program for students in last year of spec. educ.	0–2

[a]Alice Channing, *Employment of Mentally Deficient Boys and Girls*, U.S. Department of Labor, Bureau Publication No. 210, 1932. The original sample consisted of 1,018 persons. The figures on employment and earnings, however, are based on 603 males and 178 females. Excluded from these data are former students who had never worked (69) and females who were married at the time of the study. The figures for the percentage of persons never employed are based on the number in the original sample. The seven cities in the survey were Newark, Rochester, Detroit, Cincinnati, Los Angeles, San Francisco, and Oakland.

[b]Rebecca M. McKeon, "Mentally Retarded Boys in Wartime," *Mental Hygiene* (1946): 47–55. A 20% sample was selected of all boys leaving special classes between 1932 and 1942. Of 210 persons surveyed, 7 were still in school, 4 had died, and 8 were in institutions at the time of the study. Of the remainder, 76 were at work in the city, one was an invalid at home, and the rest were in the military service.

[c]W. J. McIntosh, "Follow-Up Study of One Thousand Non-Academic Boys," *Journal of Exceptional Children* (March 1949): 166–91.

[d]Harold A. Delp and Marcella Lorenz, "Follow-Up of 84 Public School Special Class Pupils with IQ's below 50," *American Journal of Mental Deficiency* (July 1953): 175–82. At the time of the study, only 41 of the former pupils were at home; 10 were working, 2 full-time, 3 regular part-time, and 5 on odd jobs.

[e]Frances Mullen, "Mentally Retarded Youth Find Jobs," *Personnel and Guidance Journal* (Oct. 1952): 20–25. This is a nonrandom sample of the more than 2,000 pupils who left ungraded classes during the 5 years prior to the evaluation. Teachers of special classes were merely asked to make informal inquiries and pool their knowledge.

[f]Harold R. Phelps, "Post-School Adjustment of Mentally Retarded Children in Selected Ohio Cities," *Exceptional Children* (Nov. 1956): 58–91. All subjects had been in special classes for a period of at least one year and median attendance was 3.4 years. The data on occupation and earnings were based on interviews with the employers of 67 males and 20 females.

[g]Allen Bobroff, "Economic Adjustment of 121 Adults Formerly Students in Classes for Mental Retardates," *American Journal of Mental Deficiency* (January 1956): 525–35. See also, Allen Bobroff, "A Survey of Social and Civic Participation of Adults Formerly in Classes for the Mentally Retarded," *American Journal of Mental Deficiency* (July 1956): 127–33. Labor market conditions were such that more than four-fifths of the employed persons in the sample found jobs within a week of looking. Seventy-two percent found jobs without help from family, friends, or agencies. Five of the seven men listed as unemployed were not actively seeking work.

[h]R. D. Collman and D. Newlyn, "Employment Success of Mentally Dull and Intellectually Normal Ex-Pupils In England," *American Journal of Mental Deficiency* (Jan. 1957): 484–90. The educationally subnormal group included children enrolled in 6 special day schools (74 subjects) and 3 residential schools (98 subjects). For the distribution of employment by IQ groups among the educationally subnormal group see R. D. Collman and D. Newlyn, "Employment Success of Educationally Subnormal Ex-Pupils in England," *American Journal of Mental Deficiency* (April 1956): 733–43.

[i]Gerhart Saenger, *The Adjustment of Severely Retarded Adults in the Community*, Report to the New York State Interdepartmental Health Resources Board, Albany, New York, 1957.

Age	Sex	IQ	Race	Unemployed (%)	Employed at time of interview (%)	Never employed (%)	Unemployed 20% of time or more (%)
16–18	Both	49–84		29.9	58.2		
16–18	Both	Trainable			28.6		
		Educable			32.1		

All subjects had, at some time, tested below IQ 50. Although a few subjects had IQs below 40, the great majority were in the 40 to 50 range. Fifteen percent of those working were at home, in a workshop or some other sheltered employment. Thirty-three percent were "on their own," or working for parents, relatives, or friends. Fifty-two percent were in regular private business or industry.

jT. Ferguson and Agnes W. Kerr, "After-Histories of Boys Educated in Special Schools for Mentally-Handicapped Children," *Scottish Medical Journal* (1958): 31–38.

kJack C. Dinger, "Former Educable Retarded Pupils," *Exceptional Children* (March 1961): 353–60.

lLouis H. Orzack, John T. Cassell, and Harry Halliday, *An Educational Work/Experience Program for Secondary School Educable Mentally Retarded Students*, Bridgeport, Connecticut: Parents and Friends of Mentally Retarded Children of Bridgeport, Inc., 1968. The employment data were obtained from a follow-up study of students who had attended special education classes in the high school, and who could be located (61 out of 174). Earnings data were obtained from a report of the earnings of students participating in a cooperative educational work/experience program.

mThelma M. McFall, "Post school Adjustment: A Survey of Fifty Former Students of Classes for the Educable Mentally Retarded," *Exceptional Children* (May 1966): 633–34.

nMerle W. Mudd, Brina B. Melemed, and Henry Wechsler, *Post-School Vocational Adjustment of Educable Mentally Retarded Boys in Massachusetts*, mimeographed copy of report. The sample includes almost all special-class students who terminated their education during 1961 and 1962 and who were still in Massachusetts at the time of the study.

oJack Tobias, Ida Alpert, and Arnold Birenbaum, *A Survey of the Employment Status of Mentally Retarded Adults in New York City*, Report to the Office of Manpower Research, Manpower Administration, U.S. Department of Labor, conducted by the Association for the Help of Retarded Children, New York City Chapter, April 1969.

pDon A. Grate, *A Work Experience Program for the Mentally Retarded in Their Last Year in School* (Portland, Oregon; Goodwill Industries of Oregon, no date). Of 30 clients employed outside the workshop (including 8 housewives), 19 were employed within the sheltered workshop setting initially and moved on to competitive employment.

qSamuel R. Sweeny, Jr., *A Work Experience Program for the Mentally Retarded in Their Last Year in School* (Wilmington, Delaware: Opportunity Center, Inc., 1968). These students were described as those with the more severe vocational problems.

rW. R. Baller, "A Study of the Present Social Status of a Group of Adults Who, When They Were in Elementary School, Were Classified as Mentally Deficient," *Genetic Psychological Monographs* (1936): 167–244; Don C. Charles, "Ability and Accomplishments of Persons Earlier Judged Mentally Deficient," *Genetic Psychological Monographs* (1953): 3–71; Warren R. Baller, Don C. Charles, and Elbert L. Miller, "Mid-Life Attainment of the Mentally Retarded: A Longitudinal Study," *Genetic Psychological Monographs* (1967): 235–329.

The original study was conducted by Baller in 1935. Included in the percentage of those relatively permanently employed were women who were employed or whose husbands were employed. Charles reported a follow-up study of 151 of the mentally retarded group identified in Baller's research. The 1964 study included as many of both groups (mentally retarded and

Footnotes to Table 32 (Continued)

controls) as could be located and interviewed. In addition, a middle group, comprised of individuals whose IQs ranged from 75 to 85 were studied by Baller in 1937 and were again followed up in the 1964 study.

[s]Channing, *Employment of Mentally Deficient Boys and Girls* (see footnote a). The percentage employed at time of interview is based on the number who had worked at least one year outside of an institution and includes married females. The percentage unemployed 20% of the time or more was based on persons for whom information on work histories was available and who had worked at least one year outside the institution. It excludes married women.

[t]Robert B. Edgerton, *The Cloak of Competence* (Berkeley: University of California Press, 1967). Edgerton emphasized that these subjects represented the releasees from Pacific State Hospital that would be most likely to succeed.

[u]Thorleif G. Hegge, "The Occupational Status of Higher-Grade Mental Defectives in the Present Emergency. A Study of Parolees from the Wayne County Training School at Northville, Michigan," *American Journal of Mental Deficiency* (July 1944): 86–98. The percentage employed at time of interview includes males in the military service and, evidently, women keeping house.

Table 33. Employment status of adults formerly in special education classes—the Baller Study

Name of study	Number in community	Year of evaluation	Place of study	Descrip. of special educ. class	Time lapse between eval. & previous contact (in years)
18. Baller study[r]		1935	Lincoln, Nebraska	Opportunity classes	
Subjects	101				4–19
	60				
Control group	124				
	78				
Subjects		1951			17–32
	70				
	43				
Subjects (low group)		1964			
	58				31–46
	44				
Middle group					31–46
	65				
	50				
High group (original control group)					31–46
	64				
	56				

Note: See footnotes following Table 32.

VRuby Jo Reeves Kennedy, *The Social Adjustment of Morons in a Connecticut City*, done under the supervision of the Governor's Commission to study the Human Resources of the State of Connecticut in collaboration with the Carnegie Institution of Washington, 1948; also, Ruby Jo Reeves Kennedy, *A Connecticut Community Revisited: A Study of the Social Adjustment of a Group of Mentally Deficient Adults in 1948 and 1960.* A report on Project No. 655 to the Office of Vocational Rehabilitation, DHEW, Washington, D.C., June 1962.

During 1936 and 1937 a Connecticut study identified some 50,000 to 60,000 mentally inadequate persons. Of these, about 27,000 were classified as morons who were living at home with parents or other relatives. Most were of school age.

For purposes of the Kennedy study, the names of 260 mentally deficient persons with IQs between 50 and 75 were obtained from the census. They were between 20 and 30 years old in 1945 and were living in a town ficticiously identified as "Millport" when originally tested. An additional 15 persons were located by a special search of special-class enrollees who met these criteria. Nineteen persons, however, were dropped from the study because neither they nor their families could be located in "Millport." About two-thirds of the subject group had attended special education classes. This study developed a control group of 129 "nonmorons" who were matched as closely as possible to the subject group, except that the control group had IQ ratings of 75 or more.

In the 1960 survey, as many of the original sample were located as possible.

Age	Sex	IQ	Relatively permanent employment (%)	Occasional employment (%)	Unemployable (%)
Over 21					
	Males	Under 70	16.8	76.3	6.9
	Females		26.7	60.0	13.3
	Males	100–120	55.6	44.4	0
	Females		56.4	43.6	0
Late 30's		Under 70	Usually empl.	No reg. empl	
Early 40's	Males		92.9	7.1	
	Females		83.7	16.3	
					Totally depend. on relatives
50's			Ent. self-sup.	Part self-sup.	
	Males	Under 70	65.5	32.8	1.7
	Females		75.0	15.9	9.1
50's		75–85			
	Males		95.4	4.6	0
	Females		94.0	2.0	4.0
50's		100–120			
	Males		96	3	1
	Females				

Table 34.   Employment status of adults formerly in residential care

Name of study	Number in community	Year of evaluation	Place of study	Type of residential care	Time lapse between eval. & previous contact (in years)
19. Channing study[s]	98 36	1925	Illinois	Public inst.	1–8
20. Edgerton study[t]	20 28	1961	California	Public inst.	3–12

Note: See footnotes following Table 32.

Table 35.   Other follow-up studies of the employment status of retarded adults

Name of study	Number in community	Year of evaluation	Place of study	Source of subjects	Time lapse between eval. & previous contact (in years)
21. Hegge study[u]	91 33 38 24	1943	Michigan	Training school	1–3
22. Kennedy study[v] Subject	143 93	1948	Connecticut	Regular classrooms and educable spec. educ. classes	11
Controls	65 49				
Subjects	113 64	1960			23
Controls	54 47				

Note: See footnotes following Table 32.

Age	Sex	IQ	Unemployed (%)	Employed at time of interview (%)	Never employed (%)	Unemployed 20% of time or more (%)
		Mostly		49.6	12.6	
	Males	50-70			6.1	28.0
	Females				30.6	43.8
Adult			22			
	Males	48-85				
	Females	Mean 65				

Age	Sex	IQ	Unemployed (%)	Employed at time of interview (%)
15-20				
	Males	50-75	11.4	88.7
		76-91	18.2	81.9
	Females	50-75	11.4	88.6
		76-91	4.8	95.2
23-33		50-75		
	Males			90.9
	Females			52.7
	Males	75+		86.2
	Females			49.0
38-48	Males			91.2
	Females			46.9
	Males			92.6
	Females			57.4

those placed in residential care or still in school, and even those who had died.

b) The number of persons reported as being in subgroups of the original sample will not always agree with the total in the sample, because the personal characteristic being described is not always known for all members of the sample.

c) The definition of unemployment used in these studies is not the same as used by the Department of Labor, since it includes all persons not working and the percentages are calculated on the entire population base. The Department of Labor counts a person as unemployed only if he is actively seeking work and computes unemployment rates as a percentage of the employed and unemployed, thus excluding students, housewives, the retired, the willingly idle, the discouraged worker, and those *unable to work.*

Factors affecting vocational success. Tables 32 to 35 present a bewildering array of employment rates among the retarded, ranging from 99.5% to 20%. Many factors explain this variance and must be assessed before we come to any conclusion about the overall vocational adjustment of the retarded.

Level of Aggregate Demand. A vigorous demand for workers opens up opportunities for the retarded which would not otherwise exist. The extraordinarily high rate of employment reported by McKeon (Table 32) was a direct consequence of the critical labor shortage during World War II. Most of these retarded adults found work with little or no outside help.

During the latter part of World War II, Coakley studied 37 retarded persons. Twenty-five had IQs between 60 and 75. In 1940 only 4 of these 25 were employed in regular factory jobs. The others, for the most part, were either unemployed or engaged in low-paying, irregular jobs. Twelve had IQs below 60, only one of whom had been employed in 1940.[14] At the time of interview, all 37 were in substantial employment.

At the other extreme, the Baller study (Table 33), conducted during the depths of the depression, found that only one in six retarded males and one in four retarded females had located relatively permanent employment. In the 1951 follow-up, however, 93% of the males and 84% of the females were usually employed (housewives were counted as usually employed) and, in 1965, 66% of the males and 75% of the females were entirely self-supporting. The lower percentages in 1964 as

[14] Frances Coakley, "Study of Feeble-Minded Wards Employed in War Industries," *American Journal of Mental Deficiency* (October 1945): 301–6.

compared to 1951 do not necessarily indicate a reduction of employ-ability among the subjects, since not all "usually employed" persons are entirely self-supporting.

Kennedy (Table 35) observed that the percentage employed among the retarded declined slightly for noninstitutionalized females between 1948 and 1960, a period during which the unemployment rate rose from 3.9% to 5.5%. The converse should have been expected, since the subjects were in the prime of their working lives in 1960, had had sufficient time to adjust to the society they lived in, and the children of retarded women would usually have been of an age where the mother could return to work. In contrast, in 1948, when the original survey took place, the labor force participation rate (LFPR) for white females 25 to 34 years old (at that time, the subjects were 23 to 33 years old) was 31.3%, and in 1960 the LFPR for white females age 35 to 44 had risen to 41.5% and the LFPR for white females age 45 to 54 was 7 percentage points higher (the subjects were 38 to 48 years old.)[15] The employment of retarded men was virtually unchanged during this period.

Changes in the level of economic activity apparently have a greater effect on the employability of the retarded than on the general popula-tion. In the Kennedy study, in contrast to the retarded subjects, em-ployment among nonretarded controls rose between the two evaluation periods, although several other factors contributed to this rise. In the Baller study, the proportion of relief recipients among the retarded (a rough proxy for the percentage unemployed) rose from 17% to 52% between 1931 and 1935, while among the nonretarded controls the comparable percentages were 5% and 16%. In addition, Baller remarked that relief recipients among the controls received less aid.

Sex. Retarded females have more difficulty finding work and are less likely to seek work than retarded males. Saenger (Table 32) ob-served that most jobs held by the subjects in his sample were unsuitable for women. He also noted that not working is more socially acceptable for women than for men and that parents may be more reluctant to expose their daughters to the harshness of the social environment than their sons. Although he was referring to the severely retarded, the same comments are also applicable to the mildly retarded. In addition, since many mildly retarded females marry, they have the option of escaping the rigors of remunerative employment by devoting their time to full-time housekeeping.

[15] U.S. Department of Labor, *Statistics on Manpower, A Supplement to the Manpower Report of the President*, March 1969, p. 5.

In the Mullen study (Table 32), unemployment among female retardates was 70% higher than among male retardates, which conforms to our expectations as to the unavailability of work for female retardates. Several studies, however, appear to contradict this hypothesis. Dinger (Table 32) found that the unemployment rate for female retardates was lower than for male retardates. Channing (Table 32) reported that unemployment rates for males and females formerly in special education classes was almost identical. These contradictions, however, are readily explainable by the demographic characteristics of the populations. Channing computed unemployment rates only for unmarried females with some history of employment.

In the Dinger study the percentage of females who were married was 61%, whereas in the Mullen study the comparable percentage was only 18%. The median age of females in the Dinger study was eight years greater than in the Mullen study, which presumably explains this divergence.

If we can generalize from these studies, unemployment rates among both mildly and severely retarded females are higher than for comparably retarded males when these persons are teenagers and in their early twenties. This relationship appears to reverse itself for the mildly retarded by the time they reach the late twenties. At the same time, however, employment among female retardates also declines, since marriage permits greater numbers to withdraw from the labor force. Presumably, this also explains the reversal of unemployment rates.

These observations may explain the decrease in employment among female retardates in the Kennedy study (Table 35), since the percentage of women retardates who were married and living with their spouse increased from 55% in 1948 to 73% in 1960. The decrease in aggregate demand may have induced some married female retardates to exercise their option to engage in full-time housekeeping.

The unwillingness or inability of female retardates to engage in the productive occupations available to them is further shown by the relative percentages never employed. In the Channing study of former special education students, females were eight times more likely to have never been employed than males, and in her study of former patients in residential facilities, the ratio was of the order of five to one. In the Bobroff study (Table 32), 21% of the females had never been employed; among males the comparable percentage could not have been more than 2% or 3%, since only 7.4% were unemployed.

Race. Mullen (Table 32) observed that the Negro retardates had a "harder time achieving adjustment than . . . white boys and girls. A larger percent of them are unemployed and a much smaller percentage are employed at jobs carrying a worthwhile salary. These youngsters obviously suffer the addition of a racial handicap to their other handicaps, and racial discrimination appears more important in determining their lack of success than their mental handicap."

In the Tobias study (Table 32), retarded Puerto Rican males had somewhat higher, and retarded Negro males significantly lower rates of employment than retarded white males. Among retarded females, Negroes had slightly higher rates of employment than whites or Puerto Ricans, although Puerto Rican retardates were more likely to have had employment at some time.

The superior employment records of Puerto Ricans leads one to suspect that because of a language handicap their test scores were less representative of their abilities than were those for the other two groups.

IQ. Some researchers assert that intellectual deficiency is not a major barrier to employment among the mentally retarded, except in the more severe cases. Kolstoe concluded that "analysis of the studies seems to indicate that any earned IQ from 40 or so up to the 80's or 90's is sufficiently high not to interfere with the employment of the individual provided job selection is carefully done, the employer is understanding, etc."[16]

Few studies have specifically dealt with the employment of the severely retarded (IQ less than 50). The most important is the Saenger study (Table 32). All of Saenger's subjects scored below 55 on the highest IQ score and the great majority had IQs between 40 and 50. Overall, only one in four of the subjects living in the community was employed. Among those over 21 years of age the percentage employed was 30%, while for those under 21 it was 16%.

Saenger observed that about 40% of the males in his sample were employed, compared to only about 10% of the females. Allowing for the age factor, therefore, we would expect between 40 and 45% of severely retarded adult males (over 21) to be employed and 11 to 12% of the females. Ferguson (Table 32) reported that six out of eleven (all males) former special education students with IQs below 50 were employed nine years after leaving school.

Sweeney (Table 32) reported that 29% of a small group of severely retarded teenagers were employed within the first two years after leaving a special work-study program for students in their last year of special education, a considerably higher rate than reported by Saenger

[16] Oliver P. Kolstoe, "An Examination of Some Characteristics Which Discriminate between Employed and Not-Employed Mentally Retarded Males," *American Journal of Mental Deficiency* (November 1961): 473.

for teenagers. Undoubtedly, intensive vocational services were a factor in their success.

In the Collman study (Table 32), 36% of the males and 23% of the females with IQs between 40 and 50 were employed after being out of special education classes for 2 to 3 years. Channing (Table 32) reported that 39% of the males and 20% of the females with IQs below 50 were employed 80% of the time or more. These subjects were evidently quite young.

The Collman and Channing studies had a greater proportion of teenagers as subjects than the Saenger study. Thus, it is not surprising that they report employment rates for severely retarded males somewhat below 40%. They are sufficiently close to the Saenger results, however, so that we can accept with some degree of confidence the conclusion that between 40 and 45% of noninstitutionalized male retardates with IQs between 40 and 50 who are over 21 have obtained some form of employment.

The Collman and Channing studies seem to indicate that the percentage of adult severely retarded females who are employed is higher than the 10–12% implied by the Saenger study. However, the number of severely retarded females in the two former studies was small compared to the Saenger study. In addition, the Channing study results would be similar to the Saenger estimates if account were taken of those never employed.

Almost all of the severely retarded who are employed have IQs in the forties. Below an IQ of 40, employment usually becomes impracticable, except in strongly sheltered situations. Although there are no follow-up studies of the employment histories of persons with IQs below 40 to bolster this statement, it can be surmised that this dearth is largely because there is little to follow up.

Our next step is to look at the employment histories of persons whose measured IQ falls in the 50 to 70 range. Although almost all of the follow-up studies encompass the retarded in this IQ range, many also include a substantial number with higher IQs. Nevertheless, few studies classify the employment histories of the retarded by IQ.

Collman reported that 76% of the males with IQs from 50 to 59, and 77% with IQs between 60 and 69, were employed at the time of interview. Among females, the comparable figures were 75% and 79%. It was not made clear whether the figures for females included married housewives but one presumes they must.

Ferguson found more substantial differences. Ninety-two percent of the males with IQs between 60 and 69 were employed at the time of interview, compared to only 62% of those with IQs between 50 and 59.

Tobias classified the subjects in his study by two IQ ranges, 50 to 65 and 66 to 75. Among Negroes of both sexes the percentage employed was identical in both IQ groups. Among whites the percentage employed at interview was substantially higher for the higher-IQ groups for both males and females. Strangely, among Puerto Ricans, the higher-IQ group was less likely to be employed at time of interview and this was true of both sexes.

Channing reported that there were no differences in the percentages of persons unemployed over 20% of the time in either of the two IQ intervals—50 to 59 and 60 to 69.

To sum up, Ferguson reported that males in the IQ range 60 to 69 had a distinct employment advantage over males in the 50 to 59 range. Collman reported a very slight advantage for the higher-IQ ranges for both sexes. Channing reported no differences in employability among persons in these IQ ranges. Tobias found a marked advantage in employment among persons in the higher-IQ range (66 to 75 as compared to 50 to 65) in the case of whites of both sexes. We can assume that the Ferguson, Collman, and Channing studies were predominantly of white subjects.

The most reasonable conclusion that we can draw is that mildly retarded whites with IQs in the sixties have a greater chance of obtaining employment than those with IQs in the fifties, but that the difference is only of the order of 8 to 10 percentage points. The contradictory findings of the Channing study should perhaps be discounted because of the selection factor.[17]

Apparently, the effect of IQ differences on the employment of the mildly retarded is less significant for nonwhites than for whites. This may be due to the unreliability of the testing instrument when applied to nonwhites, or to a lower incidence of physical handicaps among nonwhites in these IQ ranges (if a substantial part of the prevalence of mental retardation among these groups is functional rather than due to organic damage or poor genetic endowment), or both.

A number of studies have recorded a puzzling result for persons with IQs above 70. Collman reported that among the educationally sub-

---

[17] Another study of the employment adjustment of educable mentally handicapped ex-pupils in Scotland reported that the mean intelligence was higher among those with superior employment adjustment among both males and females. The criteria of success was based on the number of jobs held and number of months of unemployment. The major IQ differences were between the nonadjusted, all of whom had been unemployed twelve months or more, and the borderline or well-adjusted. IQ differences between the latter two groups were minor. See R. N. Jackson, "Employment Adjustment of Educable Mentally Handicapped Ex-Pupils in Scotland," *American Journal of Mental Deficiency* (May 1968): 924–30.

normal group (i.e., those who had been in special education classes), those with IQs above 70 were less likely to be employed than those with IQs between 50 and 70, an observation that was true for both males and females. The difference in employment rates was of the order of 20 percentage points. Hegge (Table 35) found that males (formerly in training school) with IQs between 76 and 91 were less likely than those with IQs between 50 and 75 to be employed during the peak of the war demand for labor. However, Hegge reported the opposite relationship for females. Channing also reported that males with IQs above 70 were more likely to be unemployed than those with IQs between 50 and 70 and, like Hegge, found that this "disadvantage" of high IQ did not extend to females.

A number of other studies have reported similar findings. In a study of sixty mentally retarded males, employed as construction workers, who were placed out of an English institution for the mentally retarded, O'Connor reported that the "consistent failures were usually very intelligent boys comparatively speaking, with IQs always above 70, more often nearer 90."[18]

Similarly, Hartzler studied the social adjustment of 191 women 4 to 14 years after their discharge from a state institution. Sixty-three percent were classified as having made a successful community adjustment, 12% partially successful, and 25% were unsuccessful. Success was defined in terms of ability to be self-supporting and avoidance of conflict with the law. The mean IQ of the successful girls was 70 and of the unsuccessful girls 75.[19]

Kinder compared the social adjustment of girls released from a public institution in New York State (N=50) and the New York Training School for Girls (N=50), a correctional institution. In both cases, evaluation took place at least eight years after leaving the institution. All of the subjects were over 21. Although the average IQ of the mentally retarded girls was over 20 points below that of the training school girls (84 as compared to 63), a higher proportion were satisfactorily socially adjusted (60% as compared to 50%).[20]

Although a number of writers have commented on this peculiar relationship,[21] it is not as puzzling as first appears. Only a minute percent-

[18] N. O'Connor, "Defectives Working in the Community," *American Journal of Mental Deficiency* (October 1954): 176.

[19] Ethel Hartzler, "A Ten Year Survey of Girls Discharged from the Laurelton State Village," *American Journal of Mental Deficiency* (January 1953): 512–17.

[20] Elaine F. Kinder, Annette Chase, and Elizabeth W. Buck, "Data Secured During a Follow-Up Study of Girls Discharged from Supervised Parole from Letchwork Village," *American Journal of Mental Deficiency* (April 1941): 572–77.

[21] R. N. Jackson, "Employment Adjustment of Educable Mentally Handicapped Ex-Pupils in Scotland," *American Journal of Mental Deficiency* (May 1968):

age of persons in the IQ range 70 to 90 are placed in facilities for the retarded. Those that are so placed have, in the great majority of cases, serious physical handicaps or behavioral problems or extremely poor home environments. It is not surprising, therefore, that faced with multiple impediments to employment, this group should be more handicapped than the mildly retarded.

Behavior may be the most important consideration. O'Connor commented that "in all cases their hospital behavior record was substantially worse than that for the average defective." Hartzler noted that the unsuccessful girls generally came from poorer homes and were more likely to have been actively delinquent before admission to the institution.

The combination of mental retardation *and* behavioral problems can be extremely serious. Kinder reported that only five of eighteen training school girls with IQs below 80 were satisfactorily adjusted.

Strong support for the hypothesis that this unexpected relationship between IQ and employment is due to adverse selection is derived from the Collman studies. Collman studied the employment histories of "dull students" whose IQs ranged between 70 and 89 and who should be roughly comparable to those persons among the educationally subnormal with IQs *over 70*. The major reported difference between the two groups was that the "dull" group had not been in special education classes, while the educationally subnormal had been. Collman reported that 97% of the "dull" group was employed at time of interview, as compared to about 60% of the educationally subnormal group with IQs above 70. Factors other than IQ must be the cause of this striking difference.

Age. It is unfortunate that there are so few follow-up studies of the employment history of the mentally retarded who are over age 30 and that only the Saenger study (Table 32) reported on the employment success of the retarded according to age groupings. Most studies have dealt with youthful retardates within a narrow age range.

Retardates under 21 have serious vocational difficulties. The lowest rates of employment on follow-up were recorded by the Orzack, Grate, and Sweeny studies (Table 32). The subjects in the second two studies were 16 to 18 years of age and those in the first study were also in this general age range.

On the other hand, studies dealing with retardates over age 25 consistently reported high rates of employment, generally over 90% for mildly retarded males (Bobroff [Table 32], Ferguson [Table 32], Baller [Table 33], Kennedy [Table 35]), and around 50% for mildly retarded females, although we have only the Kennedy study on which to base the latter assertion.

Studies dealing with retardates between 21 and 25 found employment rates intermediate between those of retardates under 21 and over 25 (Mudd and Tobias [Table 32]).

Many of the follow-up studies combine broad age groups, including teenagers as well as adults. With the exception of the McKeon study, which was conducted during the critical labor shortage of World War II, these studies reported, as would be hypothesized, employment rates below those of studies dealing exclusively with adults and above those dealing exclusively with teenagers. One can surmise that the unemployment rates of these studies (Channing, Mullen, Phelps, Collman, and Dinger [Table 32]) would be closely correlated with the percentage of teenagers among the subjects, if the data were available to make such calculations.

Two qualifications to this age-employment relationship are needed:

1) As we have indicated, employment among mildly retarded women will decline as they grow older and marry.

2) The combination of intellectual deficiency and the infirmities of advancing age should worsen employment prospects. It is of interest to note that the Jastak study (discussed in Chapter II) found that the combination of intellectual deficiency and social maladaptation was least frequent among retarded adults in the prime of life and increased among persons over 46 years of age.

Source of Subjects. We would expect that follow-up studies of persons formerly in residential care would report the lowest employment records, follow-up studies of persons formerly in special education classes in the community would be next, and studies of the mentally retarded in general would report the best employment records.

Channing (Tables 32 and 34) reported that employment among persons formerly in residential care was two-thirds as high as employment among persons formerly in special education classes. Edgerton (Table 34) reported that out of 27 former residents of a public institution (males and unmarried females only), 6 were unemployed at interview, which is clearly above the unemployment rates of any of the other follow-up studies, except those dealing with teenage subjects and severely retarded individuals.

The only study that included retardates who attended regular academic classes, the Kennedy study (Table 35), did not report rates of employment appreciably different from similarly aged males in the 1951 Baller study (Table 33). (Employment rates for women are not comparable because of definitional differences.) In the Kennedy study, employment rates were appreciably higher than those of other follow-up studies of former special education students, but this probably reflects age differences rather than qualitative differences among the subjects.

Apparently, contrary to expectation, mildly retarded students formerly in special education programs are as successful as those who remained in regular academic programs.

Place of Residence. Krishef studied discharges from the Owatonna State School in Minnesota and concluded that wards discharged to a rural community were more likely to adjust successfully (i.e., not be returned to institutional care) than wards discharged to an urban community. Krishef attributed this to the fact that a rural community is less competitive and more protective of the individual than an urban environment.[22] Windle, however, felt that Krishef's results might be due to chance variation.[23]

In principle, residence in a rural community has advantages and disadvantages for the employment of the mentally retarded. The advantage is that there may be agricultural employment available that requires relatively few skills and has considerable flexibility as to the speed, timing, and duration of work performed. In these latter respects, farm work is similar to housekeeping. The disadvantage is that there is usually a relatively limited range of types of jobs available in rural areas, so that the retarded with serious vocational limitations will be less likely to locate jobs that are within their vocational limitations or jobs that make the best use of their residual vocational capabilities. Other disadvantages are poor public transportation and limited access to public employment and rehabilitation agencies. This last disadvantage may be offset, however, by a greater amount of informal aid from friends and relatives. The net effect of the various advantages and disadvantages of rural areas cannot be ascertained.

Perhaps the question should be raised as to whether very large cities, characterized by a bewildering maze of streets and imposing buildings and crammed with populations that scurry about in an impersonal and impatient manner, might not be disadvantageous for the employment of the mentally retarded. This might be one explanation for the higher employment rate of educable retardates in the Mudd study (Table 32) (which encompassed all Massachusetts) as compared to the Tobias study (Table 32) (all of whose subjects lived in New York City).

[22] Curtis H. Krishef, "The Influence of Rural-Urban Environment Upon the Adjustment of Dischargees from the Owatonna State School," *American Journal of Mental Deficiency*, vol. 63 (March 1959): 860–65.

[23] Windle, "Prognosis of Mental Subnormals," pp. 94–95.

Physical and Mental Disabilities. Although none of the follow-up studies grouped the retarded according to physical or psychiatric disability, the multiply-handicapped retarded are unquestionably in an extremely disadvantageous position with respect to employment.

Mercer studied eighty-one mentally retarded patients in a public mental hospital and found extremely poor employment records.[24] Lewis reported that emotional disabilities were more prevalent among drop-outs from a work-study program for educable mentally retarded students in high school than among students remaining in the program.[25]

Windle's summary of studies evaluating the effect of physical defects on community adjustment is inconclusive. He suggested that most studies dealt with formerly institutionalized patients, and institutions are less likely to release multiply-handicapped patients unless they have favorable compensating characteristics.[26]

Collman and Newlyn (Table 32), in their study of educationally subnormal ex-pupils, reported that 10% of the failures were caused by physical defects. Among the lower-grade retarded the percentage was higher. They reported that of 27 retarded adults with IQs in the 40 to 50 range, 13 were considered unemployable. Nine suffered from marked physical defects, 7 were temperamentally unstable and dangerous, 3 were mongoloids, and 3 were cretins. The authors concluded that it was this combination of handicaps, not low-grade intelligence alone, that causes unemployability.

Saenger (Table 32) (also studying adults with IQs in the 40 to 50 range) observed that persons with physical handicaps were employed less often than those without physical handicaps, but that this seemed to be related to physical appearance rather than severity of physical handicaps. Only 7% of those with distinct mongoloid features found work, compared to 23% of those with marked speech defects or impaired motor coordination. It will be recalled that the overall employment rate was only slightly higher than 23%.

Ferguson (Table 32) observed that "None of the twenty-two boys whose physique had been described when he left school as 'poor' became a skilled manual worker, and only three were in semi-skilled work; but nine of the 114 lads whose physique had been classified as

[24] Margaret Mercer, "Why Mentally Retarded Persons Come to a Mental Hospital," *Mental Retardation* (June 1968): 8-10.

[25] Patricia F. Lewis, *A Cooperative Education/Rehabilitation Work-Study Program for Educable Mentally Retarded: The Essex Plan*, Final Report of Project RD-1743, no date, p. 38. Vocational Rehabilitation Administration Project.

[26] Windle, "Prognosis of Mental Subnormals," pp. 94-95.

'good' were in skilled manual work when the study was carried out, while nineteen were in semi-skilled work. The combination of physical handicap and mental retardation is an unhappy one."

Attitudes of the Retarded. Motivation is a term often used to explain success or failure. The word conceals more than it explains. What may appear to be lack of motivation may be a mask for fear or resentment, or it may reflect a lack of opportunity to develop habits of dress or punctuality necessary for job success. Some retarded persons are too motivated. They spend too long on a task to ensure that they do not make a mistake, or they aspire to jobs beyond their capabilities and resent the jobs that are offered. In short, the retarded may have habits and attitudes that are prejudicial to vocational and social adjustment, but that do not always reflect an absence of a desire to work. These attitudes take many forms: poor self-control, distractibility, hypersensitivity, vacillation, unreliability, etc.

Often these attitudes develop from the unfortunate life styles to which many retarded children are subjected. Some are over-indulged by parents. Others are ignored. Frequently, parents refuse to accept the limitations of their retarded children. In other cases, they fail to recognize and develop the abilities that exist in these children. Opportunities for special education were limited when many retarded adults were children. Consequently, their educational experiences and their opportunities to learn the habits and attitudes necessary for social adjustment were minimal. Too often, the retarded are rejected by siblings and other children, sometimes with great cruelty. Fortunately, not all of the retarded are encased in these life styles. But one can hardly question the psychological effects on those who are. Many researchers have concluded that the attitudes of the retarded are a major, and often the most important, factor in determining employment success.

After evaluating 38 female laundry workers at the Manitoba School for Mental Defectives with respect to age, IQ, ability, attitudes, personality, and work performance, Fry concluded that "Personality seems to be the deciding factor in establishing a cut-off point between institutional and community work success."[27]

Windle reported that 25 out of 27 failures of patients on vocational leave from Pacific State Hospital resulted from some form of inappropriate behavior.[28] Collman and Newlyn reported that 52% of the fail-

[27] Lois M. Fry, "A Predictive Measure of Work Success for High Grade Mental Defectives," *American Journal of Mental Deficiency* (October 1956): 402–6.

[28] Charles D. Windle, Elizabeth Stewart, and Sheldon J. Brown, "Reasons for Community Failure of Released Patients," *American Journal of Mental Deficiency* (September 1961): 215.

ures among the mentally retarded in their follow-up study (Table 32) were due to character defects and 10% to temperamental instability.

After studying 27 employed and 11 unemployed mentally handicapped males, Warren reported that the employed group was substantially more self-confident, cheerful and cooperative, better able to accept criticism, and tended to be more careful in their personal appearance. They also showed more initiative and were more punctual and safety conscious.[29]

This is an appropriate place to dispose of one popular misconception. Nitzberg writes: "The notion that retarded people characteristically accept simple repetitive work with docility has not been true in our experience. While some can sit for hours in one place doing the same work without visible display of boredom, others find it impossible to tolerate such work and need to move around and to have variety."[30]

Similarly, Blue writes: "The Orange Grove Workshop, for example, had a heterogeneous group of TMR clients who operated adequately and quite happily at one isolated aspect of production over a long period of time. Gradually the quality and quantity of their work began to decrease. The problem required no deep study for it was obvious that all of the workers, even the one with the lowest intellect, were overcome by boredom."[31]

Attitudes of the Nonretarded. Ultimately, the retarded must be accepted by the nonretarded if they are to be integrated into community life.

In a recent survey, 926 persons who did not have a disabled person in their home were presented with the case of Thomas B., age 20 and mentally retarded. "Outwardly normal, he has the intelligence of an average 8 year old child. He can care for himself, do simple chores, and read and write at the third grade level."

Forty-six percent of the respondents felt that Thomas B. should be institutionalized, 38% felt he should live at home, and 12% were willing to leave the decision to the parents. Forty-two percent of the respondents who had gone to college, 48% of those who had gone to high

---

[29] Fount G. Warren, "Ratings of Employed and Unemployed Mentally Handicapped Males on Personality and Work Factors," *American Journal of Mental Deficiency* (March 1961): 629–33.

[30] Jerome Nitzberg, "The Sheltered Workshop as a Treatment Center for Mentally Retarded Adults," mimeographed copy of an address delivered at a conference sponsored by the Colorado Division of Institutions, Estes Park, Colorado: Mental Health-Mental Retardation Conference on Mutual Operational Concerns, June 4, 1966, p. 5.

[31] C. Milton Blue, "Trainable Mentally Retarded in Sheltered Workshops," *Mental Retardation* (April 1964): 101.

school, and 50% of those who had not gone beyond grade school felt that Thomas should be institutionalized. Only 16% of the total sample felt that Thomas should be trained to work side-by-side with the non-handicapped (19%, 16%, and 12% among the three educational groupings) although 58% felt that he should be encouraged to get special training to work in a sheltered workshop. Twenty-three percent felt he should not work at all or only if he wanted to.[32]

Considering that there are no contraindications to employment, the percentage of the sample, even among the better educated, who felt that Thomas should be isolated from society is distressingly large. However, this is probably overly pessimistic. The respondents may have been reacting to the deadly label "mental retardation." Describe the same person as a slow learner who would have some difficulty understanding all the words in the daily newspaper, but one capable of unskilled work, who requires occasional supportive counseling, and the percentage of respondents recommending institutionalization might well decline drastically. In fact, some of these respondents are probably working "side by side" with a mildly retarded person but are unaware of the fact.

Negative attitudes toward the retarded will affect their employability if employers deny them an opportunity to work, if their coworkers refuse to work with them, or if persistent and cruel teasing impedes satisfactory job performance.

Although there are undoubtedly some employers who would refuse to hire the retarded, this is partly offset by other employers who are enthusiastic about the performance of retarded workers. Employer discrimination, to the extent that it exists, is not likely to take the form of outright rejection of the retarded, but rather of overly rigid requirements for employment, e.g., minimum levels of education.

Coworker attitudes can be devastating to job success for the retarded. The Roper survey indicates that the least educated part of society were most loath to have the retarded work side by side with normal workers. Perhaps they feared a loss of prestige if a retarded person did the same work and received the same pay as they did. The importance of coworker attitudes is well illustrated by the following story of Frank, a 20-year-old retardate with an IQ of 54:

Frank was placed by the counselor on a break-in job as a car washer. The employer was properly prepared for the project and had been advised that the

---

[32] *Summary Report of a Study on the Problems of Rehabilitation for the Disabled*, conducted by Roper Research Associates, Inc., reproduced by USDHEW, SRS, no date, pp. 20–25.

client should be left alone when working. The employer was not aware of the little pranks that other employees played. The person assigned to teach him apparently was in on the fun. They deliberately misplaced the sponge and washing cloths, they hid his hat, they turned off the hose while he was working; then mysteriously turned it on again when he tried to investigate. They called him "the dummy!" He was hurt, he was angry and he was altogether confused. It was not surprising that he stayed only 3 days.[33]

Overview of Factors Affecting Employment. A surprisingly large percentage of adult retardates are vocationally successful. When vocational failure does occur, intellectual deficiency is usually not the major cause, except in cases of relatively severe retardation. The literature abounds in statements to this effect.

For example, Kirk summarized the efforts of Peckham to find out why the mentally retarded lost or quit their jobs. It was found that they quit jobs because of teasing and ridicule of fellow workers; because they have difficulty in social and vocational sophistication, such as having difficulty in transportation, leaving work without notification, unwarranted sick leaves and so forth; because they evidence dissatisfaction with the salary; because they do a poor job in budgeting their money; because they lack initiative and job responsibility; and for impulsive reasons. They quit jobs because the job is below the dignity of the family; they quit jobs because of the inability to read directions. Rarely do they lose their jobs because of inability to do the required task.[34]

White, commenting on 150 children placed in the community from the Southbury Training School (Connecticut) observed that failure was mostly due to "lack of emotional stability, personal and social inadequacies, poor work habits, unwise use of leisure time, and poor habits of health and sanitation."[35] None failed because of lack of academic knowledge.

O'Connor and Tizard after sampling 104 high-grade male defectives argued that "ability to overcome the hazards of employment, as measured by the ability to retain jobs or meet with employers' approval or both, is partly a function of general locomotion, coordination and dex-

[33] Jane H. Potts, "Vocational Rehabilitation for the Mentally Retarded in Michigan," *Vocational Rehabilitation of the Mentally Retarded*, USDHEW, Office of Vocational Rehabilitation, Rehabilitation Service Series No. 123, p. 146.

[34] Samuel A. Kirk, "Vocational Rehabilitation: An Educator's Critique on Past, Present, and Future Programs," *Vocational Training and Rehabilitation of Exceptional Children*, Proceedings of the 1957 Spring Conference of the Woods Schools, Langhorne, Pennsylvania, 1957, p. 31.

[35] Wesley Dale White, "Education for Life Adjustment," *American Journal of Mental Deficiency* (September 1954): 405.

terity, and partly a function of emotional stability. To a lesser extent, it is also a function of cognitive ability."[36]

Liu, in a study of 618 female admissions to Brockhall Hospital (England), concluded that "a well integrated and stable personality living in conditions uncomplicated by unfavorable family or economic difficulties and having an IQ below 50 or above 30 can be trained to learn a simple repetitive type of job under sheltered conditions . . . those with an IQ over 70, who may be handicapped by emotional, psychoneurotic difficulties, or organic disorders may be untrainable."[37]

Finally, Harold concludes: "In view of the lack of a positive correlation between the intelligence quotient and either the type or calibre of the patient's performance on a job, it is clear that other factors are of greater significance in determining whether employment is satisfactory. Two of these factors appear to be the total personality adjustment of the individual and the degree of guidance which he receives from others."[38] These statements may go too far in minimizing the role of intellectual deficiency in causing vocational failure.

Intellectual deficiency may itself contribute to the development of other employment impediments. Attitudes prejudicial to work is the most obvious example of where this may occur. In addition, it is frequently the combination of intellectual deficiency with other employment impediments which causes vocational failure, not any one factor alone. There are three reasons for this.

First, most of the jobs available to the retarded require physical labor. If, in addition to mental retardation, a person suffers from a disability that excludes him from jobs requiring manual labor, the prospects of vocational success become negligible. On the other hand, a healthy retarded person, or a physically disabled person of normal intellect will usually experience relatively little difficulty locating employment.

Second, many employers are willing to hire a mentally retarded person with no physical disabilities, or a physically disabled person of normal intellect, but would hesitate to hire anyone with both of these characteristics.

---

[36] N. O'Connor and J. Tizard, "Predicting the Occupational Adequacy of Certified Mental Defectives," *Occupational Psychology* (July 1951): 205–11.

[37] M. C. Liu, "Changing Trends in the Care of the Subnormal," *American Journal of Mental Deficiency* (November 1963): 351–52.

[38] Edward C. Harold, "Employment of Patients Discharged from the St. Louis State Training School," *American Journal of Mental Deficiency* (October 1955): 397–402.

Finally, a combination of employment impediments may reduce a person's capacity to adjust to one or the other. For example, being blind and retarded, or mentally ill and mentally retarded creates serious adjustment difficulties. Obviously, the greater the number of employment impediments, the greater the difficulty in locating and retaining employment.

It is impossible to list the myriad combinations of employment impediments that occur. What it is necessary to emphasize is that when a retarded person is unable to succeed in employment, one must usually look for multiple impediments to employment.

Earlier, we observed that there is a significant relationship between level of IQ and employment. This does not necessarily contradict our conclusion that intellect by itself is not a major obstacle to employment, except in severe retardation. A more likely explanation is that the proportion of retardates with other employment impediments increases as the degree of intellectual deficit becomes more severe.

Employment of the noninstitutionalized mentally retarded. The employment of retardates with IQs below 40 was previously concluded to be negligible.[39] In our estimate of the number of noninstitutionalized adult retardates, however, this IQ range is subsumed in the broader 25 to 49 range.

The Taylor study (Table 7) reported that 0.11% of the population had an IQ between 40 and 50 and that 0.18% had an IQ between 30 and 50. If to this latter percentage we add 0.03%, to adjust for those with IQs between 25 and 30, then we can estimate that about half of the persons in the 25 to 49 IQ interval had IQs of 40 or over.

We estimated previously that among persons over age 21 with IQs between 40 and 50, 40% to 45% of the males and 10% to 12% of the females were employed. We will assume rates of 45% and 12%.

Most follow-up studies are of minimal value in ascertaining the employment success of the mildly retarded, largely because of inadequate demographic stratification. Basically, we will rely on six studies for this purpose: the Collman, Ferguson, Mudd, Tobias, Baller (1951), and Kennedy studies.

Leaving aside the Tobias study for the moment, the lowest rate of employment for mildly retarded males was reported by Collman (76%) followed by Mudd (83%), Ferguson (87%), Kennedy (1948 and 1960, 91%), and Baller (1951, 93%).

---

[39] A few are gainfully occupied under sheltered conditions. Because of their small numbers and low earnings, this will not create a significant bias in our estimate of below-average earnings.

In Figure 1, these rates are positioned according to the median age reported in the studies, or the midpoint of the age range, or my judgment of where the midpoint is. The solid line shows the age-employment profile of white males in 1967. (The subjects of these studies were predominantly Caucasian.)

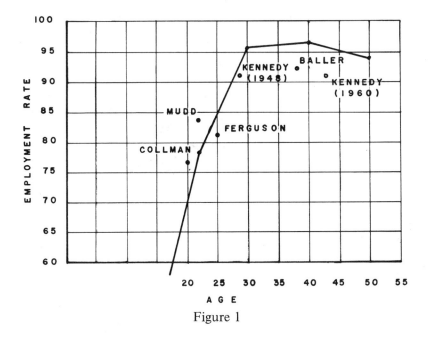

Figure 1

During youth, the percentage of mildly retarded males employed is comparable to, and perhaps slightly higher than, among their nonretarded counterparts. This is because a substantial number of nonretarded youths attend school until 21 or 22 years of age, while few retardates do so after age 18. Thus, this is not inconsistent with the conclusion that many retarded youths have unusual vocational difficulties.

After mildly retarded males reach their mid-twenties, their employment rates fall three to five percentage points below the population average, as judged by visual evaluation.[40] This employment differential appears highly consistent throughout the various age levels.

[40] The two studies which used control groups appear to contradict these conclusions. Collman reported almost universal employment among a group of nonretarded subjects; their employment rate was almost 25 percentage points higher than

We will assume that employment rates among mildly retarded males are, on the average, four percentage points below those of their nonretarded counterparts.[41] Since 91% of adult males between the ages of 20 and 65 were employed in 1967, then, if our figure of 4% is correct, about 87% of mildly retarded adult males were employed.

Now let us consider three possible objections to what some might consider an optimistic conclusion. First, the Tobias study reported considerably lower rates of employment and at the same time used a slightly higher IQ range. One critical omission in the Tobias study was a chart showing the age distribution of the sample. We are told (p. 44) that the subjects of the study were, on the average, almost five years older than the 18- to 19-year-olds whom Tobias felt would be a fair comparison group in terms of employment. However, while interviewing took place during 1966 and 1967, the sample was derived from students terminating special education classes during 1960 and 1963. Given the early age of termination of school by many retarded, it is probable that a large number of 19- and 20-year-olds were included from 1963. This would significantly depress employment rates and might suffice to explain the discrepancies between the Tobias conclusions and those of the Mudd or Collman studies. There is also a possibility that retardates in large cities have greater adjustment problems.

A second problem is that we have based these estimates of employment on surveys conducted on Caucasians, although earlier we concluded that over half of the retarded were nonwhite. Although nonwhites would face greater employment difficulties than whites, an offsetting consideration is the possibility that much of the retardation among nonwhites is culturally caused. In other words, nonwhites with cultural retardation may have greater adaptive ability. Finally, it is probable that the added infirmities of advancing age will depress employment rates among the retarded more than the nonretarded after age 50.

---

for the mildly retarded, although most were evidently in their late teens and early twenties. However, the Collman control group was derived from an English school where students were expected to leave school at 15 years of age and begin work.

Kennedy found that employment among mildly retarded males was somewhat higher in 1948 than among the controls, despite the fact that their median age was in the late twenties. This unexpected conclusion remained even after the results were adjusted for eight controls who were in school and not working. Kennedy's control group was probably atypical since the percentage employed was below the average for that age group.

[41] This does not mean that only 4% are unemployed. Normal unemployment among white males is about 2%, so that 6%, or three times this average, would be a more appropriate figure, and, for reasons to be noted below, even 6% may be too low.

Only three of these six follow-up studies reported on employment rates among mildly retarded females. The variation is remarkable. Collman found that 77% of mildly retarded females were employed at interview. By contrast, the employment rate for 20- to 24-year-old females in the United States in 1967 was 50%. No other follow-up study, regardless of age or IQ range, reported employment rates for female retardates as high as those of the Collman study.

Kennedy reported that 51% of the female retardates were employed in 1948 and 47% in 1960. The 1948 rate was about 11 percentage points *higher*, and the 1960 rate was almost identical to the national rate of comparably aged females in 1967. To further complicate matters, the nonretarded females in the Kennedy study had employment rates almost 10 percentage points above the national average. Moreover, female labor force participation has been rising since 1948 so that these differences between Kennedy's groups and the general population were even more pronounced in 1948 than indicated above. Retarded women in the Kennedy study had employment rates about 14 percentage points above the national average for women of similar age in 1948. In 1960 the comparable figure was four percentage points.

The most reasonable conclusion is that the employment histories of the females in the Kennedy and Collman studies are atypical of the United States. In the Collman study, it is probable, as noted earlier, that housewives are counted as employed.

These studies do agree, however, that the employment of mildly retarded women was considerably below that of nonretarded women controls—by 22 percentage points in the Collman study and 10 percentage points in the 1960 Kennedy study. In 1948, however, Kennedy reported slightly higher employment rates among retarded women than among nonretarded women, a finding that could not be explained by the small differences in marital status or numbers of children.

Female employment rates in the Tobias study were about 20 percentage points below those of nonretarded females of comparable age. Other studies also indicate considerably below-average employment among retarded females. Mullen reported that 22% and Dinger that 12% were unemployed. The Baller study (1948) found that 16% had no regular employment (homemakers were considered to be regularly employed). In 1960 Baller reported that 25% of the females were only partially self-supporting; 9% were totally dependent upon persons other than themselves or their spouses.

Apparently, employment rates among mildly retarded women are between 10 and 20 percentage points below those of nonretarded females, depending upon the age group being considered. The overall loss of employment should be nearer the lower figure, since the highest rates of unemployment are found among female retardates in their late teens and early twenties.

We will assume that the loss of employment among mildly retarded females age 20 to 64 is 12%. Since 45% of all adult women are employed, this implies an employment rate of 33% among mildly retarded females.

Table 36 shows the estimated number of noninstitutionalized retardates, age 20 to 64, by IQ and sex who were employed in 1968 and 1970. (col. 1); the increase in employment that would occur if the retarded had the same employment rates as the general population in 1967 (col. 2); and the number who, even if not retarded, would not be employed at a point in time because of normal unemployment and nonparticipation in the labor force.

Over 1.5 million retardates were gainfully employed in both 1968 and 1970. Loss of employment among the retarded was 340,000 in 1970. Another 892,000 would not normally be expected to be at work.

Over 90% of the employment loss occurs among the mildly retarded, a consequence of their large numbers rather than poor employment histories. Employment loss among mildly retarded women is three times that of mildly retarded men.

Table 36 must be interpreted cautiously. The estimated loss of employment due to retardation does not *represent* the number of jobs needed by the retarded. Some are too severely disabled to engage in remunerative employment. Some women have made a satisfactory adjustment as homemakers.

Even more importantly, normal nonparticipation in the labor force is largely a consequence of school attendance, homemaking (in the case of women), and early retirement. The retarded almost never attend school as adults, are less likely to be married than the nonretarded, and are less likely to have the wherewithal for early retirement.

The proportion of retardates seeking work may, therefore, be greater than the labor force participation rate of the general population.

Factors affecting earnings. The problems of estimating the earnings of retarded workers are even more formidable than estimating their employment rates. Relatively few follow-up studies provided such information. Inflation, economic growth, and regional differences in earnings combine to prevent any comparison of the earnings of retardates among these studies. A lesser, but still important, difficulty is that some studies report hourly, others weekly, and others annual earnings; some studies reported average earnings, others median earnings, and still others a distribution of earnings.

Table 36. Employment status of the noninstitutionalized retarded, age 20–64, 1968 and 1970

IQ	Number in community		Number employed		Loss of employment due to mental retardation		Normal unemployment and nonparticipation in labor force	
	Male	Female	Male	Female	Male	Female	Male	Female
1968								
0–24	26,000	30,000	0	0	23,700[a]	13,500[b]	2,300	16,500
25–39	40,500	45,500	0	0	36,900[a]	20,500[b]	3,600	25,000
40–49	40,500	45,500	18,200[c]	5,500[d]	18,600[e]	15,000[f]	3,700	25,000
50–69	1,232,500	1,243,500	1,072,300[g]	410,400[h]	49,300[i]	149,200[j]	110,900	683,900
Total	1,339,500	1,364,500	1,090,500	415,900	128,500	198,200	120,500	750,400
1970								
0–24	29,000	32,000	0	0	26,400[a]	14,400[b]	2,600	17,600
25–39	43,000	48,000	0	0	39,100[a]	21,600[b]	3,900	26,400
40–49	43,000	48,000	19,400[c]	5,800[d]	19,800[e]	15,800[f]	3,800	26,400
50–69	1,262,000	1,271,000	1,098,400[g]	419,000[h]	50,500[i]	152,500[j]	113,500	699,100
Total	1,377,000	1,399,000	1,117,400	425,200	135,800	204,300	123,800	769,500

[a] 91% of column 1.
[b] 45% of column 2.
[c] 45% of column 1.
[d] 12% of column 2.
[e] 46% (91%–45%) of column 1.
[f] 33% (45%–12%) of column 2.
[g] 87% of column 1.
[h] 33% of column 2.
[i] 4% (91%–87%) of column 1.
[j] 12% (45%–33%) of column 2.

Tables 37 and 38 summarize data on earnings from follow-up studies. The studies in Table 37 were described in the footnotes to Tables 32 to 35, while those in Table 38 have not been previously described. When a distribution of earnings was reported, median earnings were estimated.

To evaluate these data they must be compared with earnings of the nonretarded during approximately the same time period and preferably in the same geographic location. Only two studies (Kennedy and Peterson) used a control group. For most of the remaining studies, we utilized the information on earnings of production workers on manufacturing payrolls by state and selected areas published by the Bureau of Labor Statistics. The contrasting data for the Bobroff and McIntosh studies were reported directly by those studies.

These comparison data must be used cautiously. They are a reasonable approximation of the earnings of male workers (although some women are included on manufacturing payrolls). However, they have no relevance to the earnings of women workers. In addition, there is a marked age profile of earnings. Since most follow-up studies have relatively young subjects, part of the difference between the earnings reported by follow-up studies and the average earnings prevailing in the area will be due to the age composition of the subjects. This relationship may operate in reverse. In the Kennedy study (1960) the earnings of retarded males are almost exactly those prevailing in Connecticut during 1960, although below those of the control group. This is a consequence of the fact that both the retarded and the controls were in the age group where earnings are highest.

Earlier we calculated age-sex specific estimates of median earnings among employed workers. For purposes of our subsequent analysis these were combined to obtain median earnings of all males and all females age 20 to 64—$6,981 and $3,678, respectively in 1968 and $7,741 and $4,079 in 1970. As before, we will examine differences in earnings among demographic groups.

✓ *Sex.* In the general population, women's earnings were 53% of those of men. Only two studies reported ratios of women's to men's earnings among retardates lower than 53%. Both were probably atypical. The subjects of the Orzack study (Table 32) were among the youngest of any of the follow-up studies. Only fifteen retarded women were evaluated in the Peterson study (Table 38) and not all were employed.

In other studies, the ratio of female to male earnings ranged between 56% and 86%. If we exclude the Phelps study (Table 32), which included fairly young retardates, and the Hegge study (Table 35), which was conducted under wartime conditions, the range is 65% to 74%.

Table 37. Earnings reported for mentally retarded persons, selected follow-up studies

Name of study	Year of evaluation	Sex	IQ	Age	Earnings	Comparison earnings
11. Channing study	1923–24	Males	Less than 50 50–59 60–69 70 or over	17–24	$17.60/wk. 22.51/wk. 25.12/wk. 24.65/wk.	
		Females	Less than 50 50–59 60–69 70 or over		12.00/wk. 15.03/wk. 15.20/wk. 15.82/wk.	
12. McKeon study Defense workers Nondefense workers	1943	Males	52–83	16–27	M = $48.00/wk. M = $28.50/wk.	
13. McIntosh study	1947	Males		16–30	M = $29.83	$ 38.54 = Median weekly, Canada, 1948
16. Phelps study	1952	Males Females	M = 61	M = 22	M = $1.30/hr. M = $0.75/hr.	
17. Bobroff study	1953	Males Females	40–99	28–30	$2.08/hr. $1.42/hr.	$ 2.23 average/hr., mfg., Detroit
19. Saenger study	1956	Both	Less than 55	17–40	M = $14.29/wk.	$ 73.93 average weekly, New York City[a]
11. Dinger study	1960	Both	50–85	15–36	M = $3,327/yr.	$4,705 average/yr., Pennsylvania[a]
12. Orzack study	1965	Males Females			$30.74/wk. 8.75/wk.	$ 113.16 average/wk., Bridgeport, Conn., 1965[a]
14. Mudd study	1966	Males	50–79	21–22	M = $76.00/wk.	$ 103.79 average/wk., Mass., 1966[a]

Table 37. (Continued)

Name of study	Year of evaluation	Sex	IQ	Age	Earnings	Comparison earnings
15. Tobias study	1966–67	Both	50–75	early 20's	M = $1.43/hr.	$ 2.78 average/hr., New York City, 1967[a]
16. Grate study	1967	Both	49–84	16–18	M = $46.54/wk.	$122.54 average/wk., Oregon, 1967[a]
19. Channing study	1925	Males	50–70		M = $20.71/wk.	
		Females			M = $14.50/wk.	
21. Hegge study	1943	Males	51.90	15–20	M = $39.62/wk.	
		Females			M = $34.28/wk.	
22. Kennedy study	1948	Males	50–75	23–33	M = $46.30/wk.	M = $ 46.90/wk. (controls)
		Females			M = $33.30/wk.	M = $ 30.90/wk. (controls)
	1960	Males		38–48	M = $88.20/wk.	M = $102.30/wk. (controls)
		Females			M = $58.00/wk.	M = $ 66.40/wk. (controls)
						$ 88.60/wk. average/wk., Conn.[a]

Note: M = Median. The numbers assigned to these studies are the same as assigned in Tables 32 through 35.

[a]These data are taken from selected issues of *Employment and Earnings and Monthly Report on the Labor Force*, U.S. Department of Labor, Bureau of Labor Statistics. These earnings are those prevailing in April of the year of the survey, with the exception of the Harold Study which was based on the July figures.

Table 38. Earnings reported for mentally retarded persons

Name of study	Number of subjects	Year of evalua- tion	Place of study	Former status of subjects	Time lapse between eval. & follow-up (in years)	Age	Sex	IQ	Earnings	Comparison earnings
23. Coakley study[b]	37 12 25	1944	Ramsey County, Minnesota	County wards		21–45	Males	40–74 40–59 60–75	Mean = $37.95/wk. Mean = $43.31/wk.	
24. Krishef study[c]	41 42 31 24	1953	Minnesota	County wards		Mean = 39 Mean = 33 Mean = 41 Mean = 38	Males Females	Below 59 60–79 Below 59 60–79	Mean = $1850/yr. Mean = $2050/yr. Mean = $1340/yr. Mean = $1511/yr.	
25. Harold study[d]	74 50 24	1954	St. Louis, Missouri	Public instit.	1–15	15–39	Males Females	33–81		$73.63 average/wk., St. Louis[a]
Employed in industry	29								Mean = $208/mo.	
Employed as domestics or in institu- tions	45								Mean = $140/mo.	
26. Peterson study[e] Retarded group	30 15	1958	Iowa	Classes for educable mentally retarded	5–15	21–32	Males Females	Mean = 65	Mean = $54.85/wk. Mean = $19.25/wk.	$88.36 average/wk., Iowa[a]
Comparison group	30 15					21–32	Males Females	Mean=103	Mean = $89.30/wk. Mean = $55.00/wk.	

Table 38. (Continued)

Name of study	Number of subjects	Year of evalua-tion	Place of study	Former status of subjects	Time lapse between eval. & follow-up (in years)	Age	Sex	IQ	Earnings	Comparison earnings
27. Delaware study[f]	90 39	1967	Delaware	Classes for educable mentally retarded in high school	1-10	16-26	Males Females	47-93	M = $3,000/yr. M = $1.60/hr.	$6,079 average/yr., Delaware, 1967[a] $2.93, average/hr., Delaware[a]

Note: M = Median. See footnotes to Table 37.

[a]These data are taken from selected issues of *Employment and Earnings and Monthly Report on the Labor Force*, U.S. Department of Labor, Bureau of Labor Statistics. These earnings are those prevailing in April of the year of the survey, with the exception of the Harold Study which was based on the July figures.

[b]Frances Coakley, "Study of Feeble-Minded Wards Employed in War Industries," *American Journal of Mental Deficiency* (October 1945): 301–6. All were employed as a condition of being included in the study.

[c]Curtis H. Krishef and Manford A. Hall, "Employment of the Mentally Retarded in Hennepin County, Minnesota," *American Journal of Mental Deficiency* (July 1955): 182–89. All subjects were employed. All persons in the sample were on the Hennepin County active caseload, i.e., those for whom the county welfare board provides casework services.

[d]Edward C. Harold, "Employment of Patients Discharged from the St. Louis State Training School," *American Journal of Mental Defi-ciency* (October 1955): 397–402. The sample consisted of patients discharged from the St. Louis State Training School between 1939 and 1953 who: (1) had been in the institution at least 6 months; (2) were 14 years or older when discharged; (3) were living in or near St. Louis; and (4) had established themselves in the community by employment or marriage.

[e]Le Roy Peterson and Lloyd L. Smith, "A Comparison of the Post-School Adjustment of Educable Mentally Retarded Adults with that of Adults of Normal Intelligence," *Exceptional Children*, vol. 26 (April 1960): 404–8. The comparison group was obtained from families of low economic status at the time they attended school. All but three graduated from high school.

[f]Delaware Foundation for Retarded Children, "Follow-up Study of Occupational Education Work-Study Program Leavers," 1967.

There are several reasons why this ratio among retardates might be expected to be somewhat above the population average:

1) One factor contributing to the earnings disparity between men and women in the general population is the lower educational attainments of women. Among retardates there is little, if any, difference in years spent in school between men and women.

2) Another important reason for relatively low female wages is the greater tendency of women to work part time. In May 1967, 30% of employed women 20 to 64 years old, were working part time as compared to slightly less than 5% of employed men.[42] If we compared the earnings of *full-time* female and male workers, the ratio would be considerably higher. In the Kennedy study (Table 35) there were no part-time workers in 1960. The ratio of female to male earnings was 66% for retardates and 65% for the controls. In 1948 the comparable figures were 72% and 66%. It is probable that part-time workers are underrepresented in the other follow-up studies.

Age. The age profile of the earnings of the mildly retarded follows a pattern similar to that of employment. Initially, their earnings are about as high as their nonretarded counterparts. At some point, apparently in their late twenties, the earnings of the nonretarded surpass those of the retarded. Eventually, the earnings of the mildly retarded stabilize between 85% and 90% of the population average.

In the Orzack and Grate studies (Table 32), the earnings of the retarded are low, 25% to 35% of the state average. This, however, is a function of the youth of the subjects. Looking back to Table 29 shows that the earnings of teenage youth generally fall into this range.

The earnings of mildly retarded males in the Mudd study (Table 32) were 74% of the state average in manufacturing. However, the earnings of 20- to 24-year-old white males generally are about 76% of the average for all white males (the Mudd study subjects were 21 to 22 years old).

The Mudd study results are consistent with those of the 1948 Kennedy study (Table 35), where there was almost no difference in the earnings of employed retardates and employed controls. The subjects in the Kennedy study were several years older than those of the Mudd study.

By 1960, however, the earnings of the subjects of the Kennedy study had fallen to a little over 85% of those of the control group. These observations become reasonable when possible explanations are consid-

[42] U.S. Department of Labor, Bureau of Labor Statistics, *Employment and Earnings and Monthly Report of the Labor Force*, June 1967, p. 23.

ered. Because of longer school attendance, the nonretarded are more likely to have part-time and temporary work while teenagers. As young adults the retarded have more seniority and have begun their limited progress on the occupational ladder. Over time, however, the occupational advance of the nonretarded is more rapid than that of the retarded. Moreover, college graduates begin entering the labor force during their early twenties at salaries beyond what most retarded could attain. It is of interest to observe that the relative earnings of employed whites and nonwhites also follow this pattern, probably for the same reasons.

IQ. Among the *mildly* retarded there appears to be a relationship between earnings and IQ, although not a large one. The Channing (Table 32), Coakley (Table 38), and Krishef (Table 38) studies all reported slightly higher earnings for those with IQs above 60 as compared to those with IQs below 60. Bobroff (Table 32) reported a correlation between earnings and IQ of 0.32 and Dinger (Table 32) reported a similar correlation of 0.21.

There is little question of the effect of relatively severe retardation on earnings. The subjects of the Saenger study (Table 32) had median earnings only one-fifth of those prevailing in New York City.

Aggregate Demand. McKeon (Table 32) reported that the retarded working in defense industries had earnings almost 70% higher than those in nondefense industries. Hegge (Table 35) found the same relationship, although it was less pronounced. Evidently, the critical need for manpower during World War II opened up employment opportunities at skill levels that would not otherwise be available to the retarded.

Race. No information was available on the relationship between race, mental retardation, and earnings. The net effect is uncertain. The percentage decrease in earnings among nonwhites might be greater than among whites, because of the combined effect of racial discrimination and mental retardation, and it might be less if measured IQ among nonwhites is less reflective of their abilities than among whites.

Reduced earnings among noninstitutionalized retardates. It is probable that differences in the earnings reported by most follow-up studies could be reconciled if adequate information on the earnings by age, sex, IQ, and the prevailing wage rate in the community were available.[43]

The Kennedy study (Table 35) is the only study which specifically related the earnings of mildly retarded men and women in the prime of

---

[43] For example, median earnings reported by the Tobias study (Table 32) were about one-half of those prevailing in manufacturing in New York City. This, however, is not unexpected considering the youth of the subjects and the fact that the earnings of male and female subjects are not distinguished.

their lives to a control group of comparable age. However, rough adjustments to other studies indicate that, for the most part, they are consistent with the Kennedy study.

We assume, therefore, that the relative earnings of the retarded and nonretarded in Kennedy's 1960 follow-up are a reasonable approximation of the relative earnings of these two groups in the population. We estimate that in 1968 the average earnings of employed mildly retarded males were $977 below the average for all males (14% X $6,981). Among mildly retarded females the comparable figure was $515 (13% X $3,678). In 1970 the estimated amounts that earnings were below average were $1,084 in the case of mildly retarded males and $530 in the case of mildly retarded females.

Among youthful retardates, relative earnings are more favorable than indicated above, but this may serve to offset the possible biases caused by the inclusion of some persons with IQs of 70 to 74 in the Kennedy study (29%) and the probably deteriorating relative earnings of retardates past their prime working years.

The average earnings of the subjects of the Saenger study (Table 32) were 19% of average manufacturing earnings in New York City. The majority of these subjects had IQs between 40 and 50 and four-fifths were males. The earnings of the male subjects relative to the general population should be slightly greater than 19% of the average in manufacturing.

We will assume that the earnings of employed male and female retardates with IQs between 40 and 50 are 20% of the average earnings of their counterparts in the general population. We estimate that in 1968 their average earnings are $5,585 and $2,942 per year below the average for their respective sexes. In 1970 the comparable losses of earnings were $6,193 and $3,263. Because of uncertainty about the effects of race in the earnings of the retardates, no adjustment will be made for this variable.

Skill level. Even the most ardent advocates of the social usefulness of the retarded occasionally perpetuate the misconception that they are limited to routine repetitive work and that such work provides them with great satisfaction. We have already dealt with one part of this unfortunate and misleading stereotype, i.e., that all of the retarded cheerfully labor away, week after week, on monotonous tasks.

The other half is equally untrue. Table 39 presents information on the skill levels of the employed retarded from four of the follow-up studies.

Among the mildly retarded, semiskilled and even skilled employment appears to be the rule rather than the exception. The percentage work-

Table 39.   Distribution of employed retarded by skill level, selected studies

Name of study	Percentage of workers in semi-skilled work		Percentage of workers in skilled work—including clerical, sales, and mgmt.	
	Male	Female	Male	Female
8. Collman				
Normal group	30.6	21.1	53.1	71.9
Dull group	35.6	53.5	25.7	36.4
Educationally subnormal	48.2	48.8	—	1.2
10. Ferguson IQ:				
Under 50	16.7		—	
50–59	5.6		16.7	
60–69	19.8		7.4	
70–79	18.8		10.1	
18. Baller (1964)	31.7	17.7	18.8	20.6
22. Kennedy 1948:				
Subjects	47.8	67.0	24.1	7.1
Controls	34.3	26.5	47.4	63.3
1960:				
Subjects	24.8	49.0	55.0	14.2
Controls	20.0	23.3	65.5	69.7

ing at semiskilled or skilled levels ranged from about 25% in the Ferguson study (Table 32) to 80% in the 1966 Kennedy study (Table 35). Among the follow-up studies, only the Collman study (Table 32) did not find any appreciable numbers in *skilled* work, and this was probably a function of the youthfulness of the subjects.

Although it is impossible to derive firm conclusions, it is probable that at least half of the employed mildly retarded are in semiskilled work or better and that many are in skilled work.

Self-sufficiency. A basic test of the adjustment of adult retardates is the degree to which they attain self-sufficiency. Obviously, this requires employment or marriage to an employed person. In addition, earnings must be sufficient to maintain acceptable living standards. The retarded must also be able to handle money properly: pay bills on time and avoid excessive debt. Self-sufficiency also requires that they obey the law, dress properly, maintain an apartment or house, and at least 243 other things.

In one sense none of us is totally self-sufficient. In our highly specialized society we rely on one group to maintain our health, another to maintain our vehicle, still another to provide public transportation, and so on. One test of self-sufficiency is that we know to which of these specialized groups to apply to satisfy particular needs.

The fact that a retarded person cannot prepare a tax return is less important than whether he knows where to turn for help. But a rule of reason must be applied. Should a retarded adult be considered self-sufficient if he must seek aid each time a bill must be paid?

A number of follow-up studies have measured the self-sufficiency of the retarded. We will confine our attention to the Kennedy, Baller, and Fairbank studies.[44] These studies dealt with mildly retarded populations that were well into adulthood. In addition, each utilized a control population.

The Kennedy and Baller studies have been described previously. A summary of the Fairbank study is as follows:

Number of subjects: 122
Year of evaluation: 1930
Place of study: Locust Point District of Baltimore, Maryland
Source of subjects: All children in the district believed to be sufficiently subnormal to need special training
Time lapse between evaluation and previous contact: 17 years
Age: Approximately 23 to 33
IQ: Average was approximately 70
Sex: 72 males and 50 females

Table 40 summarizes the self-support status of the retarded as reported by these studies. Although the data appear inconsistent, most of these apparent inconsistencies can be resolved.

The Baller study reported that substantially fewer of the retarded are entirely self-supporting than did the Kennedy study. If, however, we combine the wholly self-supporting with the partially self-supporting, the resulting percentages become almost identical. In fact, the Baller study indicates that males are more likely to make a contribution toward their support than the Kennedy study.

The crucial difference between these studies is that Kennedy measured the self-support status of the subjects at the *time of interview*,

[44] Ruth E. Fairbank, "The Subnormal Child—Seventeen Years After," *Mental Hygiene* (April 1933): 177–208. In 1914 there were 1,502 children of school age in Locust Point, 221 of whom were at work or home. Of the remaining 1,281, 166 (13%) were sufficiently subnormal to need special training. Seventeen years later 122 of the original 166 children were located and interviewed. The original control group consisted of 145 persons, of whom 100 were located on follow-up and interviews were conducted with 90.

Table 40.   Self-support status of mentally retarded persons as reported
by three studies

Name of study	Number in sample	Degree of self-support			
		Wholly self-supporting	Partially self-supporting	Not self-supporting	Supported by spouse
		(%)	(%)	(%)	(%)
Kennedy study, 1948					
Males					
Subjects	141	95.0	2.1	2.8	
Controls	72	84.7	9.7	5.6	
Females					
Subjects	88	82.9	4.5	12.5	35.2
Controls	49	83.7	6.6	10.2	38.8
1960					
Males					
Subjects	112	92.0	4.5	4.5	0.9
Controls	55	90.9	3.6	5.5	
Females					
Subjects	64	89.1	0.0	10.9	42.2
Controls	47	93.8	0.0	6.2	36.4
Baller study, 1964					
Males					
Subjects	58	65.5	32.8	1.7	
Middle groups	65	95.4	4.6	0.0	
Females					
Subjects	44	75.0	15.9	9.1	a
Middle group	50	94.0	2.0	4.0	a
High group—males					
& females	120	96.0	3.0	1.0	a
Fairbank study					
Males					
Subjects	72	80.6	5.6	13.9	
Controls	40	87.5	2.5	10.0	
Females					
Subjects	50	74.0	4.0	22.0	58.0
Controls	40	88.0	2.0	10.0	48.0

[a]Not reported.

while Baller measured self-support status for the entire *thirteen-year
period preceding the interview.* At any point in time, a small percentage
of persons will be unable to support themselves because of recent job
loss, illness, strike, etc. Many, however, will resume work and regain
self-support status, but others will suffer similar temporary misfortune.
It is obvious that the percentage unable to support themselves entirely
over long periods will be larger than the percentage not entirely self-
supporting at a moment of time. In addition, the percentage making

some contribution toward self-support will be greater than exists at a moment of time. Both of these observations are consistent with the Kennedy and Baller studies.

Despite the high rate of self-sufficiency in the Kennedy study, 45% of the subjects had received assistance from public and private welfare agencies between 1948 and 1960. About 17% had received cash assistance (as compared to slightly over 5% among controls). By contrast, Baller reported that 16% of the subjects had received relief between 1951 and 1964, which presumably was also cash relief.

Two problems with the Fairbank study are that it was conducted during the depression and over half the subjects had IQs greater than 70. In addition, since 13% of the school-age population was included in the study, one might question the validity of some of the IQ test scores of persons scoring below 70. In effect, the Fairbank study is composed of subjects who would be comparable to the combined middle and low groups in the Baller study.

The depressed economic conditions explain why the Fairbank study reported higher rates of dependency than the Kennedy study. However, the combination of relatively high IQs and the time of interview method of evaluating self-support resulted in a greater percentage of *totally* self-supporting persons than in the Baller study.

The Baller and Fairbank studies agreed that the retarded were less likely to be self-sufficient than the controls. The contradictory 1948 Kennedy finding that male retardates were more likely to be self-sufficient than male controls was due to continued school attendance by some of the latter group. The 1960 Kennedy and Fairbank studies reported that female retardates were more likely to be supported by their spouses than nonretarded women, which is in accord with our earlier observations on labor force participation of retarded women.

The picture that emerges is that at a point in time, about 90% of the mildly retarded are entirely self-supporting, and that over a 12- to 14-year period, about two-thirds will maintain that status continuously. The first half of this scenario is probably too sanguine. In 1960, seven of the Kennedy subjects earned less than $35 per week. It is questionable whether these persons should be considered fully self-sufficient. Below IQ 50, few retardates have earnings sufficient to attain self-sufficiency.

Loss of earnings. Table 41 shows our estimates of the below average earnings of noninstitutionalized retardates in 1968 and 1970. In 1968 the nation was $3.0 billion poorer because the productivity of the retarded in the community was below average (or zero). A combination of rising productivity and price inflation (mostly price inflation) increased this loss to $3.4 billion in 1970. These estimates of loss among the noninstitutionalized retarded are over four times as great as the loss of earnings among the institutionalized mentally retarded.

LOSS OF HOMEMAKING SERVICES AND OTHER UNPAID WORK

Homemaking services. An attractive, well-organized home that provides a suitable milieu for the intellectual and social development of children is a major component of people's well-being. In homes where the wife does not seek paid employment, almost half of the families' productive capacity is devoted to this purpose.

Two approaches have been used to value a homemaker's services. One is by the wages that would have to be paid to hire a replacement, which are usually estimated by the current wage for a domestic worker. Weisbrod refined this approach by estimating the increase in cost that would be incurred as families increase in size.[45]

Although one may raise the question as to whether a housewife is more or less efficient than a "specialist"[46] more important criticisms of this approach are that it fails to take account of the importance of the management role of a housewife and the value of child care and the fact that most housewives are on the job for more than 40 hours per week.[47]

An alternative approach is to value a homemaker's services by their opportunity costs, i.e., what housewives could earn in paid jobs after taxes and other expenses (child care, extra clothing expense, possibly a maid).[48] The reasoning is that the services of a housewife must be worth at least that much or they would not forgo paid employment. Thus, it represents a minimum valuation of these services. Rigorously applied, this approach would lead to the absurd conclusion that the larger the family, the lower the value of the wife's services, because of the increased expenditure required for child care.

[45] Dorothy Rice, *Estimating the Cost of Illness*, Health Economics Series No. 5, PHS Publication No. 947–6 (Washington, D.C.: USGPO, 1966), p. 14. Burton Weisbrod, *Economics of Public Health* (Philadelphia: University of Pennsylvania Press, 1961), p. 70.

[46] Marie Geraldine Gage, *The Homemaker's Work Load and Its Value* (New York State College of Home Economics, Department of Household Economics and Management, Report 9, 1964, Reissued by the Pennsylvania State University, 1968), p. 17.

[47] Florence Turnbull Hall and Marguerite Paulsen Schroeder, "Time Spent on Household Tasks," *Journal of Home Economics* (January 1970): 23–29.

[48] A. R. Prest and R. Turvey, "Cost-Benefit Analysis: A Survey," *Economic Journal* (December 1965): 722.

Table 41. Estimated value of below average earnings of the noninstitutionalized mentally retarded aged 20–64, 1968 and 1970

	Number of persons		Average loss of earnings		Aggregate loss of earnings	
	Male	Female	Male	Female	Male	Female
			1968			
Persons not employed because of retardation, (all IQs from Table 36)	128,500	198,200	$6,981	$3,678	$ 897,000,000	$ 729,000,000
Employed retarded, IQ 40–49	18,200	5,500	5,585	2,942	102,000,000	16,000,000
Employed retarded, IQ 50–69	1,072,300	410,400	977	515	1,048,000,000	211,000,000
Loss of earnings					2,047,000,000	956,000,000
Total loss of earnings					$3,003,000,000	
			1970			
Persons not employed because of retardation, all IQs (from Table 36)	135,800	204,300	7,741	4,079	1,051,000,000	833,000,000
Employed retarded, IQ 40–49	19,400	5,800	6,193	3,263	120,000,000	19,000,000
Employed retarded, IQ 50–69	1,098,000	419,400	1,084	530	1,190,000,000	222,000,000
Loss of earnings					2,361,000,000	1,074,000,000
Total loss of earnings					$3,435,000,000	

Empirically, opportunity costs are usually estimated by assuming that housewives could earn as much as other women of similar age. This raises the obvious question of whether housewives have less innate ability or motivation than other women.

The best approach to valuing a housewife's services, if data were available, would be to value a homemaker's services by the cost of hiring a domestic worker for housekeeping duties, plus an allowance for the cost of child care, plus a management fee.

Since the necessary data are not available, we will value a housewife's services by what she could earn, if employed, less estimated tax payments. No adjustment will be made for other work-related expenses. Our calculations will be limited to the value of loss of homemaking services among female retardates.[49] We will first estimate this loss among the institutionalized population. During May 1967 the percentage of women keeping house full-time (no paid employment) was 16.3% among 18- to 19-year-olds, 52.1% among 20- to 64-year-olds, and 79.4% for those over 65.[50] The number of women not keeping house because of retardation was estimated by multiplying the percentage of women keeping house in the general population by the number of female retardates in residential care in each of these three age groups (Table 42).

Based on the earnings survey that was described previously, median earnings of 18- to 19-year-old females in 1968 were $2,651. For 20- to 64-year-old females, they were $3,678, and for those 65 and over $2,364. In 1970 the comparable figures were $2,940, $4,079, and $2,622. We will assume that take-home pay is 75% of gross earnings. Since married women's earnings are added to their husband's earnings to determine taxable income with little corresponding increase in deductions, a marginal tax rate of about 25% is not unrealistic. These estimated values of a homemaker's service are shown in Table 42. Interestingly, these estimates, based on foregone earnings, are similar to the estimates of the earnings of domestic workers.

One problem with these estimates of the value of homemaking services is that they are based on the earnings of all employed females, including those working less than 40 hours per week (as noted previously, our estimates of annual earnings have a built-in assumption of 52 weeks of continuous employment). One point of view is that if we are estimating the value of full-time homemaking in terms of foregone

[49] Almost all full-time homemakers are women. The Department of Labor reports that less than one-fifth of one percent of men (over half of whom are over 65) report themselves as keeping house full-time.

[50] U.S. Department of Labor, Bureau of Labor Statistics, *Employment and Earnings and Monthly Report on the Labor Force*, June 1967, p. 18.

earnings, then we should utilize the wages of full-time work, since, presumably, these are the earnings that are foregone. On that basis our estimates are too low.

On the other hand, women who work do not give up housekeeping activities altogether. Hall and Schroeder recently reported a study in which they found that employed women spent 42.1 hours doing household tasks, as compared to 54.1 hours for full-time homemakers. They cited an earlier study by Wiegand which found that employed homemakers spent 28.7 hours on household tasks, as compared to 51.8 hours for full-time homemakers.[51] If we adjusted for family size, the disparity would be even less. Women who work do not, therefore, forego the full value of the homemaking services that they would perform if they did not work. If a woman works, she does not reduce her homemaking efforts by 100%, but by a lesser amount. One cannot, therefore, argue that the foregone wages of a full-time homemaker represents her valuation of her homemaking services. Rather they represent her appraisal of the value of the reduction in homemaking services and leisure time that would occur if she returned to work.

The assumption that a homemaker's foregone earnings measures the minimum value, to her, of her homemaking services requires the additional assumption that the value she places on the leisure time she loses if she accepts employment is equal to the value of the homemaking services she continues to perform. If housewives were free to vary their activities among work, housekeeping, and leisure in such a way as to equate the marginal benefits of each type of activity, this would be a reasonable assumption. Under these ideal circumstances, however, it is unlikely that many would choose full-time work, especially if they had small children.

The point of the matter is that the wages homemakers forego by not undertaking full-time work probably overstate the actual value they place on their homemaking services, because part of what they are buying is leisure. Since the leisure they are buying represents only a couple of hours per day, we may anticipate that homemakers place a high value on this time and only necessity, high earnings, or the desire for a career could induce them to forego this leisure. Women who work part-time usually do so at hourly rates substantially less than they would receive if they worked full-time, again indicating the high value placed on leisure time at the end of the working day.

Our estimate of the value of a homemaker's services is about 13% less than it would be if based on the earnings of full-time women workers.[52]

[51] Hall and Schroeder, "Time Spent on Household Tasks," p. 29.

[52] The average earnings of women who work at full-time jobs for an entire year are about 13% higher than the average earnings of women who work at either

Whether this difference is too large or too small cannot be determined. It is, however, an adjustment in the right direction.

We have stressed the point that employed women continue to perform at least part of their homemaking duties. We cited two earlier studies, one of which indicated that the hours spent on homemaking tasks by employed women are 54% of the hours spent on these tasks by full-time homemakers (Wiegand), and one of which indicated that this percentage was 78%. We will utilize the more conservative estimate and assume that institutionalized females who would have worked had they not been retarded would also have provided homemaking services equal to 37.5% (50% of 75%) of their gross earnings. In short, their homemaking services are being valued at 50% of those of full-time homemakers. This approach presumes that the productivity of employed women is almost twice as high as the productivity of full-time homemakers. This is because an employed woman is in approximately the same position as a man who moonlights on a half-time job. Both are sacrificing leisure for income.

The estimated value of the loss of homemaker's services among institutionalized female retardates was slightly less than $150 million in both 1968 and 1970 (Table 42).

As before, we will restrict our discussion of the noninstitutionalized population to those between 20 and 64 years of age. We assume that female retardates with IQs below 40 do not perform any significant homemaking services.

Many retardates in the 40 to 49 IQ range perform household tasks. Saenger reported that 19% of the subjects in his study (all of whom had IQs below 50) could be considered the equivalent of regular housekeepers, and that about 80% performed *some* useful service. However, he reported that only 3% of the women were married, so that the household tasks they perform are in the homes of others and, in most cases, an offset to what others would do.[53] Moreover, performing simple household chores falls short of the vastly more complicated task of managing a home.

We will assume, therefore, that 19% of the noninstitutionalized adult females in the 40 to 49 IQ range provide homemaking services that are

---

full-time or part-time jobs for an entire year (based on data contained in U.S. Department of Commerce, Bureau of the Census, *Income in 1970 of Families and Persons in the United States*, Current Population Reports, Series P-60, No. 80, October 4, 1971. It will be recalled that our earnings estimates are based on the assumption that workers employed at a point in time will be employed for a full year. Two intermittent workers, working six months each, are treated as the equivalent of one year-around worker.

[53] In some cases other household members may be freed for paid employment.

valued at 50% of normal. The reduction in the number of full-time homemakers will be estimated at 33.1% (52.1–19.0). Among persons with IQs between 40 and 50 who are employed or who would have been employed were it not for their retardation, we will assume that the loss of homemaking services is equal to 37.5% of the loss of earnings.

In our discussion of the self-sufficiency of the retarded, we observed that mildly retarded adult women were slightly more likely to be supported by their husband's earnings than women generally. Among this group, mental retardation may actually increase the number of full-time homemakers. We assume, therefore, no loss in the provision of homemaking services in this group.

The estimated loss of the value of homemaking services among the noninstitutionalized retarded was almost $235 million in 1968 and $275 million in 1970. When combined with the loss among the institutionalized retarded, the total is $380 million and $424 million, respectively, in the two years. This probably underestimates the actual loss. By assuming no loss in the value of homemaking services among the mildly retarded, we implicitly assumed that the quality of these services was comparable to those provided by the nonretarded. There is evidence to suggest otherwise, especially in the crucial area of child care.

Unpaid work. James Morgan et al., in a survey of over 2,200 families (17% were adults living alone), concluded that the average family spends about 7 hours per week on productive activities other than paid employment and homemaking: 4 hours were attributed to home production (sewing, yard work, painting, etc.), 1.7 hours to volunteer work away from home, and 1.3 hours to taking courses and lessons.[54]

Although these figures seem low,[55] they do indicate that home production and volunteer work comprise at least 6.2% of the average family's total productive effort,[56] a not inconsiderable amount.

Much of what was defined as home production appeared to come within the normal range of duties of a housewife. The distinction between normal homemaking and other unpaid work is not always clear. Painting the exterior of a house is clearly not homemaking. But what is repainting bookcases, or putting up curtains?

[54] James N. Morgan, Ismail A. Sirageldin, and Nancy Bearwaldt, *Productive Americans* (Ann Arbor, Michigan: Institute for Social Research of the University of Michigan, 1966), pp. 125–62.

[55] Ibid., pp. 408–12. We become suspicious when we note that only 8.3% of the families claimed to perform any home services, among which was included lawn work, while 84% claimed that they did not pay to have any lawn work done.

[56] Ibid., p. 185. On the average, families spent a little less than 90 hours per week at remunerative employment, housework, or home production.

Table 42.   Estimated value of reduced homemaking services among female retardates, 1968 and 1970

Female retardates in residential care	Reduction in number of females who would normally keep house full-time		Reduction in number of females who would normally be employed		Females keeping house		Employed females		Total loss
	Number	Average home-making loss	Number	Average home-making loss	Number	Average home-making loss	Number	Average home-making loss	
1968									
Age 18–19	1,100	$1,988	2,900	$ 994					$ 5,069,000
20–64	32,800	2,758	28,500	1,379					129,764,000
65+	5,000	1,773	1,100	886					9,840,000
1970									
Age 18–19	1,000	2,205	2,700	1,102					5,180,000
20–64	30,000	3,059	26,000	1,529					131,524,000
65+	4,800	1,966	1,000	983					10,420,000
Noninstitutionalized female retardates, age 20–64									
1968									
IQ 0–39	39,100	2,758	34,000	1,379	8,600	$1,379	5,500	$1,103	154,724,000
40–49	15,100	2,758	15,000	1,379					80,257,000
1970									
IQ 0–39	41,700	3,059	36,000	1,529	9,100	1,529	5,800	1,223	182,604,000
40–49	15,900	3,059	15,800	1,529					93,804,000
Total									
1968									$379,654,000
1970									$423,532,000

In previous work, I have assumed that the value of unpaid work, other than normal homemaking services, was 25% of a person's gross earnings largely on the belief that most workers spend at least ten hours a week on miscellaneous tasks at home. The issue of the efficiency of such work at home was avoided. This applies primarily to male workers. Undoubtedly, almost all the time devoted to home activities by employed women is spent on normal household duties. The value of these activities was taken into account in the previous section.

In view of the results of the Morgan study, a figure of 25% may appear too high. There, is however, reason to believe that Morgan was unable to obtain complete information on unpaid tasks other than homemaking. We will, therefore, continue to use the 25% figure for males. Hopefully, future research will permit refinement of this estimate.[57]

The value of the loss of unpaid work among the retarded is estimated by multiplying 25% times the loss of earnings among male institutionalized retarded of all IQs and the noninstitutionalized male retarded *with IQs below 50*. This loss of earnings was previously estimated at $1 billion in 1968 and $1.1 billion in 1970. Loss of unpaid work other than normal homemaking is, therefore, estimated at $250 million and $276 million for these two years. This assumes that males with IQs between 40 and 50 perform some useful unpaid work, other than homemaking, equal to 25% of their earnings.

As in the case of homemaking, it is assumed that there are no losses of this nature among the noninstitutionalized mildly retarded. Losses among those mildly retarded males unable to carry on such activities are assumed to be offset by above-average amounts of this type of work performed by those individuals who are not remuneratively employed.

---

[57] The data used in the Morgan study were apparently reanalyzed by Sirageldin who imputed dollar values to the estimates of the amount of time families spent in various unpaid activities. These dollar values were based on the prevailing hourly wages for these different activities. Sirageldin concluded that the value of housework, plus home production, plus volunteer work came to 46% of a families' disposable income, i.e., gross income less income taxes plus imputed rent for homeowners. My approach indicates slightly over 40% of gross income for these three categories of unpaid work. Despite the divergence in the conceptual basis of disposable income as opposed to gross income, the percentages are quite close and lead me to suspect that I have understated the value of unpaid work. My reasons for not utilizing the Sirageldin conclusions were that Sirageldin did not impute any value to child care provided by the mother (except as children increased the amount of housework that is done). Moreover, I doubt whether the survey fully took account of all the unpaid work that people did around the house. See Ismail Abdel-Hamid Sirageldin, *Non-Market Components of National Income* (Ann Arbor, Michigan: Institute for Social Research of the University of Michigan, 1969).

This estimate omits the loss of unpaid work on tasks other than normal homemaking among retarded women who would have been full-time homemakers but are prevented from being so because of their retardation. One problem is that the distinction between homemaking services and other unpaid work is not clear for this group. We could for purposes of consistency increase the estimated value of homemaking services among full-time homemakers by 25% to allow for other unpaid work. However, the effect on our aggregate estimates would be small, and in view of the uncertainty surrounding the valuation of home-making services, there seems little merit in making such a questionable adjustment.

OTHER EFFECTS OF MENTAL RETARDATION

Few of the other effects of mental retardation can be quantified. Nevertheless, they are important. Many people argue that they are more important than loss of productive capacity. Therefore, if only briefly and impressionistically, some of these other effects should be discussed.

Crime. Fear of the criminal proclivities of the retarded was an important stimulus to the development of residential facilities. Estimates of the proportion of prisoners and delinquents who were retarded ran as high as 90% in the earlier literature.[58]

Because of differences in the criteria of mental retardation, in the definition of antisocial behavior, and in the time span over which anti-social behavior is measured, there is, for all practical purposes, no comparability among follow-up studies investigating these factors. Four follow-up studies, however, used comparison groups. Several important conclusions can be drawn.

First, the retarded commit acts in violation of the law more often than the nonretarded. Peterson (Table 38) reported that 62% of the retarded were involved in criminal activities compared to 31% of the controls. Ferguson (Table 32) found that 31% of ex-special-school boys had been *convicted* of a violation of law by the age of 22, as compared to 16% of a sample of 568 men who had attended normal schools.

Between 1951 and 1962, Baller (Table 33) found that 12% of the male retardates and none of the female retardates had committed a civil offense, as compared to 12% and 4% among the middle group and no such reported cases in the high group.

---

[58] Herbert Goldstein, "Social and Occupational Adjustment," in *Mental Retardation, A Review of Research*, Harvey A. Stevens and Rick Heber, eds. (Chicago: The University of Chicago Press, 1964), pp. 214–17.

Kennedy (Table 35) reported that between 1948 and 1960, male retardates and male controls had identical arrest records (16%), although female subjects were arrested more often than their control counterparts (7% to 2%). However, prior to 1948, male subjects were arrested over three times as often as male controls (29% to 9%). Among females the comparable rates were 8% and 0%.

In Chapter IV we observed that there are over twice as many retardates in state and federal prisons as would be expected on the basis of their number in the population. In addition, some retarded offenders are sent to public institutions or public mental hospitals.

A second important conclusion is that illegal acts committed by the retarded are more serious than those committed by the nonretarded. This was not readily apparent in the Baller study, where almost all of the civil offenses were drunkenness charges. In the Kennedy study, however, 42 of the arrests of subject males led to incarceration between 1948 and 1960 and 2 among the subject females (representing one person who was arrested twice). Not one control was sentenced to a prison term. Twelve of the male subjects (11%) were arrested on serious charges: sexual offenses, burglary and theft, assault, and homicide with a car (one case).

Allen found that criminal homicides constituted 39% of the crimes committed by retarded prisoners, a level significantly higher than that of other prisoners.[59] Levy, studying seventeen prisoners with IQs below 70 in Washington State found that 59% had committed violent crimes, as compared to 18% of the male prison population.[60]

A third observation is that the retarded are considerably more likely to violate the law when young. In 1935 Baller found that about one-half of the subjects had been prosecuted for a relatively serious offense. Kennedy also found a higher crime rate among retardates in the earlier phase of her study.

Finally, the great majority of the retarded, almost 90% of the males and virtually all of the females in the Kennedy study, had committed no serious illegal acts.

Few retardates with IQs below 50 are involved in crime. Saenger (Table 32) reported that a check of the police files revealed that only 5% of the subjects of his study had police records, a figure far below average. Apparently three-fourths of these cases were for sexual delin-

[59] Richard C. Allen, "Legal Norms and Practices Affecting the Mentally Deficient," *American Journal of Orthopsychiatry* (July 1968): 641.

[60] Sol Levy, "The Role of Mental Deficiency in the Causation of Criminal Behavior," *American Journal of Mental Deficiency* (January 1954): 455–64.

quency. Channing reported that only 3% of the males and none of the females with IQs below 50, formerly in special education classes, had delinquency records.

Levy noted that 15 of the 17 retarded prisoners were nonwhite, 16 came from broken homes, 8 suffered from nervous or mental diseases, most had minimal school attendance, and none had held a job for more than three months. Their criminal activities need not necessarily be regarded as a consequence of their intellectual deficiency.

Psychic effects. Only a few of what appear to be the more important of the psychic effects of retardation will be described.

Mental retardation affects all household members. Meyer and Schreiber report that parents frequently express concern that the siblings of the retarded may feel overburdened by the care of the retarded, responsible for the retardation, obligated to make up to the parents for what the retarded child could not give them, and guilty for being the normal children. Normal siblings become apprehensive of their prospects for marriage. Some fear that they themselves may be someday called upon to provide care for an aging retarded sibling. Many wonder if they will have a retarded child.

Perhaps the most important psychic effect of having a retarded sibling is the shame felt by a normal child. Meyer and Schreiber observed that almost every normal sibling of a retarded person eventually asked: "Why did it have to happen in my family, to us, to me?" One of the most difficult tasks that a normal sibling must face is to tell his friends about his retarded brother or sister.[61]

Parental reactions to mental retardation encompass every known emotion. Among the more commonly reported are guilt, shame, anger, and fear of the future: Will someone care for their child when they die; will their child ever work?

Olshansky has described what he regards as the most important psychic effect on parents: ". . . most parents who have a mentally retarded child suffer from a pervasive, psychological reaction, chronic sorrow. . . . The parents of a normal child have to endure many woes, many trials, and many moments of despair. Almost all these parents know, however, that ultimately the child will become a self-sufficient adult. By contrast, the parents of a mentally defective child have little to look forward to; they will always be burdened by the child's unrelenting demands and unabated dependency. The woes, the trials, the

---

[61] Meyer Schreiber and Mary Feeley, "Siblings of the Retarded: I. A Guided Group Experience," *Children* (November–December 1965): 221–25. See also Jane O'Neill, "Siblings of the Retarded: II. Individual Counseling," *Children* (November–December 1965): 226–29.

moments of despair will continue until either their own death or the child's death."[62]

Perhaps Olshansky overstates the case. Many retardates are employable and self-sufficient. Olshansky himself reported that less than one-third of the parents of a group of former special-class students considered their children retarded.[63]

Among the retarded, isolation, rejection, and repeated frustrations are bound to combine to produce serious psychic effects: bitterness, hostility, fearfulness, irascibility, and more. The most important psychic effect may well be loneliness, which itself is intertwined with, and may be the proximate cause of, many other psychic reactions. Loneliness and isolation are difficult to measure. Kennedy (Table 35) reported that membership in clubs and participation in group activities was only slightly less frequent for the retarded in 1960 than for the controls. However, membership in groups does not imply active participation, and the groups were defined broadly to include organizations such as unions, PTAs, etc.

The Baller study (Table 33) gives a more accurate picture. Over 40% of the subjects of this study reported *no* friendship among their peers while attending school, and another 40% reported little interaction with the friends they had. As adults, 60% of the retarded reported no membership in community clubs or similar organizations as compared to 48% among the middle group and 23% among the high group. Only 4% of the retarded actively participated in group activities, as compared to 17% among the middle group and 33% among the high group. Another study found that 23 out of 44 retarded adolescents had essentially no social activities, interests, or contacts. [64]

Of the many psychic losses associated with mental retardation, we have stressed shame among the siblings of the retarded, sorrow among their parents, and loneliness among the retarded themselves. Others may disagree with this emphasis.[65] This is less important than establish-

---

[62] Simon Olshansky, "Chronic Sorrow: A Response to Having a Mentally Defective Child," *Social Casework* (April 1962): 190–93.

[63] Simon Olshansky and Jacob Schonfield, "Parental Perceptions of the Mental Status of Graduates of Special Classes," *Mental Retardation* (October 1965): 16–20.

[64] S. L. Hammer and K. E. Barnard, "The Mentally Retarded Adolescent," *Pediatrics* (November 1966): 845–57.

[65] Wolf Wolfensberger, "Counseling the Parents of the Retarded," in *Mental Retardation, Appraisal, Education, and Rehabilitation*, Alfred A. Baumeister, ed. (Chicago: Aldine Publishing Company, 1967), pp. 330–35. Wolfensberger has summarized the literature on the reactions of parents of retarded children and finds that different researchers stress a wide variety of reactions.

ing the fact that psychic losses are of major importance. The inadequacies of measures of productive losses are fully apparent in the comment of a retarded girl after being placed on a job: "For the first time in my life, I can give my mother a Christmas gift."[66]

Mental retardation does not invariably lead to these psychic losses. Some retarded lead socially well-rounded lives, many normal children respond to their retarded siblings affectionately and even with pride, and many parents have a mature and understanding acceptance of their child's limitations. To a large extent, these psychic losses are not a direct consequence of mental retardation, but rather a consequence of community misunderstanding, occasional intolerance, lack of needed services, etc.

Military service. Anyone who scores below the 10th percentile on the Armed Forces Qualification Test (AFQT) is automatically rejected. Few retardates could score above this level. High school drop-outs scoring between the 10th and 30th percentiles are accepted only if they pass additional aptitude requirements.

In 1968, 7.3% of all examinees scored below the 10th percentile of the AFQT; another 1.4% were rejected because they scored below the 30th percentile, were nonhigh school graduates, and failed to pass the aptitude test. Many of these failures had IQs in the seventies and eighties. Most of the severely retarded are never examined.

There is nothing surprising in these figures, since, by definition, about 10% of the population must fall below the 10th percentile of the AFQT. These rejections become more significant when examined by race. Nationally, 26% of Negroes compared to less than 5% of the rest of the population fell below the 10th percentile of the AFQT; 5% of Negroes as compared to 1% of all others were rejected because of limited aptitudes, even though they scored above the 10th percentile.

When looked at by state, the data are even more startling. Among Negroes, the percentage of draftees who failed the mental requirements ranged from 16% (Kansas) to 54% (Mississippi). Among all others, the corresponding percentages were 1.4% (South Dakota) and 12% (Tennessee). The southern states had the highest percentages of disqualifications among both whites and Negroes. If one believes that intellectual differences between Negroes and whites and between the poor and the affluent are primarily culturally determined, then the price of neglect may come high, especially in times of lethal military operations.

Curiously, there was an inverse relationship between the percentage of inductees medically unqualified and the percentage mentally unqual-

---

[66] Reported by John W. Macy, *Federal Employment of the Mentally Retarded*, The President's Committee on Mental Retardation, August 1966, p. 6.

ified. In 1968, 22% of Negroes were medically unqualified compared to 34% of the rest of the population, and southern Negroes tended to have the lowest rates of medical disqualifications. This led to the peculiar result that states as diverse as Mississippi and Oregon had similar rates of Negro disqualifications (between 65% and 70%), and New York, Massachusetts, Alabama, and Louisiana had similar rates of white disqualifications (45% to 50%). There is no satisfactory explanation of this inverse relationship.[67]

Effects on families. The existence of a retarded child may have tangible effects on families going beyond, but partly caused by, the psychic effects of mental retardation.

Parents. It is often asserted that serious marital discord, sometimes leading to the extreme of separation or divorce, may result after parents learn that their child is retarded. One study of 69 infants recommended for institutional care found that marital difficulties developed in sixteen cases although only two divorces resulted.[68]

Wolfensberger, on the other hand, reviewed the literature and concluded that there is no strong evidence that marital difficulties are more frequent among the parents of the retarded than among the general population. Such problems are not, it should be noted, infrequent occurrences. Moreover, broken and unstable families are usually presented as a cause of retardation and maladjustment rather than as an effect of retardation.[69] Wolfensberger cites several authors who concluded that poor family adjustment was not caused by the retarded child, but was symptomatic of existing problems which were displaced to the child. He also cited studies which suggested that instead of causing family instability a retarded child tended to pull the family together as they mobilized their efforts to deal with a common problem. It was also noted that the birth of a retarded child tended to reduce family size, because of the fear of additional retarded children and perhaps because of the financial burden of caring for the existing child.

A retarded child may also place a severe financial strain on the family, especially if placed in a private facility or if the mother is unable to work. In extreme cases normal siblings may even be compelled to forgo advanced education.

[67] All statistics used in this section are from Bernard D. Karpinos, *Results of Examination of Youths for Military Service, 1968. Supplement to Health of the Army*, June 1969, Medical Statistics Agency, Office of the Surgeon General, Department of the Army.

[68] Betty V. Graliker and Richard Koch, "A Study of Factors Influencing Placement of Retarded Children in a State Residential Institution," *American Journal of Mental Deficiency* (January 1965): 555.

[69] Wolfensberger, "Counseling the Parents of the Retarded," pp. 329–400.

Marriage among retardates. Table 43 summarizes the marital status of the retarded as reported by the Fairbank, Baller, Kennedy, and Saenger studies.

The following observations are made:

1) Among the mildly retarded, about three-fourths of the males and three-fifths of the females are married and living with their spouses as they approach middle age.

2) Baller and Kennedy reported that female retardates are less likely to be married as mature adults than male retardates. Apparently, although the number of cases in these studies are too few to be conclusive, female retardates have more difficulty in finding a spouse, are more prone to divorce, and probably are more likely to have a deceased spouse.[70]

3) During youth, female retardates are more likely to be married than male retardates. It is doubtful, however, if this has any particular significance. In the general population, women under 35 are more likely to be married and over 35 are less likely to be married than men.

4) Kennedy reported that retardates of both sexes were more likely to be married, less likely to have been divorced (the major cause of retardates being in the "other" category), and slightly less likely to have never married than the subjects of the Baller study. This may reflect the influence of a slightly higher level of intellectual functioning by the subjects of the Kennedy study. (Note the high proportion of married subjects in the Baller middle group.) In addition, the lower divorce rate in the Kennedy study may be due to cultural differences between the two groups—three-fourths of the Kennedy subjects professed to be Roman Catholics.[71]

5) Baller reported unusually high divorce rates among the retarded, with 24% of the men and 30% of the women in the low group being divorced, as compared to 7% and 6% among the middle group, and 8% (combined percentage for males and females) in the high group. Unusually high divorce rates were not apparent in the Kennedy study.

Children of the retarded. The fear that persons of limited intelligence will engulf the population with an avalanche of children is not supported by the facts. Kennedy reported almost identical procreation rates between controls and retardates of both sexes who had married. The Baller and Fairbank studies reported a similar finding for male retardates, although female retardates had considerably more children than the controls. Little can be inferred from the Baller and Fairbank

---

[70] Undoubtedly a result of the tendency of women to marry men older than themselves and the higher mortality among males.

[71] Goldstein, "Social and Occupational Adjustment," p. 241.

Table 43.   Marital status of retardates as reported in selected follow-up
studies

Name of study and characteristics of retardates	Married, living with husband	Never married	Other	Number of children divided by number of retardates ever married
Fairbank study				
Subjects: Males	50.0%	33.3%	16.7%	1.1
Females	70.0	4.0	26.0	1.8
Controls: Males	50.0	47.5	2.5	1.2
Females	50.0	38.0	12.0	1.2
Kennedy study				
1948				
Subjects: Males	44.7	52.8	2.5	1.3
Females	54.6	41.2	4.2	1.6
Controls: Males	40.0	58.8	1.2	1.4
Females	49.0	49.0	2.0	1.5
1960				
Subjects: Males	81.7	13.0	5.3	2.1
Females	73.4	15.6	11.0	2.1
Controls: Males	83.7	9.1	7.2	2.1
Females	80.9	10.6	8.5	2.2
Baller study				
1935				
Subjects: Males	33.3	n/a	n/a	1.3
Females	58.9	n/a	n/a	1.4
Controls: Males	52.4	n/a	n/a	1.3
Females	59.0	n/a	n/a	0.7
1951				
Subjects: Males	72.6	21.9	5.5	2.0
Females	58.0	22.9	19.1	2.4
1964				
Subjects: Males	71.2	15.2	13.6	n/a
Females	54.7	20.8	24.5	n/a
Middle group:				
Males	85.2	n/a	n/a	n/a
Females	80.7	n/a	n/a	n/a
High group (males & females combined)	90.0	n/a	n/a	n/a
Saenger study				
Males	2.0	98.0	0.0	1.0
Females	3.0	94.0	3.0	1.0

studies, since the retardates were young and the families incomplete when this information was collected. In a study of 1,016 families it was reported that the average IQ of parents with six or more children declined drastically, as compared to parents with fewer children.[72]

In sum, mildly retarded adults appear to have no fewer, but probably not significantly more, children than the average. However, the proportion of unusually large families may be above average among retardates.

In 1960 Kennedy found that the retarded were less likely than the controls to have never married. Similarly, in the above-mentioned study of 1,016 families it was found that the siblings of low-IQ parents were less often married than the siblings of high-IQ parents.

If account is taken of the below-average marriage rates of the retarded, then the number of children per retardate would be below average in the Kennedy study. Other writers have concluded that the effect of lower marriage and somewhat higher birth rates roughly offset each other.

A more important consequence of mental retardation among parents is the catastrophic effects it may have on the intellectual development of their children. Here we rely on the reported results of the 1960 Kennedy study. These subjects were relatively well-adjusted in that they had relatively high rates of employment, earnings, marriage, and marital stability. Nevertheless, they were two and one-half times more likely to have a child with an IQ below 75 than the controls (4.3% to 1.7%), and four times as likely to have a child with an IQ below 90 (23.2% to 6%). These relationships were even more pronounced among female retardates (who presumably had the primary responsibility for the care of their children), the comparable ratios being 3.8 to 1 and 5.4 to 1. Similarly, the proportion of children of retarded parents who failed to advance one grade per year was twice as high as among the children of the control parents (24.2% to 12.0%), and when the comparison was restricted to female parents the comparable ratio was almost three to one (32.5% to 11.8%).

Kennedy grouped the children according to three IQ levels (less than 90, 90 to 110, and 111 and over). Even within these IQ ranges the subject children were more likely to be academically retarded than control children. Thus, poor environment may depress IQ and then further depress academic achievement through failure to inculcate in students attitudes and work habits conducive to academic progress.

[72] Sheldon C. Reed, Elizabeth W. Reed, and James V. Higgins, "The Relationship of Human Welfare to Marriage Selection," *Journal of Heredity* (July–August 1962): 154–55.

SOCIAL COST OF MENTAL RETARDATION

The effects of mental retardation are numerous, diverse, and in many cases severe. Economists occasionally refer to these effects as indirect costs (as opposed to the direct costs of care and treatment). This is grossly misleading. There is nothing indirect about the effects of mental retardation on the people most concerned—the retarded and their families.

The social cost of mental retardation is defined as the increase in well-being that would occur if the retarded had the same level of vocational and social attainment and required the same developmental expenditures as the general population. In principle, it is the sum of the "excess cost" of services provided to the retarded and the effects of mental retardation. In practice, we are unable to measure and place a quantitative value on all the costs and effects of mental retardation. Any estimate that is derived is, therefore, a *partial* estimate.

Our estimate is comprised of the "excess cost" of services derived in the preceding chapter and the estimates of the loss of earnings, homemaking services, and other unpaid work that were developed in this chapter. In 1968 this estimate is $5.6 billion or $5.9 billion, depending upon whether one wishes to include current research, training, and construction expenses. In 1970 these estimates had risen to $6.7 billion and $7 billion.

A large part of this cost was borne by the general population, largely through increased taxes. About 25% of the earnings loss would have been used to pay taxes to federal, state, and local governments (approximately the ratio of total tax receipts to all levels of government to national income). Presumably, this tax loss must be compensated for by higher taxes on the general population. To this must be added income maintenance payments ($264 million in 1968, $365 million in 1970) which are financed by tax payments, to estimate the portion of this part of the loss of productivity among the retarded borne by the general population—about $1.184 billion in 1968 and $1.401 billion in 1970.

Earlier, we estimated that over 95% of the costs of services were paid by persons other than the retarded or their families. Applying this percentage to the "excess cost" of retardation services (excluding research, training, and construction funds) and adding 100% of the cost of research, training, and construction yields a total of $1.533 billion in 1968 and $2.081 billion in 1970 of excess costs of mental retardation services that must be borne by the general population.

Adding these two figures together indicates that the general population bore $2.7 billion of the social cost of mental retardation in 1968 and $3.5 billion in 1970. In 1970 exactly one-half of the social cost of mental retardation was borne by the general population. This distribution of cost would be sharply altered if it were possible to derive a measure of *total* social cost. Psychic costs are borne almost entirely by the retarded and their families.

	1968	1970
	(in 000,000's)	
Loss of earnings	$3,680	$4,142
Loss of homemaking services	380	424
Loss of other unpaid work	250	276
Excess cost of retardation services		
(excluding research, construction, and training)	1,319	1,835
Research, construction, and training	280	338
Total social cost of mental retardation	$5,909	$7,015

This measure of the social cost of mental retardation must be interpreted and used cautiously. It includes the effects of all factors which inhibit the productivity of the retarded and create service needs—physical handicaps, emotional handicaps, unstable families, etc., and not the effects of intellectual deficiency alone. In addition, it includes the effect of errors in our assumptions and measurements. There is no way to disentangle these effects, especially since it is often the *combination* of employment impediments which create major problems.

It measures loss of earnings only among living retardates. Many retardates die prematurely, so that the loss of output due to retardation is greater than estimated.

Our dissatisfaction with the concept of "excess costs" of services was expressed in the previous chapter. "Excess costs" were only about one-half of the developmental expenditures on the retarded.

The concept of social cost assumes that mental retardation is abnormal. But it is, in fact, quite normal for human intelligence to vary over a broad range. Computing social cost for this group does not measure the cost of an abnormal condition, but the consequence of normal genetic variation in intelligence. One could just as well measure the social cost of persons with IQs between 70 and 80, or 80 and 90. We would hardly want to infer that there is a cost only if IQ falls below an arbitrarily designated threshold, especially since environmental circumstances may have a depressing effect on IQ along the entire intellectual spectrum.

In the case of brain-damaged retardates, it is more correct to say that we are measuring the cost of the agent causing the damage rather than of retardation.

An estimate of the social cost of mental retardation cannot be used to justify expanding programs for the retarded. Increased efforts are justified only if it can be shown that they will generate benefits that exceed their costs.

The major uses of a measure of social cost are to describe the scope and dimensions of the problem—i.e., what types of costs are being incurred, who bears the burden, and what is being done about it—and so to stress the importance of seeking ways of reducing these costs.

At least two-thirds, and probably more, of the increase in the social cost of retardation between 1968 and 1970 can be attributed to rising prices rather than increased or improved care.

SUMMARY

1. Mental retardation has many adverse effects. They were classified as: (a) loss of productive capacity, which includes remunerated work, homemaking, other unpaid work, and use of leisure time; (b) illegal and undesirable behavior and accidents; (c) psychic effects; and (d) other effects. The extent of these effects will vary immensely among retardates.

2. All effects of mental retardation are measurable, although they cannot be expressed in terms of a common *numeraire*.

3. If institutionalized and noninstitutionalized retardates had the same employment and earnings rates as their noninstitutionalized age, sex, and race counterparts in 1967, total output would have increased by $4.1 billion in 1970.

4. Loss of homemaking and other unpaid work in 1970 was estimated at about $0.7 billion.

5. A partial estimate of the social cost of mental retardation in 1970 was $7 billion. This included the productivity losses among retardates and the excess costs of services and represents the increase in well-being that would occur if the retarded had the same level of vocational and social attainment as the general population.

6. An estimated 87% of mildly retarded adult males are employed, a rate that is only 4 percentage points below that of males in the general population. Their earnings were estimated at 86% of the average. An estimated 33% of mildly retarded females are working at wages that are

87% of average. The estimated employment rate was 12 percentage points below females in the general population, which is explainable by the greater tendency of mildly retarded females to be full-time home-makers.

7. Among persons with IQs between 40 and 50, an estimated 45% of the males and 12% of the females are employed at wages that are 19% of the average. Very few retardates with IQs below 40 are employed.

8. Intellectual deficiency alone does not cause vocational failure among retardates with IQs above 40. When vocational failure occurs, it is usually associated with other impediments to employment, such as adverse attitudes toward work, physical or emotional disabilities, job discrimination, etc.

9. Although the great majority of retardates commit no serious crimes, youthful mildly retarded adults apparently violate the law about twice as often as their nonretarded counterparts and the crimes they commit are more serious.

10. The psychic effects of mental retardation are large—perhaps more important than all other effects combined. Among these effects are the sorrow felt by retarded parents, shame felt by siblings, and loneliness felt by the retarded.

11. Most mildly retarded adults marry, although the rate of marriage appears a little below average. Very few persons with IQs below 50 marry.

12. Children of retarded parents tend to be behind the children of the nonretarded intellectually and academically. Apparently this is due to adverse environmental circumstances.

VI

Benefit-Cost Analysis

THEORETICAL CONSIDERATIONS

Introductory remarks. In benefit-cost analysis we compare the improvement in the well-being of people that results from a particular program with its cost, or we compare the differences in the improvement in well-being that results from various programs with the differences in the costs of these programs. In this section we will examine basic principles and techniques that must be understood to effectively utilize this tool. In many cases the theory will be far more sophisticated than our subsequent empirical discussion.

Benefit-cost considerations are crucial to decisionmaking. No decision on the use of resources should ever be made without some estimate, even if crude and subjective, of benefits and costs over time. Ultimately, benefit-cost considerations are the basis for determining whether a particular project should be adopted, how large it should be, and the composition of the resources that are utilized.

Clearly, the first step is to identify the relevant decision unit or units to be evaluated. It almost always is a service—educational, vocational rehabilitation, etc. In some cases we can evaluate a specific subset of the population receiving such services (e.g., mentally retarded rehabilitants). In other cases the entire service must be evaluated, since the efficiency of the service itself may be dependent upon having a number of different types of people (e.g., sheltered workshops that serve persons with various types of disabilities).

241

In principle, benefits are interpreted broadly to include any change in well-being. Sometimes these changes are negative, as when returning an institutionalized retardate to the community will create hardships on his family.

Costs are the value of the resources that would be available for alternative uses if a service was not provided.

There is a close conceptual relationship between the "cost" of mental retardation, discussed in the previous chapter, and a benefit-cost analysis of programs. These programs, if worthwhile, will reduce the effects (indirect costs) of mental retardation by more than they increase the direct costs.

The benefits used in benefit-cost analysis of mental retardation programs are in most cases a mirror image of the effects of retardation. The relevant costs, however, are developmental costs, and *not* "excess" costs, since we are concerned with all resources used to support a program.

Discounting. In benefit-cost analysis all future benefits and costs must be discounted to present value. Present value refers to the price that people would be willing to pay today for a future benefit, or, alternatively, it refers to how much they must set aside today to meet a future cost. For example, if the benefit was a $1.05 increase in earnings one year hence, and the rate of discount was 5%, then the present value would be $1.00 (since $1.00 placed in the bank would be worth $1.05 one year hence).

In general, a present benefit of P will be worth $P(1 + r)^n$ n years in the future (r is the rate of interest). Algebraic manipulation shows that a future benefit Pn will be worth $Pn/(1 + r)^n$ today. A stream of future benefits, therefore, has a present value (PV) of:

$$PV = \frac{P_1}{1 + r} + \frac{P_2}{(1 + r)^2} + \cdots + \frac{P_n}{(1 + r)^n}$$

Marginal analysis. Decisions to spend on people are always marginal where we compare the increase in benefits (marginal benefits) with the increase in costs (marginal costs). Several points need to be made.

1) Marginal benefits and marginal costs should not be confused with average benefits or average costs. Marginal values refer to the changes that occur when the services provided by a program are increased or decreased slightly.

2) Marginal costs are usually greater than average costs, and marginal benefits are usually less than average benefits. This is because

project directors usually select the most promising cases for services. As programs expand and more difficult cases are selected, marginal costs will rise, pulling up average costs, and marginal benefits will fall, pulling down average benefits. In consequence, we cannot always forecast the effect of expanding a program by its past performance. This is not always true. If services tend to be on a first come, first served basis, or if services have not been available to large groups because of geographic location or conditions of eligibility, then the past may well be predictive of the future. In addition, there are special situations when the general statement concerning the relationship between marginal and average values must be modified.

3) The determination of which costs are marginal must be made on a case-by-case basis. When services are first initiated, even construction costs are marginal. Once the facility is established, however, these costs become fixed and no longer relevant in decisions to increase the number of people served in a given facility, unless the facility itself must be expanded.

Need for ranking projects. In order to use benefit-cost analysis to determine the optimal allocation of resources, various spending opportunities must be ranked in order of their contribution to people's well-being. There are two reasons for this.

In many cases one spending opportunity will preclude the other. A new institution for the retarded may be located in any *one* of *many* different sites, or, to take another example, a retarded person may be trained for any *one* of several different vocational pursuits. In addition, more programs have been proposed for the mentally retarded than can be funded. We must select the best of these.

Methods of comparing benefits and costs. Three basic approaches to benefit-cost analysis may be distinguished: (1) comparison of a program with the alternative of no program; (2) comparison of programs with benefit-cost analyses of each program carried out against the alternative of no program and then compared with each other; and (3) comparison of the differential benefits and costs of programs. The third approach is usually termed "cost-effectiveness" analysis and will be dealt with in greater depth in the next chapter. However, much of the discussion in this chapter is relevant to this third approach and there will be frequent references to it, although the emphasis is on the first two approaches.

In general the third approach determines whether one program is superior to another, but does not make an overall determination of whether either program is worthwhile. The advantage of the third approach is its greater simplicity for many purposes, as will be noted.

The first approach is "classic" benefit-cost analysis, which determines whether a program is worthwhile. It does not, however, determine whether a particular program is the best of the possible alternative programs.

The second approach combines the function of both the first and third approaches—it determines which programs are socially desirable and which of alternative programs have the greatest return. The second approach is, as one would expect, the most difficult to implement. The most important of the procedural methods that have been used to compare the benefits and costs of programs will be described in this section. Each of these approaches will be presented as if a program were being compared with the alternative of no program; then these approaches will be evaluated on the basis of their reliability in comparing the benefits and costs of analyses carried out for different programs, i.e., the second of the three basic approaches to benefit-cost analysis described above.

The following discussion does not distinguish between whether we are considering an evaluation of the entire program (which would yield the average benefit-cost ratio) or a change in the program (which would yield the marginal benefit-cost ratio). However, the procedures would be identical in either case. As a practical matter, most empirical benefit-cost analyses have been of entire programs. From a decision-making standpoint, however, it is the marginal benefit-cost ratio which must be greater than "1" to justify expanding a program and which must be compared with the marginal benefit-cost ratios of other programs to ascertain which should be expanded.

1) The total net benefits approach measures the present value of total benefits minus the present value of total costs. If,

V =   total net benefits,

b_i =   benefits in the ith year.

c_i =   costs in the ith year,

r =   the rate of discount,

n =   the number of years over which benefits will be received,

m =   the number of years over which costs will be incurred,

then, this approach can be represented symbolically as follows:

$$V = \sum_{i=m+1}^{n} \left(\frac{b_{m+1}}{(1+r)^{m+1}} + \cdots + \frac{b_n}{(1+r)^n} \right)$$

$$- \sum_{i=1}^{m} c_o + \left(\frac{c_1}{1+r} + \cdots + \frac{c_m}{(1+r)^m} \right).$$

2) The benefit-cost ratio approach divides the present value of total benefits by the present value of total costs. If,

$$g \quad = \quad \text{the benefit-cost ratio}$$

$$g = \frac{\displaystyle\sum_{i=m+1}^{n} \frac{b_{m+1}}{(1+r)^{m+1}} + \cdots + \frac{b_n}{(1+r)^n}}{\displaystyle\sum_{i=1}^{m} c_o + \frac{c_1}{1+r} + \cdots + \frac{c_m}{(1+r)^m}}.$$

The benefit-cost ratio approach shows the average benefits for each dollar spent.

3) The internal-rate-of-return approach determines the rate of discount that equates the value of a stream of benefits to the present value of cost. If,

$$s \quad = \quad \text{the internal rate of return}$$

then

$$c_o + \frac{C_1}{1+r} + \cdots + \frac{C_m}{(1+r)^m}$$

$$= \frac{b_{m+1}}{(1+s)^{m+1}} + \cdots + \frac{b_n}{(1+s)^n},$$

where all variables but s are predetermined. In effect, s represents the rate of return on invested capital.

This formulation of the internal-rate-of-return approach differs from the usual one in that costs are discounted to present value by r, the market rate of discount, rather than s, the internal rate of return, as is usually done. This is because we feel that investment costs should be discounted by the rate at which capital funds can be obtained, rather than the subsequent rate of return on these funds. If borrowing occurs, it will be at the former rate. It has the further advantage that the present value of costs in the internal-rate-of-return approach will be identical to that used in the benefit-cost ratio approach.

The effect of this alteration, when s is greater than r (as it must be if the investment is worthwhile), is to increase the present value of costs (since the rate of discount of these costs is less), and consequently to decrease s (since benefits will have to be discounted at a lower rate in order to equal the present value of costs). In a few cases this may affect the relative ranking of spending opportunities.

EXAMPLE 1

Project	Costs			Benefits		
	Year 0	Year 1	Year 2	Year 3	Year 4	Year 5
X	100	110	121	133.10	146.41	161.05
Y	300	0	0	133.10	146.41	161.05

In example 1 the internal rate of return would be 10% for both projects if both costs and benefits were discounted by the internal rate of return. If costs are discounted at 6%, however, the internal rate of return would still be 10% for project Y, but it would fall to 8.9% for project X. This is because the present value of the cost of investment for project X in year 0 would be \$311.45, which can be described as the amount that would have to be set aside in year 0 in order to fund the project for the next two years.

4) The payback-period approach shows the number of months or years required before the accumulated present value of benefits will equal the present value of costs. If,

$$p \;=\; \text{the payback period,}$$

then:

$$1 \;=\; \frac{C_o + \dfrac{C_1}{1 + r} + \cdots + \dfrac{C_m}{(1 + r)^m}}{\dfrac{b_m}{(1 + r)^m} + \cdots + \dfrac{b_p}{(1 + r)^p}}\,.$$

For purposes of ranking alternative projects, the *payback-period approach* is of limited value. It can be used to rank projects only by the shortness of the payback period. But this is clearly prejudicial in favor of projects with immediate benefits, as opposed to those with a longer gestation period, and could lead to absurd results.

EXAMPLE 2

Project	Cost	Benefit Year 1	Year 2
X	100	106.00	0
Y	100	0	224.72

In example 2 the payback period for project X is one year, while that for project Y is approximately one and one-half years (assuming the benefit is spread evenly throughout the year). Yet assuming a discount rate of 6%, project Y has a present value twice that of project X ($106.00/106 = 100$; $224.72/(1.06)^2 = 200$). The advantage of the payback-period approach is that it requires less information than the other approaches, since future benefits need be known only for as long as it takes them to equal costs.

The problem with the total-net-benefits approach is that it fails to take account of the effect of the size of the investment. In example 3 it is preferable to fund *two* project Y's, where for the same use of resources total net benefits would be 80% higher, rather than one project Y, even though the total net benefits of project X are greater than the total net benefits of a single project Y.

EXAMPLE 3

Project	Cost	Benefit Year 1	Year 2	Present value of benefits (discounted at 6%)	Benefits less cost
X	100	60.00	72.00	120.67	20.67
Y	50	32.50	42.50	68.26	18.26

By computing the return for each dollar of cost, the benefit-cost ratio adjusts for differences in size of expenditure, but may lead to misleading results because it does not take account of the length of time that benefits will be received.

EXAMPLE 4

Project	Cost	Benefit Year 1	Year 2	Present value of benefits (discounted at 6%)	Benefit-cost ratio
X	100	0	118.81	105.74	1.06
Y	100	110.00	0	103.77	1.04

If in example 4 the benefits of project Y at the end of the first year were reinvested for another year at the same rate of return (10%), then the total benefits for the sacrifice of 100 for two years would be 121.00, the benefit-cost ratio would be 1.08, and this project would clearly be superior to project X, despite the fact that the benefit-cost ratio for project X is greater than for a single project Y.

The internal-rate-of-return approach calculates the average net *yearly* percentage return per dòllar of cost, and will not be affected by differences in the number of years over which benefits will be realized or the size of the original expenditure. However, it also can be misleading because of failure to take account of differences in the rate of capital recovery.

EXAMPLE 5

Project	Cost	Benefit		Internal rate of return	Present value of benefits (discounted at 6%)	Benefit-cost ratio
		Year 1	Year 2			
X	100	55.00	60.50	10%	105.73	1.06
Y	100	0	119.90	9.5%	106.71	1.07

The internal-rate-of-return approach indicates that project X is superior to project Y in example 5, although the benefit-cost-ratio approach comes to the opposite conclusion. The difficulty is that almost half of the cost of the original investment in project X was recovered in the first year. The problems caused by differences in the rate of capital recovery and differences in the time span over which benefits will be received, both reflect the fact that capital investment is not being uniformly employed over the same time span. The differences between the benefit-cost-ratio and the internal-rate-of-return approaches could be resolved if all benefits of all projects were reinvested in such a way that all projects would terminate simultaneously. In the last example, if the 55.00 benefit of project X in the first period were reinvested at 10%, the total benefit at the end of year 2 would be 121.00. The internal rate of return would still be 10%, but the benefit-cost ratio would rise to 1.08 and both approaches would rank project X ahead of project Y.

Which of these two sometimes contradictory approaches should decision makers rely on? The key to the matter is whether or not benefits can be reinvested. In the business world almost all net revenues are returned to the spending agent and are available to be reinvested. Thus, the internal-rate-of-return approach is probably the most relevant.

When spending on people, however, the reverse is true. Whether received as earnings or in some other form, most benefits are used for consumption. Thus, the benefit-cost-ratio approach is the more relevant and will be utilized in our subsequent analysis.

This discussion assumes considerable relevance when it is noted that decisions based on the rate-of-return approach would tend to favor projects serving older people, and decisions based on the benefit-cost-ratio approach would favor projects serving younger people.[1]

A definitional problem. In some projects both benefits and costs occur in the same period.

EXAMPLE 6

	Cost		Benefits	
Project	Year 0	Year 1	Year 1	Year 2
X	100	0	55.00	60.50
Y	100	106	161.00	60.50

In example 6 the internal rate of return for project X is 10% and the benefit-cost ratio (using a discount rate of 6%) is 1.06; for project Y the comparable figures are slightly over 9% and 1.03. Yet the *net* cash outlay is identical in all three years for these projects.

Is there any reason to prefer project X to project Y? If the entire 200 had to be committed at the onset of project Y, and there were to be no reinvestment of benefits, two project Xs are better than one project Y, since the former would yield total undiscounted benefits of 232, while the latter would yield equivalent benefits of only 221.50. But if the 106 cost in year 1 could be paid out of the benefits of year 1, there would be no basis for choosing between the two projects. Since, in most cases, physical resources that are needed for investments do not need to be purchased until near the time of use, the second possibility appears to be the more relevant one.

In most cases, therefore, when benefits and costs occur in the same year, they should be considered on a net basis rather than considered separately. In effect, costs are considered negative benefits.

How do we treat the cases where costs are greater than benefits? As long as these losses occur before any net benefits are realized it is probably best to consider the net loss as part of the initial expenditure.

If they occur in the middle or at the end of a benefit stream, they probably should be considered as negative benefits and subtracted from

---

[1] The benefit-cost ratio approach would accumulate benefits over the working lifetime of people, clearly favoring the young, while the rate-of-return approach gives the average annual return over the years worked, which would favor older people nearing the peak of their earnings potential.

the benefits stream rather than added to costs. These are the reasons why our formulae represented all costs as occurring in the first m periods and all benefits as occurring in the $m + 1$ to n periods.

In some cases, however, it may not be desirable to net out benefits and costs. In an earlier evaluation of the vocational rehabilitation program, for example, I added the cost of "repeat" rehabilitations to the cost of the original rehabilitation rather than subtracting this cost from the increased earnings of clients. The reasons for doing so were that: (1) the subsequent costs were usually not paid for out of increased earnings; (2) costs were defined as the resources that society would save if the rehabilitation program did not exist; and (3) the program was being compared with the alternative of no program rather than with other programs. If comparisons were being made between programs, however, it would be preferable to net out the costs of subsequent rehabilitations against the benefits of the original rehabilitation.

There is no "absolutely right" way of handling the costs of "repeat" rehabilitations. The problem illustrates the difficulties of benefit-cost analysis and shows how the same data might be differently treated for different purposes.[2]

How does the distinction between gross benefits and costs and net benefits affect the four approaches to benefit-cost analysis? It is of no importance to the payback period or total-net-benefit approaches, since in neither case does the end result depend upon whether a particular item is counted as a cost or a negative benefit.

It becomes extremely important for the benefit-cost ratio and rate-of-return approaches, since benefits are often considerably greater than costs. Counting an item as a negative benefit and subtracting it from the numerator will result in a higher benefit-cost ratio than if it is counted as a cost and added to the denominator. Similarly, the way an item is treated will effect the rate of return.[3]

Conceptually, the distinction between the "net" approach and the "gross" approach to measuring benefits and costs is that the net approach measures the increase in well-being resulting from an initial

[2] I am not certain which procedure is preferable for an evaluation of the rehabilitation program.

[3] A unique problem of the rate-of-return approach is that "if there are any negative terms after the first positive one, an attempt to solve this sequence for its implied over-all rate of return may give multiple solutions or no real solutions." (Martin J. Bailey, "Formal Criteria for Investment Decisions," *Journal of Political Economy* [October 1959]: 477). This, of course, occurs only if subsequent costs are treated as negative benefits. And it can be avoided if some way of offsetting these negative benefits with positive net benefits that exist before or after the negative benefit is devised. Of course, there may be unusual situations where this is not possible, but they are rare.

sacrifice of well-being while the "gross" approach compares the total benefits resulting from the total resources employed by a project. A similar problem occurs when the provision of one type of service (e.g., education) may lead to a decrease in the provision of another type of service (e.g., institutional care). Usually savings in other treatment costs are treated as a benefit and added to the numerator in benefit-cost calculations. This procedure is correct if (1) we are evaluating a program independently of any other program and are primarily concerned with identifying all of its favorable effects, or (2) if these programmatic savings occur in years subsequent to those of the service being evaluated (thus we can treat this case in a fashion parallel to that of negative benefits discussed above). However, if the savings in other program costs are concurrent with the program being evaluated, then these cost savings must be subtracted from the cost of the program being evaluated, for only the net figure would represent the increase in the use of resources caused by the program.

Maximizing well-being. The goal of resource allocation decisions is to maximize the contribution to human well-being of the use of available resources. This requires selecting those projects which provide the highest returns per dollar expended at the margin. We must consider two situations: one where one type of investment precludes another, and one where this is not the case.

Consider the second situation. Society requires both M.D.s and plumbers. Suppose training an additional M.D. generated lifetime benefits of $500,000, and training an additional plumber generated lifetime benefits of $300,000. If training costs were $100,000 and $50,000 respectively, the marginal benefit-cost ratios would be 5 and 6.

Training in both professions is justified by economic considerations. The greatest return per dollar invested, however, is for training plumbers. If resources are too limited to provide training in both occupations, training for plumbers would be the choice, based on economic principles.

In the short run, the goal of investing in people is to allocate scarce resources in such a way that the marginal benefit-cost ratios of the various ways of investing in people are roughly equal. Training additional plumbers would spread the market for their services more thinly, reducing their earnings (and the cost of training would also presumably rise). The marginal benefit-cost ratio would decline and eventually approach the corresponding ratio of training additional M.D.s. At this point, training of persons in both occupations would commence.

Suppose funds were inadequate to train enough plumbers to drive their marginal benefit-cost ratio to the level of that of training additional M.D.s. In that case, fewer physicians should be trained and the freed resources diverted to training additional plumbers, which would lower the marginal benefit-cost ratio of plumbers and raise that of physicians. This process should continue until the ratios are brought into equality.

In general, if spending in one type of training or activity offers a greater benefit-cost ratio than elsewhere, funds should be shifted to the activity with the higher ratio until the marginal benefit-cost ratios of each type of expenditure are equalized. If they are not equalized, total benefits could be increased by shifting funds from lower return services to those of higher return. Presumably, the marginal benefits of the higher return services would then fall and the marginal costs would rise, and the marginal benefits of the lower return services would rise and the marginal costs fall, until the marginal benefit-cost ratios are brought into equality.

The whole point of the matter is that dollars are invested where the greatest returns can be realized. We must avoid the common and futile effort to bolster lagging activities by pumping additional resources into them (further lowering marginal benefits and raising average costs).

The ultimate goal is to achieve a marginal benefit-cost ratio of one for the different ways of investing in people. Any ratio greater than one usually means that worthwhile spending opportunities are being forgone. In terms of the other three approaches to benefit-cost analysis, the same point is reached when marginal net benefits are zero, the marginal rate of return equals the rate of discount, or as long as there is some determinate payback period for marginal cost. Thus, as long as they are expressed in marginal terms, any one of the four approaches to benefit-cost analysis will give the same solution for the ideal ultimate allocation of resources. Differences in the approaches become critical only when we are forced to choose among competing worthwhile expenditures because funds are not adequate for both.[4]

Now consider the second situation where one investment precludes another. For example, a person may be trained as either a plumber or an M.D., but not both. If the benefit-cost ratio for training a person as a plumber were greater than the benefit-cost ratio of training a person as an M.D., would this mean that the person should be trained as a

[4] In effect, this means that socially we are allocating resources to activities with rates of return below what could be attained. One way to resolve this problem is to force a transfer of resources by increasing taxes to pay for social programs. The fact that such a solution must be attained by coercion, however, may indicate that we are using too low a rate of discount for future benefits, so that an excess of worthwhile expenditures is a statistical artifact, and in fact the pain of transferring resources would be greater than the benefits received. This brings us to the question of comparing benefits and costs among people, a topic which will be discussed

plumber. Not necessarily. In order to make this decision we must calculate the marginal benefit-cost ratio of choosing one profession over another by dividing the difference in benefits of the two professions by the difference in costs. In the case of our example, the marginal benefit-cost ratio of selecting a medical career would be $200,000/50,000 = 4$. It is this marginal benefit-cost ratio which must be compared with other spending opportunities to determine whether the person should be trained as an M.D. or a plumber.

If the benefit-cost ratio of the best alternative uses of the additional funds required to become an M.D. was greater than 4, then the person should be trained as a plumber (and the money savings used for one of the higher yielding alternative uses of funds); if it was less than 4 then he should be trained as an M.D.

This distinction between the relevant marginal benefit-cost ratios, when investments are mutually exclusive and when they are not, and, in this case, between the relevant decisionmaking criteria for the individual and for society is crucial to an understanding of benefit-cost analysis.

It should be emphasized that benefit-cost ratios for the same training or activity will differ among people because of differences in talents and inclinations. In principle, this requires the evaluation of the relative benefits and costs of preparing for many different occupations for each person. One could visualize a theoretical situation where for a given level of costs, the different benefits associated with different ways of using these resources were ranked. As costs increased, it can be assumed that the highest level of benefits attainable will also increase. For each increase in costs, the change in benefits for the best possible use of the funds could be estimated and the resulting marginal benefit-cost ratios calculated. In practice, few people have a clear picture of more than a few of these differences when choosing a career. However, when the differences become sufficiently large, they do make a difference in people's choices.

For mutually exclusive investments, we can envisage the same type of short- and long-run optimizing criteria as in the case of nonexclusive investments. In the long run, individuals would prepare for occupations where their marginal benefit-cost ratio equaled one—i.e., where the increase in benefits just equaled the increase in costs. In the short run, the

---

below. It is worth emphasizing, however, that each individual may have a different viewpoint on the extent to which we are sacrificing worthwhile investments, and that this difference in part reflects differences in the degree of concern and responsibility felt for other members of society, as well as differences in the assessment of the gains to be achieved from these activities.

marginal benefit-cost ratio for persons considering one form of training over another should equal the marginal benefit-cost ratio established throughout society, assuming that there are inadequate resources to drive this ratio down to one.

Our earlier example is obviously a disequilibrium situation. Additional investment in the training of plumbers will reduce the marginal benefit-cost ratio for that occupation to 5, at which time the marginal benefit-cost ratio for both occupations and between these occupations would be equal. Unless additional resources were available this would represent a short-term equilibrium.

Because the marginal benefit-cost schedule would differ for each person, there would be a distribution of persons among different occupations. Market forces would correct deviations from an optimal distribution of the populace among occupations. If these criteria for maximizing well-being operated perfectly, the optimal number of persons in each occupation and the most economically suitable occupation for which each person should train would be determined. Any deviations from this equilibrium would automatically establish pressures to return society to the equilibrium point.

It should be stressed that the term "marginal benefit-cost ratio" has different meanings in different contexts. In the preceding comments it was used in two different ways. In one case we referred to the marginal benefit-cost ratio of training an additional M.D., where we were considering the total cost of training an additional person in each profession, as compared to total subsequent benefits. In the other case, we used the term to refer to the increased benefits resulting from the differential use of resources involved in training a person as an M.D. rather than as a plumber. The same type of analysis would be required if we were considering different ways of providing educational services to the retarded, or different ways of creating employment opportunities, each of which involves mutually exclusive alternatives.

The distinction between mutually exclusive and nonmutually exclusive investments forced us into using benefit-cost ratios based on differences in benefits and costs. However, these ratios were used in a way that required prior knowledge of marginal benefits and costs for each occupation. Our discussion of analyses of investments using the "difference" method in Chapter 7 will not be restricted to mutually exclusive investments, nor will it require prior knowledge of benefits and costs for each program.

It may be surprising to some that our criterion for maximizing well-being does not always maximize well-being for each individual. In our example we might not prepare a person as an M.D. even though the marginal benefit-cost ratio is extremely favorable. This is because of limited resources. Society may prefer to train one person as a plumber and one as an M.D. Because of limited resources, however, the choice may be between training two plumbers or one M.D. The first alternative will often be the preferable one.

Special situations. There are several situations where allocation of resources might not be guided strictly by benefit-cost evaluations of projects. One such situation would be the "once chance only" project that must be made at a particular time. It may be justifiable to invest in "one chance only" projects and forgo investments that offer higher rates of return but which are deferable. Medical conditions which will progress to more severe disabilities are a common situation where this could occur.

Still another such situation arises when rates of return vary over time. Then we must ascertain the combination of spending opportunities over time that yield the highest return, an exceedingly complex problem,[5] especially if rates of capital recovery differ over time.

Problems of measurement. In this section we will describe some of the major empirical difficulties in benefit-cost analysis.

The Approach. In benefit-cost analysis, we often seek to compare what happens if services are rendered with what would happen if services were not rendered.[6] There is, unfortunately, no method by which we can make a direct comparison, since one state of affairs obviously precludes the other.

Three methods have been used to estimate the effects of services provided to people. One is to compare two groups of individuals, one of which receives services and one of which does not ("with and without" studies). Another is to compare the social adjustment of people before and after services are rendered ("before and after" studies). Finally, it is sometimes *inferred* that the social adjustment of people is due to the provision of a particular service (e.g., relating differences in earnings among adults to differences in educational attainments). The validity of "with and without" studies depends upon the selection of a control

---

[5] Bailey, "Formal Criteria for Investment Decisions," pp. 476–88.

[6] The importance of being rigorous about this requirement can be illustrated by my earlier work on vocational rehabilitation. It is sometimes asserted that it is less economically beneficial to serve clients with low earnings at closure than those with higher earnings. However, clients with the lowest earnings at closure also tended to have the lowest earnings at acceptance and the lowest costs of services, so that increased earnings per case service dollar tended to be about as high for less productive rehabilitants as for the more productive. From the standpoint of economic efficiency, it appeared as worthwhile to serve low productivity clients as high productivity clients (R. Conley, *The Economics of Vocational Rehabilitation* [Baltimore: The Johns Hopkins Press, 1965], pp. 108–22).

group that is similar to the treatment group in every respect, except for the provision of services. This requirement can rarely be achieved.

A rigorously defined control group would be one where people are randomly assigned to receive treatment or not receive treatment. Denial of services is rarely acceptable or even possible, since those denied will often find comparable services elsewhere. Many control groups, therefore, consist of persons who have opted not to receive services or who have been denied services. Persons who choose not to receive services sometimes do not need them and sometimes lack motivation. Persons who are denied services usually are not able to benefit from them. Because of differences between the control and treatment groups, some effort to standardize for these differences must be made.

The number of variables which affect social adjustment is large and control or treatment groups are rarely large enough to permit standardization for all of these factors. In addition, because of the combination effect of many of these variables (e.g., mental retardation and physical disability), it is sometimes necessary to adjust for combinations of variables.

Even when the sample is large and the data copious there are no variables which can unequivocally measure differences in motivation, innate ability, and opportunity. Moreover, we are not always certain which variables should be controlled. For example, marital status can be looked upon as an effect of mental retardation, or a motivational variable, or both. In the first case we should not control for this variable, in the second we should, and the last case is ambiguous.

It should be pointed out that when two programs are being compared, the problem of a control group is much easier to resolve. However, participants in programs are often selected on suitability grounds, and when such selection occurs, one group cannot be used as a control for another. A valid comparison group can be derived only by randomly assigning clients to one kind of treatment or the other.

The difficulties of obtaining a suitable control group often force researchers to rely on "before and after" studies. The assumption is that there would be no change in the client if services were not rendered. Often this is not true. (1) Such an approach is usually inapplicable in the case of young people, since they lack any experience which can be used to estimate their adult adjustment. (2) In addition, many people seek services, especially medical and vocational, in order to forestall the social maladjustment (e.g., the prospect of job loss) that they anticipate. Their pre-service adjustment will appear more satisfactory than it would be if services were not rendered. (3) Another problem is that some persons overstate social maladjustment (especially lack of earnings) in order to qualify for publicly or philanthropically provided services. (4) Finally, most adults seek vocational services only when they become unemployed. Many, if left to their own devices, would eventually have located employment.

Even when "before and after" studies may be applicable, there is the serious problem of determining the length of time prior to acceptance that is most indicative of the future adjustment of clients without special services. Too short a time period understates the capabilities of many who are seeking assistance precisely because of a sudden worsening of their social adjustment (e.g., becoming unemployed, see 4 above). Too long a time period would overstate their potential capabilities, since it would include their social adjustment prior to the onset of the circumstances which created a need for special services. Presumably, there is a period of time prior to acceptance for each program where these errors just offset each other, but we have few a priori conceptions as to how long this is.

"Before and after" studies are probably most satisfactory when used to measure the change in the physical or mental condition of the client. They are least satisfactory when used to measure changes in social adjustment. The results of "before and after" studies are usually less reliable than those of "with and without" studies. However, we are far more likely to be able to obtain the data necessary for the former form of analysis. The use of inference to determine the effect of a service would appear to be the least satisfactory of the three methods but is often the only one possible.

These are very general statements concerning the difficulty of evaluating the effects of programs. The biases that have been described are conflicting, in that some would cause an overstatement and some an understatement of program benefits. These biases will vary among benefit-cost studies and must be carefully explored and defined on a project-by-project basis. One can be assured that biases will exist in almost every case.

The problem of relating benefits to services is the Achilles' heel of benefit-cost analysis and is often used as a basis for discounting the results of these analyses. To illustrate, manpower programs have often been accused of "creaming," i.e., accepting the most promising applicants for services, many of whom might have done quite well on their own. This problem is of sufficient importance that one economist has contended "that the experience of the great majority of the trainees in the early years of MDTA. . . . is therefore of minor interest to the poverty program."[7]

---

[7] David O. Sewell, "Critique of Cost-Benefit Analyses of Training," *Monthly Labor Review* (September 1967): 48.

Benefits. The measurement of benefits is one of the unsolved problems in most evaluations of investments in people. Data is scanty. Measuring instruments are imperfect or nonexistent for many benefits. By their very nature, many benefits cannot be expressed in terms that are directly comparable.

In addition, although it is not too difficult to enumerate the main benefits of these programs, there are many ripple effects that reverberate through society and may extend many years into the future. For example, investing in the retarded will help them to become better parents, which will pay social dividends for generations. These ripple effects are not always of minor importance. Their identification and measurement is, however, usually dismissed with a helpless shrug (or a highly abstract mathematical model with no empirical content).

Costs. We must distinguish between reported program costs and social costs. Social costs are the value of those resources that would be available for other uses if a particular service were not provided. Marginal social costs refer to the change in social costs as the size of a program is changed. It is social costs or marginal social costs that are the relevant costs for benefit-cost purposes. The identification and measurement of social costs is more difficult than appears at first glance. Many of the issues here parallel the issues that were raised in our earlier discussion (Chapter IV) of the aggregate resources being devoted to the care of the retarded.

In most cases, the only cost information that is available is current program expenditures. Often these costs include consumption expenditures (food, clothing, etc.) which are not a part of social cost, since they would be provided whether the persons received the service or not. More important, however, are the following cost elements which are a part of social cost, but always, or almost always, are excluded from program costs.

1) Direct services may be received from several different sources so that costs reported by a single agency would understate the total costs of a service. Retarded children in school may go to mental retardation clinics or private practitioners for other services. Retarded adults may simultaneously receive services from employment agencies, vocational rehabilitation agencies, sheltered workshops, and other sources as well, all assisting the person to prepare for gainful employment.

2) Sometimes the persons being served, or their families, pay part of the cost of services.

3) Agencies serving people depend upon the provision of many indirect services by other agencies—fire protection, police protection, highway systems, etc. A part of the cost of providing these indirect

services should be considered as part of the cost of providing direct services. The issue becomes relevant, since public and private nonprofit agencies are usually exempted from paying property, sales, or excise taxes, which are the customary means of funding these indirect services.

In principle the correct way to handle this problem would be to add a pro-rated share of the cost of providing these services to the cost of agencies. Agencies that were not exempt from property, sales, or excise taxes would have their tax payments subtracted from their operating costs, since these taxes do not represent a use of resources that is necessary for agency operations. In most cases, however, this is an impossible statistical task. The calculations could be greatly simplified if it is assumed that the value of free government services received by agencies could be measured by the sales, excise, and property taxes paid by these agencies, or the imputed value of these taxes in the case of exempt agencies.[8] Although statistically convenient, there is little to justify such an assumption.

If the cost of these indirect services cannot be estimated, then it must be emphasized that in comparing private, profit-seeking agencies with public or private nonprofit agencies, the value of the tax exemption should either be added to the costs of the nonprofit agencies or subtracted from the costs of the profit-seeking ones. Otherwise cost differences arise that give a misleading view of the relative social costs of these programs.

4) Many agencies are at the bottom of an administrative hierarchy that includes county, city, state, regional, and federal offices. A part of the costs of higher administration should be allocated to the provision of services.

5) Many agencies utilize professionals whose training has been subsidized by private or public funds. A part of these prior training costs should be allocated to the current cost of services.

6) Similarly, most research designed to improve methods of serving people is available for public use without charge. A portion of the costs of prior research should be allocated to the current cost of services.

7) Many agencies do not pay rent for the offices and treatment facilities they use. A fair rental value composed of the implicit interest on the capital investment, depreciation, and a management fee should be charged against the current costs of services.

[8] E.g., Rudolph Blitz, "The Nation's Educational Outlay," *Economics of Higher Education*, Selma Mushkin, ed. (Washington: U.S. Department of Health, Education, and Welfare, Office of Education, 1962), p. 153.

8) Most persons receiving services must incur some transportation expense in traveling to and from the facilities where the services are provided. In the case of residential facilities, friends and relatives of the client will incur transportation costs. Such expenses are often over-looked; yet they may be crucial when evaluating alternative sites for facilities.

9) Forgone earnings are a major component of the cost of develop-mental services.[9] Mothers who elect to remain home forgo substantial earnings. Beyond elementary school, students must choose between paid employment and continued school attendance.

10) Costs must include an allowance for the possibility that serv-ices will not always achieve their goal. If total program costs are used, this does not normally become a problem, since this includes costs to both successful and unsuccessful clients. But if actual case service costs per individual are calculated, then an allowance for the risk of failure must be incorporated.

Obviously, it is difficult, and sometimes impossible, to obtain mean-ingful data on many of these cost categories; frequently they are ig-nored in evaluative studies. The importance of these cost categories will vary from study to study. Much depends upon the scope of the evalua-tive effort, since this will determine which of these cost elements will be increased if a service is provided, i.e., marginal social cost. If a proposed program change would utilize existing buildings and person-nel, the marginal costs of construction, training, and usually indirect services are zero. Larger program changes will have to consider these variables. Usually the results of past research can be considered a free resource with a zero marginal cost. If, however, an entire program, of which research is an integral part, is considered, then this variable must also be brought into the analysis, since cessation of the program would free the resources used for this purpose. In those cases where alternative programs are being evaluated, the task of measuring costs and benefits may be simplified, since it is frequently possible to make decisions by measuring only the differential benefits and costs of programs and not their total benefits and costs.

One final note. Some program budgets include expenditures for re-search, construction, and/or training. It should be clear that these ex-penditures are not part of the costs of current services but of future services and should be pro-rated accordingly. Sometimes, however,

---

[9] For example, one economist estimates that forgone earnings comprise three-fifths of the total cost of secondary and higher education in the United States. Theodore W. Schultz, *The Economic Value of Schooling* (New York: Columbia University Press, 1963), p. 29.

these costs are used as proxy variables for the portion of past research, construction, and training costs that should be allocated to the costs of current services.

Special problems. There are a number of controversial areas in benefit-cost analysis, some of which will be dealt with here.

Multiplier Effect. It is sometimes argued that increasing the earnings of workers will have a multiplier effect on output, greatly increasing the benefits that can be attributed to the original expenditure. The argument is that as these increased earnings are spent for goods and services, other workers will be hired to produce these items, and they, in turn, will spend a portion of their increased wages.

Such an argument is entirely fallacious. If the economy is operating at full employment, it is manifestly impossible to significantly increase output. If the economy is operating at less than full employment, the increase in aggregate demand is approximately counterbalanced by an increase in the aggregate supply of goods and services that these workers produce, so there is no net inducement for manufacturers to increase output. The multiplier effect assumes an autonomous increase in spending, not one that results from an increase in earnings due to greater production. Of course, one could hypothesize unlikely situations where a multiplier effect would operate, but they are of little relevance for serious benefit-cost studies.[10]

Consumption. It has been suggested that changes in consumption should be subtracted from changes in earnings to determine the net value of investing in people. In effect, this procedure measures the benefits of programs to everyone but the person the program is trying to help. It would, however, be difficult to justify a benefit-cost model that did not take full account of the improvement in well-being of the retarded.

The issue of consumption in benefit-cost analysis resolves into a question of distribution. However, rather than consider the distribution of benefits between the retarded and everyone else, the approach used in this analysis will be to consider the distribution of benefits between the retarded and their families and everyone else. From a decisionmaking standpoint this seems more relevant.

There is one situation where consumption expenditures assume more than distributional significance. Maintenance of employment may require expenditures on special clothing, tools, transportation, etc. In

---

[10] For example, one could assume that the original project was financed by deficit spending. At full employment, this would be fiscally irresponsible. At less than full employment it would be short-term and only one among many ways of achieving economic stimulation, and not necessarily the best way.

principle, these work-related expenses should be subtracted from earnings to determine the net effect of increased earnings on well-being.[11] In practice, we lack data for this refinement. Work-related expenses can be an important consideration to persons who must choose between public maintenance and marginal employment.

Technical Progress. Over time, the earnings of workers will gradually increase because of rising productivity. These increases should be considered as part of the benefits of preparing people for gainful work, even though they are independent of the efforts of the workers or the original training. If not assisted to find gainful employment, these workers would presumably be either unemployed or working on less skilled jobs with correspondingly lower productivity gains. In the former case, none of the benefits of productivity change would be realized, and in the latter case, only part would be realized.[12]

Between 1947 and 1970, output per man hour in the United States in the private sector grew at an annual rate of 3.1%. During the same period, national income per person employed increased 2.2% annually. Because of depressed conditions, these figures are somewhat lower than they would have been had 1968 been chosen as a terminal year. Many factors determine the rate of economic growth—improvements in the educational attainment of the population (including improvements in the quality of education), capital accumulation, reduction of discrimination, vacation and holiday policies, etc. Ultimately, the one crucial factor is technological change. The other factors are eventually self-limiting, since the educational attainments of the population cannot be indefinitely upgraded, discrimination will ultimately vanish, even capital could become redundant (although there appears to be considerable scope for further economic expansion through changes in these variables). Although either a higher or lower rate of economic growth is possible in the future, we will assume that it will average 2.5% per worker. This rate is a rough extrapolation of the post-World War II experience. If anything, it may be low. As will be noted below, statistical growth rates have probably understated the true growth rate of output.

[11] In not all cases by their full amount. Purchasing clothing for work may reduce expenditures on clothing for other purposes or these clothes may serve a joint purpose. It is the marginal increase in expenditures that is relevant.

[12] In some occupations, earnings will rise even though productivity does not increase (e.g., teaching). Increased earnings in these jobs are the way in which productivity gains are shared throughout the economy, are necessary to keep workers in these occupations, and represent an increasingly higher valuation of these services by the rest of society. Because of this last factor, even these increased earnings should be included in benefit-cost calculations.

Inflation. Earnings will also increase over time because of inflation-ary tendencies in the economy.[13] Increases in earnings that are due to inflationary price increases clearly do not contribute to individual well-being and are *not* a benefit in preparing people for gainful employment. Our subsequent calculations will, therefore, be expressed in terms of the prices prevailing in 1970.

It is worth noting, however, that existing methods of adjusting for price level changes over time may have the effect of understating the growth of real output—i.e., the actual increase in well-being over time. For one thing, they take inadequate account of quality change—a 1960 black and white television set is assumed to be worth no more than a 1970 one. In addition, it is assumed that there is no increase in productivity in many service occupations—government secretaries with electric typewriters are assumed to be no more efficient that they were with manual ones.

On the other hand, smog control devices are included in measures of GNP, although they should probably be considered a cost of an expand-ing economy—at least we must recognize that some production is used to rectify problems that arise and not to *add* to the total stock of *well-being.*

There is no way to take account of these conflicting influences on the growth of well-being over time in order to make an adjustment to our assumed rate of growth. It is possible that the statistical growth rate will overstate the true growth rate in the future, largely because of the effects of environmental pollution.

Determination of the Appropriate Discount Rate. The choice of dis-count rate has an important and sometimes dominating effect on the conclusions of benefit-cost analyses. The higher the rate of discount, the lower the present value of future benefits and the lower the benefit-cost ratio. This can cause projects which are worthwhile at one discount rate to have a benefit-cost ratio below the critical level of "1" at an-other. In addition, since increasing the rate of discount will have a smaller proportionate effect on the present value of the benefits of projects whose benefits are in the near future rather than spread over many years, changing the rate of discount can reverse the relative desir-ability of projects. For example, high discount rates would favor invest-ments in people who are in the prime of their working lives as opposed to the young whose best earning years are considerably in the future.

---

[13] It is generally assumed that both prices and wages are flexible upward, but rigid downward. Each new price or wage increase becomes locked in the economy until the next upward movement. Prices of goods and services are usually less rigid than wages.

The choice of discount rates is one of the most critical tasks confronting the benefit-cost analyst. There is no satisfactory method of making this choice. Various criteria for selecting a discount rate have been suggested. The most common are: (1) the rate at which people are willing to sacrifice present consumption for future consumption (time preference), usually measured by the rate of interest on long term government bonds; and (2) the expected rate of return on private investment (marginal productivity of capital).

Neither of these approaches is satisfactory for our purposes. The marginal productivity approach faces the problem that expected returns on investment vary widely, depending upon the degree of risk involved. The rate on government securities is substantially determined by federal monetary policy, so that use of this rate would cause evaluations of services to the retarded to be partly determined by short-run stabilization policy. One could, however, argue for the use of the average rate on long-term government securities over a period of time.

In any event, since tax payments are drawn from funds which would have been partly used for consumption, and partly saved, neither of the two approaches is applicable, since they do not represent what would have been the alternative use of funds. Also, some economists feel that a social rate of discount should attach more weight to the future than the private rate and therefore should be lower. Moreover, relatively few people are engaged in capital investment or in purchasing government securities and their preferences as to discounting the future may not be generally valid for the entire population. Finally, most services are financed by taxes, and the discount rate that people would use in evaluating investments on their own behalf may differ from the discount rate they would use when evaluating the payment of taxes for the purpose of spending for the benefit of others. Economists frequently argue that public programs are underfunded because benefits appear high relative to costs. The failure of society to give greater support to public programs may well be due to people discounting benefits received by others much higher than benefits received by themselves. This raises the question of whether a social rate of discount should reflect individual preference or, in some way, be independent of people's attitudes about discounting the future benefits of public programs.

A number of benefit-cost studies have used two rates of interest, partly to evaluate the sensitivity of the results to the interest rate chosen, and partly to reflect divergent views on which rate is appropriate.[14] In the subsequent analysis, we will use only one discount rate because it has the great advantage of reducing the number of calcula-

[14] Burton Weisbrod, "The Valuation of Human Capital," *Journal of Political Economy* (October 1961): 431.

tions, and because an intermediate rate probably yields results that are acceptable to more economists than rates chosen as the upper and lower bounds of acceptable discount rates.[15]

Subsequent calculations will use a discount rate of 7%. This is slightly higher than the rate which most frequently appears in the literature (6%),[16] but is probably justified in view of interest rate increases in the last few years.[17] Economists sometimes argue for a relatively high rate on the grounds that investments in people are highly risky. However, in most evaluations the risk factor is handled separately through estimates of the number of clients with which the programs will not be successful. The discount rate, therefore, should probably be on the low side. Another reason for utilizing a relatively low discount rate is that existing interest rates incorporate, to an unknown degree, societal estimates as to the future rate of inflation.

Another discounting problem. In principle, future benefits and costs should be discounted to the year in which the initial expenditure occurred. Since different services are initiated at various stages in the life cycle, this could lead to evaluations of services that are discounted to widely varying ages among retardates, including time of birth and even before. This would be cumbersome to calculate, confusing to interpret, empirically almost impossible, and would require innumerable tables.

Another problem is that if discounting is begun at a young age, the present value of future benefits will be surprisingly small and could be misleading to persons not thoroughly familiar with the interpretation of discounted data. Few persons have significant earnings before age eighteen, but the present value of a dollar eighteen years hence is low, and thirty years hence is insignificant.

The effect of discounting can lead to unexpected results. Using a discount rate of 5% and assuming an annual productivity increase of 0%, Miller and Hormouth found that the present value of the expected lifetime earnings of males in the experienced labor force increased steadily from age 18 to age 28, and did not fall below the level of 18-year-olds until age 40 (although the *undiscounted* value of lifetime earnings increased steadily after age 18).[18] Similarly, below age 18 the

[15] In this decision I have been greatly influenced by Klarman (see Herbert E. Klarman, *The Economics of Health* [New York: Columbia University Press, 1965], pp. 164–66.)

[16] Herbert E. Klarman, "Economic Aspects of Mental Health Manpower" (mimeographed), p. 33.

[17] Of course, interest rates may also decline. Since 1950 declines in interest rates have usually been less than the preceding increases.

[18] Herman P. Miller and Richard A. Hormouth, *Present Value of Lifetime Earnings*, U.S. Bureau of the Census, Technical Paper No. 16 (Washington: US GPO, 1967), p. 7.

earlier a specific service was rendered the lower would be the discounted value of future benefits and, consequently, the lower the benefit-cost ratio. Whether persons other than economists, or even economists, would be willing to allocate resources differently on the basis of such findings is dubious.

To deal with these problems, two sets of calculations will be presented in the subsequent analysis, one using a discount rate of 7% and one showing undiscounted values. In addition, age 18 will be used as a base age to which subsequent benefits and costs of providing services to the retarded will be discounted to present value. Benefits and costs incurred prior to age 18 will be compounded, i.e., multiplied by $(1.07)^{18-n}$ where n represents the age at which the benefits or costs are realized. This procedure will simplify the calculations and present a fairer perspective of the productive abilities of the retarded. Even if we cannot resolve all of the problems of discounting, this comparison of discounted and undiscounted data will give a clear view of the effects of discounting. In our subsequent work we will not present undiscounted benefit-cost ratios, since they are clearly improper. Undiscounted earnings and cost data, however, have purposes that extend beyond the calculation of benefit-cost ratios.

Although the procedure of compounding benefits and costs rather than discounting them is unorthodox, it can be shown that this procedure yields the same benefit-cost ratio as would be obtained if benefits and costs were discounted to the year of the initial expenditure. Consider the simplest case, where a single cost is incurred in year 0 and a single benefit in year n. Then, the resulting benefit-cost ratio is:

$$\frac{b/(1 + r)^n}{c}$$

Suppose that the year m (less than n) is used as the base year. Then the benefit-cost ratio under our procedure equals:

$$\frac{b/(1 + r)^{n - m}}{c(1 + r)^m}$$

which equals: $\dfrac{b/(1 + r)^{n - m} \cdot 1/(1 + r)^m}{c}$ or $\dfrac{b/(1 + r)^n}{-c}$.

In the general case where benefits and costs extend over a number of years and are variable in amount, it can also be shown, although it requires much more complicated equations, that the benefit-cost ratio is independent of the year which is chosen as a base.

Although the procedure of using age 18 as a pivotal age for discounting future earnings and costs and compounding benefits and costs incurred at an earlier age is atypical and will undoubtedly be critically appraised by some economists, it represents, I believe, the only manageable procedure for discounting future benefits when these benefits result from a variety of services provided at different ages.

Interdependence of Services. Benefit-cost studies must give some consideration to the principle of diminishing returns, which states that as increasing amounts of resources are devoted to a particular use, marginal benefits become progressively smaller. This applies on both an individual and a program basis. For example, at some point, continued special education of the retarded becomes of minor value to the adult adjustment of the individual. If special education is expanded to encompass more retarded children, greater numbers of the more severely handicapped will be enrolled, increasing costs per child and decreasing the expected level of adult adjustment.

It is the reality of diminishing returns that imposes limits on the amounts that should be invested in developmental services. As the term is being used here, it includes the increasing marginal costs of serving more severely handicapped persons, as well as the decrease in the future effects of these services. (It costs more to provide special education to the severely retarded than to the mildly retarded, and the future earnings of the severely retarded will be less.)

The principle of diminishing returns assumes that all other factors are constant. In evaluating expenditures on people this is usually not a valid inference. There is ample reason to support the assertion that the better educated in the United States also had superior diets and medical care and were given more parental and professional guidance. It can be assumed that at least part of the superior earnings position of the better educated is due to all of these factors and not to education alone.

This brings us to the crucial issue of interdependence among services to people. A single investment, such as education, may be necessary to satisfactory adult adjustment, but it is by no means sufficient. Although it is possible that a part of the total adult adjustment of a person can be attributed to a single service, it is probable that a large part depends upon the *combined* effect of numerous services.

This raises two possibilities for benefit-cost analysis of services to a defined group of people, such as the mentally retarded. We can consider a single benefit, such as earnings, and compare this benefit with the cost of all the services that are needed to generate this benefit. Or we can look at each service separately and estimate the difference in the benefits on a "with and without" basis.

The first approach runs into almost insoluble problems of what services are necessary and how they can be measured, but is the more relevant from a policy standpoint. The second approach presents the problem that if several services are evaluated, then the same benefits will be counted more than once, since each service was necessary to generate those benefits. In the second case, great care is needed in the interpretation of evaluative studies, especially since the expansion of one service, without the concurrent expansion of complementary services, may lead to disappointing results.

Redistributive problem. Most programs for the retarded are financed by taxes on the general population. This divergence between those who bear the burden of providing services and those who reap the benefits results in what may be called the redistribution problem.

From a very technical standpoint, a project cannot be said to be justified on the basis of benefit-cost analysis *unless no one* is made worse off as a result of the expenditure.[19] This is because we do not know if the utility to taxpayers of the dollars they sacrifice is less than the benefits to the recipients of the services, even though in dollar terms the latter may be larger than the former.

In many cases, the problem does not arise, since taxpayers may gain substantially from services rendered to retardates. If services are instrumental in vocational adjustment, then their tax burden will decline because of increased taxes paid by retardates, and because of a reduction in taxes needed to fund public income maintenance programs. There are many other possible ways in which taxpayers may benefit: crime and accidents may decrease, they may be less discomforted if poverty is alleviated, etc.

When the redistribution problem does arise, it can be resolved if the gainers compensate the losers. A practical example of this is loans to students in higher education, where students repay the costs of their education.

This solution must not be pushed too far in the case of the mentally retarded. Most retarded adults would be understandably reluctant to incur a large debt on the basis of a little-understood and obviously uncertain estimate of increased future productivity.

When the redistributive problem does arise, there are several grounds on which the provision of publicly provided services can be defended:

[19] And more technically, even this is not sufficient if the economy is undergoing change, since there is no assurance that after the change is made the condition that no one is worse off would still hold (see John V. Krutilla, "Welfare Aspects of Benefit-Cost Analysis," *Journal of Political Economy* (June 1961): 226–35. Such

1) In the case of education, most people will eventually pay back in support of the educational system about as much as was expended on them. This can be termed the lifetime averaging approach.

2) In the case of special groups, such as the mentally retarded, publicly provided services can be regarded as a type of social insurance, and possibly even self-insurance, against the risk of unpredictable, unpreventable, and catastrophic conditions.

3) Certain goals, among which are that all people have a right to services that will enable them to achieve social and vocational adequacy, as well as a right to a minimum standard of living, may be defined as social or collective goals.

The actual allocation of the cost burden between the public and private sector is a matter that must be socially determined for each service and often may differentiate between different people receiving that service, especially when there are differences in ability to pay. There is no right or wrong, or even optimal, method of allocating costs. This matter will be discussed further in the next chapter.

In regard to the distributive problem, it is worthwhile noting that none of us has a truly unique claim to the value of what we produce by our individual efforts. Our great wealth depends not only upon these efforts but also upon the vast store of technical knowledge, the accumulated capital goods, and the rich and fertile land to which we have fortuitously fallen heir. Few Americans could have attained their present affluence as citizens of one of the less advanced economies of the world. If, then, we owe so much to the past, perhaps we should not resent being asked to share a part of our affluence with those among us who, for reasons beyond their control, are unable to fully exploit their heritage.

General observations. Quantification of the benefits and costs of programs for the retarded present many difficulties. Lack of data, lack of comparability among existing data, measurement errors, and the necessity for arbitrary decisions on conceptually obscure issues (e.g., determination of the appropriate discount rate) combine to produce a degree of uncertainty and confusion in benefit-cost studies that most researchers find highly unsettling. It is important to keep the following observations in mind:

1) Comparisons of one benefit-cost study with another are difficult and often impossible. To begin with, error margins are uncomfortably wide. In addition, different assumptions about discount rates and other methodological considerations can cause wide variation in results.

---

esoteric considerations need not hinder the benefit-cost analyst. We accept the world as it is and adjust to change if and when necessary.

Another problem is that the composition of benefits that may be expected from different programs will vary broadly. Since many of these benefits cannot be reduced to the common denominator of dollars, there is often no objective basis for comparison.

Even when benefits can be expressed in monetary magnitudes, they are often not comparable. Small increments of income may have more meaning to the poor than larger increments of income have to the more affluent, so that we cannot always assume that those programs which result in the greatest increase in earnings make the greatest contribution to social well-being.[20]

Finally, benefit-cost analyses themselves must be interpreted differently in different contexts. Vocational rehabilitation programs usually have higher benefit-cost ratios than general educational programs. This cannot be used to urge concentration of resources in vocational rehabilitation at the expense of general education however, since the benefits of rehabilitation are themselves dependent on the prior provision of educational services.

2) Measurement problems often lead researchers to emphasize a conservative approach to empirical quantification, usually taking the form of a generous estimate of costs and a minimal estimate of benefits, and, typically, concentrating on those empirical magnitudes which can be substantiated by "hard" data. Such underestimation can be as misleading as overestimation and may have the unfortunate consequence that worthwhile programs are insufficiently funded. It is preferable to make a reasoned "best" judgment as to the most probable levels of benefits and costs rather than commit the "error" of conservatism. Footnoted qualifications are, after all, quickly forgotten, while existing numbers are misinterpreted and etched irretrievably into abbreviated summaries.

3) Because of the many limitations and uncertainties inherent in benefit-cost studies, they can never completely obviate the need for subjective decisionmaking; they can only provide better information on which to make decisions. It is important, therefore, that each study present a detailed explanation of the importance of missing information, possible errors in the data, and the assumptions underlying the study.

4) Many benefit-cost studies will, due to data limitations, be far less sophisticated than anticipated at the time these projects are initiated. We must not insist on perfection. We may insist on more rigorous measures of the costs of programs and at least an effort to measure benefits.

[20] This, to economists, represents the familiar problem of interpersonal utility comparisons.

5) We must not be overwhelmed by the problems of benefit-cost studies. Assistance to the retarded cannot wait until more refined data are available. For all their uncertainties, benefit-cost studies that make maximum use of existing information are a better basis for the decisions that must be made than the alternative of intuitive judgments.

6) Future research should concentrate not only on obtaining improved data but also on developing a more refined theory for evaluating investments in people. Most previous economic efforts have evaluated a particular service—education, medical care, etc. The economics of mental retardation requires a theory that focuses on a group of people who need a wide variety of services and for whom there is a wide variety of outcomes. This complex task is in a rudimentary stage.

Special problems in evaluating services for the retarded. No single benefit-cost analysis will suffice for the mentally retarded. Mental retardation is a complex syndrome that has many causes, creates many different service needs, and results in levels of social adjustment ranging from complete dependency to virtual self-sufficiency. An evaluation of the problem requires a highly structured approach that separates the mentally retarded into relatively homogeneous groups. Because of data limitations, however, we will consider only sex and two IQ levels—40–49 and 50–69.

Although the ultimate test of programs for the retarded is the degree to which they assist their clients to improve their social and vocational adjustment, this chapter will consider only the improvement in earnings and the reduction in institutional care that can be expected if adequate developmental services are provided. Although this is only a partial measure of the benefits of these programs, it can be positively asserted that without earnings, many of the other benefits of treatment would not be realized. In most cases, a retarded person's earnings symbolize for him his usefulness to society, bolster his self-respect, maintain his image in the eyes of others, create security, and help achieve a satisfactory standard of living. It is unfortunate that the constraints of time and data prevent an adequate evaluation of the economic effects of increasing the capability of self-care for the more severely retarded. The savings in attendant cost alone may be considerable.

What should be included as the costs of generating these benefits? The resources expended on raising children are enormous. If future earnings were the sole criterion for the decision to have children, it is probable that there would be many fewer children than currently exist. In point of fact, future earnings have little relevance to people's desire to have children. With the exception of families whose religious beliefs or ignorance preclude family planning, children must be considered a form of consumption to the parents, and not an investment.

If children are considered as consumption items to families, it can be argued that many of the costs necessary to the proper development of children should not enter into benefit-cost calculations. Most parents willingly accept these costs (and in fact have a legal obligation to do so), and many of these costs will be unaffected by policy decisions that might be made (and thus become tantamount to fixed costs where marginal costs are zero). These omitted costs are large. They include the forgone earnings of mothers, and the food, medical care, recreation, and clothing expenses of a child. It can even be argued that elementary and secondary education expenses should be excluded from consideration, if a social judgment is made that *all* children are entitled to publicly provided education. Such an extreme view would consider only the costs of the further development and eventual employment of persons after they have completed public school education.

This is too idealistic. Unfortunately, not all retarded children have the opportunity to enroll in public education classes, and even more do not have the opportunity to enroll in those types of classes that would be of maximum benefit to them. Nor is it universally accepted that the government has an obligation to provide special education. In addition, not all children enjoy the quality of home care that is required for full intellectual and social development. Additional resources will have to be expended to correct these conditions, and it is probable that these additional expenditures will have to be justified by benefit-cost considerations.

There is no single "correct" solution to the problem of determining which costs should be compared with benefits. Each analysis must deal with this problem within its own frame of reference.

Two benefit-cost analyses will be presented in this chapter. One will be of the vocational rehabilitation program, in which childhood developmental expenditures are omitted. The other will be of educational programs, where we will consider as given all other childhood developmental costs.

LIFETIME PRODUCTIVITY

Table 44 contains estimates of median earnings of workers by age and sex in the United States in 1970.[21] Subsequent calculations will assume that earnings are constant within these age intervals.[22] In addi-

---

[21] These data are taken from Table 29.

[22] It would be possible to derive single-year estimates by interpolation. However this would not significantly affect our results, and there is no reason to expect that these slight changes would be in the direction of greater accuracy.

tion, we will not attempt to distinguish between the earnings of whites and nonwhites. To begin with, we have no empirical basis for doing so as far as the retarded are concerned. In addition, differential earnings between whites and nonwhites are largely due to employment discrimination, differences in educational attainment, and average levels of intellectual functioning. The last consideration is not relevant when comparing white and nonwhite retardates, since all have IQs below 70. If anything, nonwhite retardates may have a slight employment advantage over white retardates, since they are more likely to be functionally retarded than brain damaged or the recipients of poor genes. Differences in educational attainment, if any, will be much less pronounced between white and nonwhite retardates than between whites and nonwhites generally. Employment discrimination, the final consideration, is probably not widespread in the types of jobs that retardates are likely to obtain. In any event, employment discrimination and cultural deprivation are intolerable situations and social policy should not be based on the assumption that these situations will continue indefinitely.

In Chapter V we estimated that the earnings of mildly retarded workers were comparable to the earnings of the general population up to the age of 25. Earnings then declined to 86% of normal for males and 87% of normal for females. The earnings of workers with IQs in the 40 to 49 range were considerably lower, about one-fifth of the average in each age group. The earnings of mildly and moderately retarded workers, also shown in Table 44, are based on these percentages.

Table 44 shows the estimated earnings of workers at a point in time. Table 45 shows the estimated earnings of a worker, age 18 in 1970, as he enters into successive age groups in the future. Thus, an 18-year-old male will be 45 years old in 1997, and his average earnings will be almost $18,000 per year. These estimates are based on an assumed productivity growth of 2.5% and are expressed in 1970 dollars—i.e., as if there were no inflation.

Table 46 shows the same earnings discounted to present value in 1970 using a discount rate of 7%.

Suppose a person began work in 1970 at age 18 and worked continuously until age 69. Table 47 shows the estimated aggregate earnings over the worker's lifetime and the present value of these earnings. The lifetime earnings of Table 47 assume a continuous work history. Not all adults work however; some are unemployed and some do not wish to work.

Table 48 shows the estimated *average* lifetime earnings of persons in the specified sex and diagnostic categories on a discounted and undiscounted basis. It was calculated by multiplying the estimated percent-

Table 44. Estimated median earnings of workers in the United States, 1970

				Age			
	18–19	20–24	25–34	35–44	45–54	55–64	65–69
General population							
Men	$2,996	$5,721	$7,779	$8,481	$8,211	$7,220	$4,552
Women	2,940	4,274	4,163	4,057	4,041	3,877	2,622
Mildly retarded							
Men	2,996	5,721	6,690	7,294	7,061	6,209	3,915
Women	2,940	4,274	3,622	3,530	3,516	3,373	2,281
Moderately retarded (IQ 40–49)							
Men	599	1,144	1,556	1,696	1,642	1,444	910
Women	588	855	833	811	808	775	524

Table 45. Estimated future median earnings of a worker, age 18 in 1970, as he moves into successive age groups (1970 prices)

	Age						
	18–19	20–24	25–34	35–44	45–54	55–64	65–69
General population							
Men	$3,033	$6,321	$10,363	$14,462	$17,921	$20,166	$13,502
Women	2,976	4,724	5,546	6,918	8,820	10,828	7,776
Mildly retarded							
Men	3,033	6,321	8,912	12,437	15,412	17,343	11,612
Women	2,976	4,724	4,825	6,019	7,673	9,420	6,765
Moderately retarded (IQ 40–49)							
Men	607	1,264	2,073	2,892	3,584	4,033	2,700
Women	595	945	1,109	1,384	1,764	2,166	1,555

Note: These estimated earnings were computed by the formula:

$$V = \frac{A\,(1.025)^{n-18}\,[1 + 1.025 + (1.025)^2 + \ldots + (1.025)^{i-1}]}{i}$$

where: A = earnings in age interval in 1970

n = lowest age in interval

i = number of years in interval

275

Table 46. Present value of estimated future median earnings of a worker, age 18 in 1970, as he moves into successive age groups, discounted at 7% (1970 prices)

	Age						
	18–19	20–24	25–34	35–44	45–54	55–64	65–69
General population							
Men	$2,934	$4,844	$4,850	$3,440	$2,167	$1,240	$ 691
Women	2,879	3,620	2,596	1,646	1,066	666	398
Mildly retarded							
Men	2,934	4,844	4,171	2,958	1,864	1,066	594
Women	2,879	3,620	2,259	1,432	927	579	346
Moderately retarded (IQ 40–49)							
Men	587	969	970	688	433	248	138
Women	576	724	519	329	213	133	80

Note: These present values were computed in the same way as the estimated future median earnings in Table 45, except that: (1) "A" represents the undiscounted value of future earnings; and (2) the inverse of the discount rate was used in place of the productivity growth factor.

276

Table 47. Estimated lifetime earnings of workers employed
continuously from age 18 to 69 (1970 to 2021,
1970 prices)

	Undiscounted earnings	Discounted earnings
General population		
Men	$734,000	$151,000
Women	390,000	86,000
Mildly retarded		
Men	637,000	134,000
Women	343,000	78,000
Moderately retarded (IQ 40–49)		
Men	147,000	30,000
Women	78,000	17,000

Table 48. Estimated average lifetime earnings of workers. adjusted for
probability of employment from age 18 to 69 (1970 to
2021, 1970 prices)

	Undiscounted	Discounted
General population		
Men	$630,000	$134,000
Women	164,000	38,000
Mildly retarded		
Men	522,000	114,000
Women	103,000	25,000
Moderately retarded (IQ 40–49)		
Men	66,000	14,000
Women	9,000	2,000

[23] U.S. Department of Labor, Bureau of Labor Statistics, *Employment, Earnings and Monthly Report on the Labor Force* (June 1967): 17–18.

age of persons employed in each age, sex, and diagnostic category in 1967 by the estimated earnings of workers in that category.

The percentage employed among the general population by age and sex was obtained from Department of Labor data for May 1967.[23] Based on the discussion contained in Chapter V, it was assumed that employment rates among mildly retarded males are the same as for the general population up to age 25, and thereafter are 4 percentage points below average, and that mildly retarded females had employment rates 12 percentage points below average. Among persons with IQs from 40 to 49, it was assumed that the employment rate was 45% for males and 12% for females.

Table 49 shows the estimated lifetime earnings of workers after an adjustment is made for the probability of death after age 18. On the basis of the discussion in Chapter II, it was assumed that mortality rates among the mildly retarded were 25% higher than their age and sex counterparts in the general population, and the corresponding percentage among persons with IQs between 40 and 49 was assumed to be 75%.[24]

Table 50 shows the estimated total lifetime productivity of paid workers, i.e., earnings plus the value of unpaid work other than that performed by full-time homemakers. Following Chapter VI it was assumed that the value of unpaid work was 25% of gross earnings in the case of men and 37.5% in the case of women (representing homemaking services performed in addition to paid employment).

Table 51 shows the estimates of the lifetime value of homemaking services provided by full-time homemakers. These estimates are based on the conclusions of Chapter V. The services of homemakers in the general population were valued at 75% of the gross income of employed women. Homemaking services by the mildly retarded were assumed to be equal in value to those provided by women in the general population, and homemaking services provided by women in the lower-IQ group were assumed to be one-half as valuable. The slight difference in the estimated value of lifetime homemaking services between women in the general population and the mildly retarded results solely from the higher mortality of the latter.

The percentage of women who are full-time homemakers was derived from the Department of Labor source previously cited. The percentage of mildly retarded women who were full-time homemakers was assumed to be equal to the general population. In the lower-IQ range, it was assumed that 19% of the women were full-time homemakers.

To place the productivity of women in better perspective, estimates of the average total productivity of women over their lifetime are presented in Table 52. Average total lifetime productivity is the sum of the average lifetime value of homemaking service among full-time homemakers, average earnings, and the average value of homemaking services

---

[24] Mortality rates for the general population for 1967 by sex and corresponding to our age intervals were obtained from USDHEW, PHS, National Center for Health Statistics, *Vital Statistics of the United States, 1967*, Volume II—*Mortality*, Part A, pp. I–8 and I–9. Average survival rates were computed in each age-sex grouping by subtracting one-half of the percentage dying during the period from the percentage surviving at the beginning of the period.

Table 49. Estimated lifetime earnings of workers, adjusted for probability of death, from age 18 to 69 (1970 to 2021, 1970 prices)

	Adjusted for percentage employed		Assuming continuous employment	
	Undiscounted	Discounted	Undiscounted	Discounted
General population				
Men	$612,000	$132,000	$710,000	$148,000
Women	161,000	37,000	383,000	85,000
Mildly retarded				
Men	503,000	112,000	611,000	131,000
Women	101,000	25,000	335,000	77,000
Moderately retarded (IQ 40–49)				
Men	62,000	13,000	138,000	29,000
Women	9,000	2,000	76,000	17,000

Table 50. Estimated lifetime earnings of workers, adjusted for unpaid work, from age 18 to 69 (1970 to 2021, 1970 prices)

	Adjusted for percentage employed		Assuming continuous employment	
	Undiscounted	Discounted	Undiscounted	Discounted
		(Adjusted for mortality)		
General population				
Men	$764,000	$165,000	$887,000	$185,000
Women	222,000	51,000	526,000	117,000
Mildly retarded				
Men	629,000	140,000	763,000	164,000
Women	139,000	34,000	461,000	106,000
Moderately retarded (IQ 40–49)				
Men	78,000	16,000	173,000	37,000
Women	12,000	3,000	104,000	23,000

Table 51. Estimated lifetime value of homemaking services provided by full-time homemakers, from 18 to 69 (1970 to 2021, 1970 prices)

	Adjusted for percentage who are full-time homemakers		Assuming continuous homemaking	
	Undiscounted	Discounted	Undiscounted	Discounted
		(Adjusted for mortality)		
General population	$153,000	$31,000	$287,000	$64,000
Mildly retarded	152,000	31,000	286,000	64,000
Moderately retarded (IQ 40–49)	27,000	6,000	142,000	32,000

281

Table 52. Estimated average productivity of women, taking account
of remunerative employment and homemaking services,
from age 18 to 69 (1970 to 2021, 1970 prices)

	Undiscounted	Discounted
General population	$375,000	$82,000
Mildly retarded	291,000	65,000
Moderately retarded (IQ 40–49)	39,000	9,000

provided by employed women. This in effect assumes a composite
woman who spends about half her lifetime in paid employment and
half in keeping house full-time.

Qualifications to estimates. These estimates represent the values of
the productive efforts of people and, as has been previously emphasized, are a partial measure of the activities that contribute to well-
being. In addition, they are based on a particular set of estimates and
assumptions (e.g., discount rates, mortality rates, economic growth
rates), most of which could be modified in numerous ways to produce
varying results. There is no overwhelming indication that the values we
have used for these variables are the most appropriate ones.

These estimates are based on the assumption that a particular set of
employment and earnings relationships existing in 1967 will continue
into the future. Among the more probable of the changes in these
relationships that would affect these estimates are: (1) the labor force
participation rate of women will presumably continue its historic rise in
the future; (2) the earnings of women relative to men will probably
improve; and (3) improved services to the retarded, especially the more
severely retarded, will undoubtedly increase both their labor force participation rates and average earnings in the future. If anything, our
assumptions concerning these variables would cause us to underestimate
the lifetime productivity of the retarded, especially in the cases of
female retardates and the severely retarded.

The employment rates used to estimate average productivity are
those estimated for the noninstitutionalized population in Chapter V.
Our estimates of lifetime earnings are valid, therefore, only for retardates who avoid institutionalization during their lifetimes. In the case of
the mildly retarded, the bias is so small as to be irrelevant. It is somewhat more important in the case of persons in the lower-IQ range.
However, if we took account of the institutional population, we would

need to consider the utilization of the retarded in institution work, and it is uncertain as to whether our final estimates would be higher or lower than those presented in this chapter.

Although we estimated that the average value of homemaking services among full-time homemakers was 75% of the earnings of women in remunerative employment for the general population, the relative value of homemaking services to remunerated employment will be higher in the case of retarded women; in the case of women with IQs between 40 and 49, our estimate of the value of homemaking services they perform is higher than our estimate of the earnings of women in this IQ range.

As mentioned previously, I feel uncomfortable with the assumption that the quality of the homemaking services provided by mildly retarded women is the same as those provided by nonretarded housewives. It may well be true, however, that moderately retarded women are being more effectively utilized as housekeepers than in remunerative employment. Many of the moderately retarded are marginally employed on a part-time or irregular basis, often on makeshift jobs. However, this relationship would not be expected to hold for moderately retarded women in stable full-time employment.

It should also be stressed that there is great variation in productive effort within the various demographic groups that we have examined. One glaring, but statistically unavoidable gap in our calculations thus far has been employment and earnings information on the physically or emotionally handicapped mentally retarded.

Conclusions. (1) The earnings of most retardates are substantial. On the average (adjusted for the probability of employment), mildly retarded men who were 18 years old in 1970 will earn more than $500,000 during their lifetimes and mildly retarded women will earn about $101,000. If we take account of the value of homemaking services and other unpaid work, average lifetime productivity is over $600,000 for mildly retarded men and is almost $300,000 for mildly retarded women. When discounted at 7%, these measures of total lifetime productivity have a present value of $140,000 and $65,000.

2) The average earnings of the moderately retarded are considerably lower—$62,000 for men and $9,000 for women. When adjusted to take account of unpaid work and homemaking, these estimates rise to $78,000 and $39,000, with present values of $16,000 and $9,000.

3) These averages values may be misleadingly low as an indication of the potential productivity of the retarded, especially the moderately retarded. Many are economically idle or economically under-used, because of a lack of appropriate training and supportive services. Our estimates of lifetime earnings, based on the assumption of continuous

employment, may provide a better measure of the productive *potential* of most retardates.

In the case of mildly retarded males and females, an assumption of continuous remunerative employment would increase our estimates of lifetime earnings to about $600,000 and $300,000. If we take account of unpaid work among continuously employed retardates, lifetime productivity increases to almost $760,000 and $460,000 with present values of $164,000 and $106,000. In the case of women keeping house full-time, the comparable estimates are $286,000 (undiscounted) and $64,000 (discounted).

More importantly, in the case of moderately retarded males and females, average total lifetime productivity is $173,000 and $104,000, if continuously employed, with present values of $37,000 and $23,000. For moderately retarded women keeping house, the comparable estimates are $142,000 and $32,000.

4) The unexpectedly high level of economic success of the retarded may surprise many, especially those whose stereotype of the retarded is based on those in the lower-IQ ranges. More critically, it may be asked how the mildly retarded could achieve a slightly greater measure of economic success than many of the more intellectually endowed, but culturally maladapted (or "deprived," or "disadvantaged") in our society.

In Chapter V, it was concluded that intellectual deficiency was not a major barrier to employment for persons with IQs above 50, and that vocational failure was usually a consequence of negative attitudes about jobs, authority, people, etc. It is precisely in this area that the culturally maladapted are most apt to be deficient. Negative attitudes and job discrimination may explain the relatively poorer vocational adjustment of this group.

VOCATIONAL REHABILITATION

Costs. Unpublished data from the Rehabilitation Services Administration reports that case service costs for mildly, moderately, and severely retarded rehabilitants were $573, $780, and $888 respectively in 1970 (including cases with and without case service costs). In Chapter IV, we estimated that the average *total* cost (case service costs plus counseling plus other agency overhead) for *all* retarded rehabilitants was $2,830 for the same year. It was assumed that average total rehabilitation costs for each level of retardation bore the same relationship to average total costs for all retarded rehabilitants as average case service costs for each level of retardation bore to average case service costs for all retarded rehabilitants ($709 in 1970). Our estimates of average total costs are $2,468 for the mildly retarded, $3,361 for the moderately retarded, and $3,830 for the severely retarded.[25]

These are the costs of a single rehabilitation. Previous rehabilitations were reported by 5.5% of retarded rehabilitants in 1969 (as compared to 9.5% of all rehabilitants).[26] However, only one-third of the retarded rehabilitants in 1969 were 20 years of age or over. Presumably, most "repeat" rehabilitations were in this older group. We would expect, therefore, that at least 16.5% of retarded rehabilitants would require services more than once (2 X 5.5% to account for those under 20, and 5.5% to account for those who already received services more than once).

We will increase our estimates of the cost of rehabilitation for a retarded client by 50% to allow for the possibility of "repeat" rehabilitations, as well as for other omitted costs which should be attributed to rehabilitation, such as costs of direct or indirect services incurred by other public or private agencies, earnings forgone while undergoing rehabilitation, and prior research, training, and construction costs. On this assumption, the average total lifetime rehabilitation costs would be $3,703 for the mildly retarded, $5,044 for the moderately retarded, and $5,746 for the severely retarded.

Benefits. A priori, we would expect that the average lifetime productivity of retarded rehabilitants would be less than our estimate for retarded workers generally, since the very fact of referral for vocational rehabilitation is a manifestation of some vocational difficulties. However, the data do not support this hypothesis. The average weekly earnings, at closure, of retarded rehabilitants with earnings (91% of all retarded rehabilitants) in 1969 was $56.09 per week at closure, or about $2,920 per year.[27] Although this is less than half of our estimate of average productivity among employed adult retardates, it is almost identical to our earlier estimate of median earnings among mildly retarded 18- and 19-year-olds (Table 44). As already observed, almost two-thirds of the retarded rehabilitants are in this age range. Of course, one-third of the retarded rehabilitants were in an age range where we

[25] In effect, this assumes that the more severely retarded required more counseling effort than the less severely retarded. For example, for the mildly retarded this calculation would be $\frac{572}{656}$ × $2,830 = $2,468.

[26] USDHEW, SRS, RSA, *A Profile of Mentally Retarded Clients Rehabilitated During Fiscal Year 1969*, September 1971.

[27] Ibid.

would expect substantially higher earnings, but this is partly offset by the fact that almost 40% of the retarded rehabilitants were reported as being in the moderate or severe range of retardation.

We will assume, therefore, that the lifetime earnings of retarded rehabilitants follow the same profile and are of the same magnitude as those calculated for all employed retardates.

But which measure of lifetime earnings is most appropriate? Our measure of average earnings among *all* retardates is too low, since it is pulled down by nonworking retardates. The rehabilitated retarded, in contrast, have demonstrated both an ability and a commitment to work.

Our measure of lifetime earnings based on the assumption of continuous employment from age 18 to 69 is too high, since it is inconceivable that rehabilitants will escape any form of subsequent unemployment and many will certainly withdraw from the labor market as they approach the age of normal retirement. The last of these considerations is of minor importance. When future earnings are discounted, earnings received between the ages of 65 and 69 have an almost imperceptible effect on the present value of total earnings.

The problem of the subsequent unemployment of retarded rehabilitants is more serious. In an earlier study of the vocational rehabilitation program, I concluded, on the basis of existing follow-up studies, that about 20% of the rehabilitants closed into remunerative employment were not employed five years after closure.[28]

We will assume that retarded rehabilitants have the same job-retention success. The lifetime earnings of retarded rehabilitants will, therefore, be estimated by reducing our estimates of lifetime earnings among continuously employed retardates by 20%.

The critical question is what retarded rehabilitants would have earned in the absence of rehabilitation services. Earnings prior to rehabilitation, one frequently used method of estimating what would have happened, are of little value for predicting the future success of this group because of the large proportion of teenage referrals.

In my previous study of the vocational rehabilitation program I concluded, on the basis of earnings during the year before referral for rehabilitation, that two-thirds of the earnings of rehabilitants after closure were due to rehabilitation services. However, because of the large number of youthful mildly retarded persons among retarded rehabilitants, I suspect that retarded rehabilitants would have had a better

---

[28] Ronald W. Conley, "A Benefit-Cost Analysis of the Vocational Rehabilitation Program," *Journal of Human Resources*, vol. IV, no. 2 (Spring 1969): 234.

chance of vocational success in the absence of rehabilitation than would other rehabilitants.

We will, therefore, assume that 50% (rather than two-thirds) of the estimated lifetime earnings of retarded rehabilitants can be ascribed to the effects of rehabilitation services. In view of the excellent employment histories of the mildly retarded reported by follow-up studies, this may still appear to ascribe too much to vocational rehabilitation. However, many of the retarded in these follow-up studies received assistance in locating work, if not from rehabilitation agencies, then from the state employment service or some other public or private agency, or, if nowhere else, from friends or relatives. The question of who provides the service is of little importance compared to whether these services contribute to vocational adjustment. Moreover, those retardates seeking rehabilitation services presumably had above average vocational difficulties.

Although our estimate of 50% must be viewed as a reasoned guess, it represents as good an estimate as is used in most benefit-cost analyses, and is probably close to the true percentage.

Benefit-cost ratios. Table 53 shows our estimates of the benefit-cost ratios of rehabilitation services. It is perhaps best interpreted as showing the present value of increased future earnings generated by each dollar expended in rehabilitating the retarded.

Increased future earnings were calculated as 40% of the lifetime earnings of continuously employed retardates (adjusted for mortality).[29]

Costs were estimated at $3,703 for the mildly retarded and $5,395 for the moderately retarded (IQ 40 to 49). The latter figure is an average of our estimates of the rehabilitation costs of the moderately and severely retarded.[30] These costs are estimates of all resources used

---

[29] Estimates of future earnings were specially calculated for retarded rehabilitants assumed to be older than 18 in 1970 and will not be found in preceding tables. It was assumed that their earnings were comparable to those of other retardates, adjusted for age, sex, and level of retardation. Future earnings were then adjusted to allow for productivity change and discounting. Readers who may question the assumption that 50% of future lifetime earnings can be attributed to rehabilitation can modify the results of Table 53 by the formula:

$$b' = b(x/.50)$$

where:

  b' = the adjusted benefit-cost ratio
  b = the benefit-cost ratio reported in Table 53
  x = a different estimate for the percentage of future
        earnings attributable to vocational rehabilitation

[30] Some persons reported as moderately retarded by vocational rehabilitation agencies undoubtedly had IQs above 50, so that our previous estimate of the cost of

Table 53.   Value of future earnings generated by each dollar spent on the vocational rehabilitation of the retarded at different ages, discounted at 7%, 1970

	Age of retardates when rehabilitated				
	18 yrs.	20 yrs.	25 yrs.	35 yrs.	45 yrs.
Mildly retarded					
Male	$14.2	$14.8	$14.8	$13.5	$10.7
Female	8.3	8.4	7.8	6.9	5.7
Moderately Retarded (IQ 40 to 49)					
Male	2.2	2.3	2.3	2.1	1.7
Female	1.3	1.3	1.2	1.1	0.9

for the rehabilitation process during the working years of the rehabilitant.[31]

The following observations are made: (1) Our estimates indicate that rehabilitation of the retarded is worthwhile in most cases on the grounds of increased earnings alone.

2) The benefits of rehabilitation are substantial. Eighty-five percent of retarded rehabilitants are under 25 years of age and about 60% are mildly retarded; about half, therefore, are mildly retarded and under age 25. Each dollar expended on the vocational rehabilitation of males in this demographic group increases the present value of estimated future earnings by over $14. Among mildly retarded youthful women, the comparable figure is about $8.[32] These ratios decline among older mildly retarded rehabilitants, but are many times greater than the critical value of "1."

3) The ratio of the present value of increased earnings to rehabilitation costs among moderately retarded rehabilitants under age 25 were about $2.20 in the case of males, and $1.30 in the case of females. Among older, moderately retarded rehabilitants, the ratios are lower and after age 45 are less than "1" for females. These estimates for older rehabilitants may be low, since one could question the assumption that

---

persons described as moderately retarded would be somewhat below the cost of serving persons with IQs between 40 and 50. It is also probable that many of those listed as severely retarded had IQs in the forties. A simple average, therefore, appeared to be the most reasonable approach.

[31] It should be noted that we have added the costs of subsequent rehabilitations into the denominator instead of subtracting them from the numerator as we earlier argued would be more theoretically correct. Had we subtracted these costs from the numerator, the benefit-cost ratios would be higher.

[32] These figures are a rough average of the ratios reported for the three groups under age 25.

only 40% of future earnings is attributable to vocational rehabilitation among older, moderately retarded rehabilitants. Vocational problems can be especially severe among this group and their capacity for independent adjustment is limited.[33]

4) These estimates take account of only part of the benefits of rehabilitation. Increased homemaking services and other unpaid work and psychic gains would further raise these ratios.

EDUCATION

Costs. To estimate the value of the resources expended on the education of the retarded requires knowledge of the number of years they remain in school and the types of classes they attend, as well as the annual costs of these classes. Until recently, special education classes for retardates beyond the elementary level were rare. Since few retardates could benefit from attending regular academic classes at a secondary level, most dropped out of school at an early age. Kennedy reported that fewer than 9% of her sample of mildly retarded persons went beyond the eighth grade. She also reported that 94% of these subjects repeated at least one grade, and almost four-fifths repeated two or more grades.[34] Three-fourths of the mildly retarded subjects of the more recent Mudd study had left school by the age of 16 or shortly thereafter.[35]

We will assume that most mildly retarded adults attended school for ten years, which corresponds to the usual age span of compulsory school attendance (6 to 16) and is also in general agreement with the results of the Mudd and Kennedy studies.[36] Kennedy reported that

[33] This method of evaluating increased earnings due to rehabilitation differs in several ways from that employed in my earlier work. (1) Previously, I did not incorporate a factor for increasing productivity. It is worth noting, however, that using an assumed annual productivity change of 2.5% and a discount rate of 7% is equivalent to using a discount rate of 4.4% and zero productivity change. Previously I used discount factors of 4% and 8%. (2) In my earlier work I did not develop a lifetime profile of earnings for rehabilitants. I assumed that earnings reported for 20-year-olds remain constant throughout their lives rather than rise to the higher earnings of older workers. After reviewing the results of follow-up studies of retardates, I am convinced that the approach used here is more appropriate.

[34] Ruby Jo Reeves Kennedy, *The Social Adjustment of Morons in a Connecticut City*, Report by the Commission to Survey the Human Resources of Connecticut, June 1948, p. 16.

[35] Merle W. Mudd, Brina B. Melemed, and Henry Wechsler, *Post School Vocational Adjustment of Educable Mentally Retarded Boys in Massachusetts*, mimeographed copy of report issued by the Medical Foundation, Inc., Boston, December 1968, p. 46.

[36] Recent developments in work-study programs may increase the number of years the retarded remain in school.

56% of her sample had attended special education classes. Mudd reported a comparable figure of 85%. Median years of special education were about 3 years in the former case and 4 years in the latter case. The greater percentage of special education students and the longer time spent in special education classes in the Mudd study is attributable to the fact that the subjects of this study attended school almost 25 years after those of the Kennedy study.

Tobias reported that the median age at which mildly retarded individuals were placed in special education classes was between nine and ten.[37] This would indicate a somewhat longer period of attendance in special education classes than reported by the Mudd or Kennedy studies.

Three measures of the costs of education will be developed for the mildly retarded: one will be based on the assumption that the retardate spends *ten years in regular academic classes*; one on the assumption that the retardate spends *ten years in special education classes* for the educable retarded; and one on the assumption that the retardate spends the *first five years* in regular academic classes and the *last five years* in special education classes. The third of the three measures is probably the most realistic for the majority of the mildly retarded.

Saenger reported that the moderately retarded adults in his sample spent a median of 5 years in special education classes and 1.7 years in regular classes. A few attended private classes or had private tutors. The median age of school enrollment was about 8, and the median age of leaving school was about 16. Most of those who left earlier than age 16 were committed to institutional care.[38]

We will assume that the moderately retarded spend eight years in school. To simplify our subsequent analysis, we will assume that the entire time is spent in classes for the trainable retarded. This should cause a slight overstatement of the educational resources used for the moderately retarded. Along with the cost information developed in Chapter IV, this provides us with sufficient information to estimate the value of the educational resources utilized for the average retardate.

Table 54 shows our estimate of the total educational costs of retardates who in 1970 were 18 years old. Since we have not estimated

[37] Jack Tobias, Ida Alpert, and Arnold Birenbaum, *Survey of the Employment Status of Mentally Retarded Adults in New York City*, Report to the Office of Manpower Research, Manpower Administration, U.S. Department of Labor (New York: Associated Educational Services Corporation, April 1969), p. 9.

[38] Gerhart Saenger, *The Adjustment of Severely Retarded Adults in the Community*, A Report to the New York State Interdepartmental Health Resources Board, October 1957, pp. 34–35.

Table 54.   Estimated lifetime educational costs of retardates,
            age 18 in 1970

	Total costs	
	Not discounted	Discounted (compounded)
Mildly retarded assuming:		
All regular academic classes	$ 8,700	$13,500
All special education classes	16,500	25,800
5 years in each type of class	12,800	19,000
Moderately retarded	26,000	37,800

educational costs by type of special education class for years prior to 1970, it was necessary to extrapolate the 1970 data backward. The following observations are necessary:

1) These cost figures are in terms of the price levels prevailing in 1970 and are based on those developed in Chapter IV ($1,003 for regular academic classes, $1,936 for special class programs for the educable retarded, and $3,494 for special class programs for the trainable retarded).

2) In forecasting earnings, we had to consider rising worker productivity. We must expect a symmetrical downward movement as we move backward in time. Thus, our estimate of the annual per capita cost of classes for the educable retarded was $1,936/ (1.025)^2$ in 1966 and $1,936/ (1.025)^3$ in 1965, etc.

3) As previously explained, age 18 is the base year for purposes of computing present values. In order to do so, costs incurred prior to age 18 must be compounded. Thus our present value estimate of the cost of education of the mildly retarded in 1966 is $(\$1,936) (1.07)^2 / (1.025)^2$ and for 1965 $(\$1,936) (1.07)^3 / (1.025),^3$ which is just the reverse of the previous discounting procedure.

4) Since our estimates of educational costs are for persons who were age 18 in 1970 the years that they would have attended school are 1958 to 1968 in the case of the mildly retarded, and 1960 to 1968 in the case of the moderately retarded.

5) Theoretically, these cost estimates should be adjusted for the probability of death among school-age retardates. This would not, however, cause a significant increase in estimated educational cost. Such a minor adjustment did not appear to warrant the increased calculations that it would necessitate or the philosophical hackles that it would raise.

Benefit-cost ratios. Tables 55 to 57 show the ratios of the lifetime productivity of retardates (adjusted for mortality), age 18 in 1970, divided by their lifetime educational costs.

In order to interpret these ratios as benefit-cost ratios, we must assume that in the absence of educational service, retardates would have had no earnings. But even a total lack of formal education does not constitute an overwhelming barrier to vocational success *unless* combined with other impediments to employment. In the case of the retarded, however, at least one other employment impediment exists by definition—intellectual deficiency. Lack of schooling to a retardate who cannot compensate for this deficiency with innate cleverness, and complicated by the virtual certainty of emotional problems caused by social isolation, would probably be vocationally disastrous in technologically advanced economies. Thus, the assumption that education of some type is essential to the achievement of any level of vocational success by the retarded appears reasonable.

We do not have sufficient data to develop estimates of the differences in earnings between retardates who attended special education classes and those who remained in regular education. Our ratios are greater, therefore, for retardates who attended regular education classes, since costs decline but the same rate of earnings is attributed to each approach to providing education.

In principle, the earnings of special education students should be higher than their earnings would have been had they remained in regular classes. Presumably, the curricula of special education classes was better suited to their needs.

Empirically, however, we would probably find that the earnings of retardates in regular education classes were higher because of a selection factor. The students placed in special education classes were those with the highest risk of future vocational difficulties.

Given these considerations, it is probably true that the ratio of benefits to costs is lower for students who attend special education classes than for students who attend regular education classes, as our figures indicate. However, one cannot conclude that regular education is superior to special education. This will be true for some retardates but not all. To make such judgments, we require carefully controlled experiments with random assignment of similar students to each type of class and long-term follow-up. The results of such experiments would undoubtedly be an improved knowledge of what types of students are best served in special education classes and what types should be kept in regular education classes.

We also lack data by which to estimate the effect of increased years of schooling on the lifetime earnings of retardates. These types of anal-

Table 55. Estimated lifetime productivity of retarded workers divided by costs of education, discounted at 7%

	Adjusted for percentage employed		Assuming continuous employment	
	Earnings only	Earnings plus unpaid work other than homemaking	Earnings only	Earnings plus unpaid work other than homemaking
Mildly retarded				
Males				
All regular education	8.3	10.4	9.7	12.1
All special education	4.3	5.4	5.1	6.4
Combination	5.9	7.4	6.9	8.6
Females				
All regular education	1.8	2.5	5.7	7.8
All special education	1.0	1.3	3.0	4.1
Combination	1.3	1.8	4.0	5.6
Moderately retarded				
Males	0.3	0.4	0.8	1.0
Females	0.1	0.1	0.4	0.6

Table 56. Estimated lifetime value of homemaking services provided
by retarded full-time homemakers divided by costs of
education, discounted at 7%

	Adjusted for percentage in homemaking	Assuming continuous homemaking
Mildly retarded		
All regular education	2.3	4.7
All special education	1.2	2.5
Combination	1.6	3.3
Moderately retarded	0.2	0.8

yses are important in the determination of what would be the optimum
number of years of schooling for retardates.

Our ratios are gross estimates of the relationship between the resources used in the education of the retarded and a part of the resulting
benefits. They are insufficiently refined to show how much education
should be provided to retardates or what form their education provision
should take. Perhaps the best way of expressing the matter is that our
figures show the ratio of average benefits and costs, but not of marginal
benefits and costs.

As we have emphasized, education is essential to, but not sufficient
for, vocational success. Many other services are needed: parental care
during childhood, medical care, etc. Why are the costs of these additional services not included in the cost portion of our benefit-cost
ratios? In most cases these additional services are essential to life and, as
long as euthanasia is rejected, will be provided regardless of whether
education is provided to the retarded. Our analysis implicitly assumes
that the provision of education to retarded children is the only additional use of resources that must be justified on the basis of outcomes.

Table 57. Estimated average productivity of retarded women, taking
account of remunerative employment and homemaking
services, divided by lifetime costs of education,
discounted at 7%

Mildly retarded	
All regular education	4.8
All special education	2.5
Combination	3.4
Moderately retarded	0.2

Therefore, we need only estimate what would have happened to earnings if education were not provided and compare that with what earnings actually were. Educational costs are variable costs and all other costs are fixed costs, essential to the outcome of education, but not relevant to the decision to provide education.

If, however, we are assessing the variable costs of the lifetime earnings of retardates two additional cost elements must be considered: clinical services to retarded children and rehabilitation services to retarded adults. Clinical services may assist the child to progress in school and adjust at home, and rehabilitation services to adults protect the substantial investment in childhood education. These services become an interrelated package, usually publicly funded, assisting the retardate to a successful adult adjustment.

The costs of vocational rehabilitation have been estimated in the previous section of this chapter.[39] In Chapter IV we estimated that (1) the average charge for a thorough initial clinical evaluation of a retardate was $575 in 1970; (2) the average age of evaluation was 7; and (3) about twelve additional annual visits would be required. Assuming an average annual cost of $50 (after the initial evaluation) and using previously explained methods, we estimated that clinical services for an 18-year-old in 1970 would have cost $1,100 and the present value of these resources would have been almost $1,800 (since they are assumed to have been incurred prior to age 18).

Table 58 shows what the sum of educational, clinical, and rehabilitation expenditures would be for retardates who receive each of these services, and the percentage decreases that would occur in the ratios in Tables 55 to 57, if these combined costs were used rather than educational costs alone.

The benefit-cost ratios of Tables 55 to 57 were not lowered as indicated by the data in Table 58, because a relatively small proportion of retardates received clinical or rehabilitation services. If we calculated the average amount spent on these services per retardate, the effect on the benefit-cost ratios would be small.

It should be noted that no allowance for the risk of failure has been built into our estimate of the cost of special education. A risk factor is automatically included in our ratios that are based on the percentage employed. Ratios based on the assumption of continuous, uninterrupted employment represent an ideal but improbable situation which hypothesizes the absence of any significant unemployment.

[39] In the previous section, the vocational rehabilitation of the retarded was evaluated on the assumption that all other developmental services were given. Here it is being integrated into a broader concept of developmental services.

Table 58.   Combined costs of educational, clinical, and rehabilitation
services to retardates, age 18 in 1970

	Not Compounded	Compounded
Mildly retarded		
All regular education	$13,500	$19,000
All special education	21,300	31,300
Combination	17,600	24,500
Moderately retarded	32,500	45,000
	Decrease in benefit-cost ratios of Tables 55 to 57 if combined costs were used in denominator	
Mildly retarded		
All regular education	29%	
All special education	18%	
Combination	22%	
Moderately retarded	16%	

The following observations are made: (1) The lifetime earnings of mildly retarded adults are many times the cost of their education. The present value of the future earnings of continuously employed mildly retarded males who divide their school years between regular academic and special education classes is almost seven times the present value of the cost of their education. Adjusting this figure for the percentage employed reduces the ratio of the present value of future earnings to the present value of costs to a little less than six. This lower figure may represent a more realistic appraisal of the actual ratio of earnings to costs. Adjusting these ratios for this value of unpaid work would, of course, raise them about 25%.

These ratios increase if it is assumed that the retarded attend all regular academic classes and decrease if it is assumed that they attend all special education classes. Although these ratios can be used to represent high and low estimates of the benefits and costs of providing education to the retarded, the intermediate case is the more typical one. Whatever the combination of assumptions used to represent the benefits and costs of educating mildly retarded males, the benefit-cost ratio greatly exceeds the critical value of "1."

2) In the case of continuously employed mildly retarded women, the present value of lifetime earnings was four times the present value of educational costs. If women were assumed to be full-time home-makers, the ratio was over three to one. The lower benefit-cost ratios for mildly retarded women reflect the less favorable earnings position of women in general and probably, also, an under evaluation of home-

making services and should not be considered an effect of mental retardation.

These ratios fall sharply when adjusted to reflect the percentage employed in remunerative work or homemaking. However, since either of the ratios represents less than half of women's productive efforts, we should look to the ratios of Table 57 where average productivity in remunerative work and homemaking is taken into account. Here the most probable ratio falls between three and four. As in the case of men, whatever combination of assumptions is used to represent the costs of educating mildly retarded women, the value of their subsequent productivity substantially exceeds the critical value of "1," if a reasonably complete measure of benefits is used.

3) The benefit-cost outlook is much less favorable for the moderately retarded. In only one case, that of continuously employed males, did the benefit-cost ratio reach the critical value of "1," and then only when other unpaid work was included. Although a separate analysis was not possible for multiply-handicapped retardates, one suspects that the results of such an analysis would be comparable to those of the moderately retarded.

Perhaps it should be noted that on an undiscounted basis our measures of benefits exceed costs in all cases and that our measure of benefits is only a partial measure of total benefits. For example, the benefits of averting institutional care have not been included.

In any event these ratios represent our estimate of the present situation. Educational efforts on behalf of the moderately retarded have long been recognized as inadequate and only in recent years has there been significant improvement in this area. In addition, supportive services for retarded adults are virtually nonexistent, a subject to which we will return in the last chapter. The benefit-cost outlook would probably be greatly improved if moderately retarded adults had early and continuing assistance in their vocational and community adjustment.

4) The high level of vocational success of the mildly retarded makes me suspect that lengthened educational programs are not the primary need for most.

5) Educational services provided to the mildly retarded can be justified on the basis of earnings alone. It is, in fact, self-defeating not to provide these services, since this would sacrifice a large long-run gain for a small short-run gain.

INSTITUTIONALIZATION

Institutional care is expensive. Average annual per patient costs (including capital costs) in public institutions were $5,865 in 1970 (Chapter IV). Not all of this would be saved if a person were not institutionalized. About 20% of this total was attributed to normal consumption expenditures. In addition, about 50% of the population of these institutions were children under age 20 in 1970. If we assume that about $2,500 per year was spent on educational and other developmental activities for children and that no funds were spent for this purpose among adults, then about $3,450 is left as the custodial cost (i.e., what is left after consumption expenditures and developmental costs are subtracted from the total costs of care) that society would save annually if institutionalization could be avoided.[40]

Consider a retardate who is placed in a public institution at birth, remains there until death, and is age 18 in 1970. Table 59 shows the estimated value of the resources that would be used for custodial purposes (i.e., net of consumption and developmental care) during the person's lifetime.

Table 59. Custodial costs of lifetime institutional care, for a retardate born in 1952 (1970 prices)

	Not discounted	Discounted (compounded prior to age 18)
Mildly retarded		
Males	$392,000	$169,000
Females	400,000	170,000
Moderately retarded		
Males	386,000	168,000
Females	397,000	169,000

The estimates are expressed in 1970 prices, assume a cost increase of 2.5% per year (corresponding to the assumed productivity change), and after age 18 are adjusted for mortality. The minor differences by sex and level of retardation are solely due to differential death rates. Table 60 shows the estimated custodial costs of lifetime institutionalization divided by the estimated educational costs of retardates.

Of course, even if no education programs were available to the retarded, not all of the mildly retarded or moderately retarded would be placed in residential care, and, in any event, relatively few would be

---

[40] This calculation is 80% of $5,865 less 50% of $2,500. In Chapter IV we concluded, on the basis of regression analysis, that the additional cost of serving children (as opposed to adults) was $2,100 in 1968. This estimate was increased by the percentage increase in the operating cost per student in regular academic classrooms between 1968 and 1970.

placed in residential care at birth. There is, however, another way to interpret Table 60. If education reduces the rate of institutionalization among the mildly retarded by about 12% *at a point in time*, then savings in institutional costs alone would justify the provision of school programs, even if all these individuals had to be supported by public assistance (since maintenance costs are excluded from our calculations). Among the moderately retarded this ratio rises to 25%.[41]

Although it has been frequently observed that educational programs have reduced the rate of institutionalization among higher-grade retardates,[42] it is, for all practical purposes, impossible to estimate by how

[41] There is a slight methodological imprecision in applying to discounted data this method of estimating the percentage reduction in the institutional population needed to justify educational programs. Discounted costs decline over time as shown by the curve *AB*. The method used above sums a constant percentage of each year's costs (*CD*). However, in the real world, institutionalization at birth is

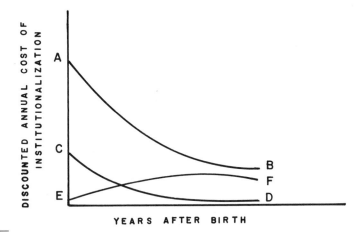

YEARS AFTER BIRTH

rare, increases gradually during early childhood, reaches a peak at an age that depends upon the severity of retardation and declines rapidly among adults. A 3% reduction in the overall rate of institutionalization would therefore be represented by a higher percentage reduction in these later years and a lower percentage reduction in the earlier years. The relevant savings in institution costs would be represented by the area under a curve such as *EF*. Since these later dollars are worth less, on a discounted basis, than dollars spent in earlier years, the decrease in the institutional population needed to justify educational programs would be slightly greater than indicated in the text above.

[42] E.g., Herbert Goldstein, "Population Trends in U.S. Public Institutions for the Mentally Deficient," *American Journal of Mental Deficiency* (January 1959): 599; Robert E. Patton and Abbot S. Weinstein, "Changing Characteristics of the Population in the New York State Schools for Mental Defectives," *American Journal of Mental Deficiency* (January 1960): 634.

Table 60.   Custodial costs of lifetime institutionalization divided by costs of education, discounted at 7%

Mildly retarded	
Males	
All regular education classes	12.5
All special education classes	6.5
Combination	8.9
Females	
All regular education classes	12.5
All special education classes	6.6
Combination	8.9
Moderately retarded	
Males	4.4
Females	4.5

much. However, considering the fact that only about one in three persons among the profoundly retarded is institutionalized, a group for whom schooling is rare, it can be reasonably surmised that a lower proportion of the moderately retarded and a far lower proportion of the mildly retarded would be institutionalized if no educational facilities were available. These proportions make it doubtful if savings in institutional costs alone would justify education programs. However, this is a highly speculative matter.

Readers who wish to pursue benefit-cost analysis to its ultimate goal may multiply the data in Table 60 times the percentages of retardates that they believe avoid institutionalization as a result of educational programs, and add these products to the ratios of lifetime earnings and education costs (Tables 55 to 57). A similar calculation could be made for the benefit-cost ratios of the rehabilitation program.

DISTRIBUTION OF BENEFITS

Most services to the retarded are publicly financed. The general public shares in the increased productivity due to these services to the extent that the retarded pay taxes to federal, state, and local governments and to the extent that income maintenance and residential care costs are reduced. At current tax and income-maintenance rates, it can be crudely estimated that, on the average, about one-half of the productivity of the retarded accrues to the benefit of the general public—about one-fourth of their income is used to pay taxes and, if they were not working, income-maintenance payments would equal about one-fourth of their income.

Surprisingly, the lower the earnings of the retarded, the greater the public share becomes. This is because income-maintenance payments are relatively stable and become an increasingly large share of earnings as earnings decline. A person earning $1,500 would pay relatively little in taxes, about $85 in federal income taxes if unmarried. If the person were not working, however, income maintenance would be of the order of $1,000. Combined income taxes paid and income-maintenance savings would be over 70% of gross earnings. In contrast, a person earning $5,000 would pay about $750 in federal income taxes. Since the income maintenance part of the public benefit is unchanged, the combined benefit to the general public would be 35% of gross earnings.

Altruism need not always be the motivating factor in providing developmental and supportive services to the retarded.

ECONOMICS OF PREVENTION

However good the social adjustment of most retardates, there are few people who wouldn't prefer prevention to treatment—at least until confronted with its costs.

The prevention of mental retardation is not an activity that will be undertaken regardless of costs. Although most people argue that physical and mental health cannot be valued, there are, in fact, implicit social judgments placed on the value of these aspects of our lives. Who doubts, for example, that the absurd number of traffic injuries and fatalities could be reduced if more resources were devoted to better roads, traffic control, and safer cars. But when the people involved in these fatalities are nameless and faceless, there are limits to the amount that will be used for their safety.

Types of Prevention. Methods of preventing mental retardation can be divided into three broad categories:

1. those which prevent brain damage that occurs after conception;

2. those which prevent the *birth* of a defective child (infanticide is assumed to be unacceptable). This breaks down into two additional cases.

a. the total number of children born to a family declines by the number of prevented births;

b. the number of children born to a family remains constant; the defective fetus is, in effect, replaced by a normal child.

3. those which through environmental modification or specialized care prevent a child's IQ from falling below the defined threshold of mental retardation.

Prevention possibilities. In Chapter III we observed that if all demo graphic groups had the same rate of mental retardation as exists among middle- and upper-class white children, the prevalence of mental retardation would decrease almost 80%. Unless one wishes to argue that there are important genetic differences among demographic groups with respect to intellectual potential, this represents the extent to which it is possible to prevent mental retardation. Much of the overall prevalence of mental retardation is probably due to cultural deprivation. However, it is generally believed that most people with IQs below 50 have suffered some degree of brain damage.

Imre reported that the rate of severe retardation (IQ below 50) was only 0.18% among middle- and upper-class white children; among lower-class nonwhite children the comparable rate was 1.89%. If we assume that this astonishing difference was due to a greater probability of neurological damage among lower-class nonwhites (because of diet, the quality of prenatal and pediatric care, etc.), then the importance of preventing brain damage assumes major proportions.

Assume that the results of the Imre study by race and social class can be generalized to the United States. If, among all 5- to 19-year-olds, there were the same percentage of children with IQs below 50 as among upper- and middle-class white children, there would have been in 1970 only 108,000 school-age children in this IQ range, instead of an estimated 241,000. On the other hand, if among all children there were the same percentage of these low IQs as among lower-class nonwhite children, the total number would rise to 1,138,000. In other words, in this age group a combination of preventive factors has resulted in preventing about 897,000 cases of severe retardation. There is evidently scope for an additional reduction of 133,000 cases.

These are minimal estimates. Upper- and middle-class whites by no means avail themselves of all preventive possibilities, nor are lower-class nonwhites completely devoid of any preventive efforts. Moreover, new preventive techniques have been developed since 1967 or are being developed (measles vaccines, intrauterine chromosome analysis, etc.).

These figures are based on extrapolation from a single county, and the numbers of severely retarded children in the study are small, especially among middle- and upper-class whites. One more or one less case would have had a noticeable impact on our empirical magnitudes. Nevertheless, the results of the Imre study are consistent with those of other studies. Moreover, as noted, our estimates may understate the importance of preventive efforts and possibilities, and, in any event, are of such large empirical magnitude that subsequent modifications based on more comprehensive data are unlikely to alter our general conclusions.

Not all people share this optimistic outlook concerning preventive possibilities. The fear is occasionally expressed that improved and more extensive prenatal, obstetrical, and pediatric care will increase the number of retarded infants that survive.[43] In view of the large number of retarded infants who die in the first year of life, such concern would appear to be well founded.

Two points cast doubt on this hypothesis. First, medical changes that reduce infant mortality often also reduce infant morbidity,[44] e.g., congenital syphilis. Morbidity is a far more common occurence than infant mortality. Although some retarded children may survive who would otherwise have died, the number of infants for whom serious brain damage is prevented is probably considerably greater. Second, and in partial support of the previous point, the prevalence of both mild and severe retardation is greatest among the lowest socioeconomic classes that typically receive the least adequate medical care—the opposite of what one would expect on the basis of the original premise.

Concern is also sometimes expressed over the possibilities that (1) medical advances will enable persons with defective genes to survive and transmit their defects to future generations; and (2) modern contraceptive techniques will lead women to defer some births until they are past their prime child-bearing years, say age 35, when the chances of a defective infant increase. It is, however, doubtful if either of these possibilities will exert a significant impact on the prevalence of retardation. There has, in fact, been a significant decrease (over 35%) in the rate of child-bearing among women over 35 in the last fifteen years.

Theoretical considerations. Our discussion of the economics of prevention will be limited primarily to the first two methods of preventing mental retardation mentioned above (i.e., prevention of brain damage and prevention of the birth of a child known to be or likely to be defective). Although the prevention of intellectual loss due to cultural deprivation is a task that should be given an urgent social priority, empirical limitations preclude an extended analysis.

From an economic standpoint, the cases where brain damage is prevented and where a defective fetus is replaced by a normal one are almost identical. In both cases the intellectual distribution of persons

---

[43] E.g., USDHEW, The Secretary's Committee on Mental Retardation, *An Introduction to Mental Retardation, Problems, Plans and Programs,* June 1965, p. 13.

[44] N. Goodman and J. Tizard, "Prevalence of Imbecility and Idiocy Among Children," *British Medical Journal* (January 27, 1962): 218–19.

actually born approximates that of the general population. For purposes of our subsequent analysis, these two cases will be combined and termed the "replacement" case.

In these days of widespread family planning the second possibility (replacing a defective fetus with a normal fetus) merits more attention than may be apparent at first glance. Ways in which it may be accomplished are: (1) interuterine detection of birth defects, with subsequent abortion if indicated; (2) completing family during the optimal child-bearing years; and (3) adoption in the case of families for whom the genetic risk of bearing defective children has been determined to be very high. It could be plausibly argued that the adoption situation belongs in the case where the number of children in a family declines. This is largely a matter of judgment and will not affect our subsequent analysis.

When the number of children per family declines as a result of efforts to prevent mental retardation, this will be called the "nonreplacement" case. It occurs when families voluntarily forgo having children because of a high risk of defect, and when families do not practice family planning, although they seek an abortion if they suspect or know that an unborn child is defective.

To estimate the value of prevention in the replacement case we compare differences in earnings, custodial costs, developmental expenditures, and other relevant variables between a mentally retarded person and an "average" person in society.

In the "nonreplacement" case, the matter becomes considerably more complicated and, in fact, our model develops serious contradictions. Normally, we consider any earnings by a retarded person as a net benefit to society, and refuse to regard their consumption as a social loss; at most, when financed by others, we will regard their consumption as a redistribution of income.

But the converse does not hold true. If we prevent retardates from being born, we usually are reluctant to regard the loss in future productivity as a social loss and almost always point to the savings in institutional costs, which include consumption expenditures, as a social gain. This problem only arises in the "nonreplacement" case where population decreases. In the "replacement" case, where population is unaffected, we make a direct comparison between a retardate and an "average" person.

From a social standpoint, these "inherent" contradictions can be resolved. If our concern is with maintaining and improving the *average* quality of life, then clearly the world must make the best use of the capabilities of its existing population. The productive efforts of the retarded clearly add to the resources available to improve the average quality of life. The birth of additional retardates, however, will not necessarily raise the average standard of living of society.

Thus, it is *reasonable* to consider as beneficial any and all productive efforts by an existing population, and it is, at the same time, *reasonable* to not count as a loss the potential productive capability of persons who are not born. In effect, these persons are not considered as a part of society, present or future.

The value of prevention in the "nonreplacement" case is: (1) the savings in the custodial costs of institutional care; (2) the savings in developmental costs; and (3) the difference between what the retarded would have consumed and would have produced if the former exceeds the latter (since this would lower the average quality of life for the rest of the population); (4) the potentially enormous psychic gains to the rest of the population; and (5) other savings (crime, accidents, etc.).

Two points must be made: (1) Most prevention efforts have prevented brain damage so that this conceptually difficult case of nonreplacement, although not insignificant, is of far less importance than the replacement case. (2) Benefit-cost ratios based on these different approaches are in no way comparable and cannot be used to rank alternatives.

Several other points should be mentioned:

1) It is not always certain that a fetus is defective. This creates analytical problems which must be dealt with on a case-by-case basis. In general, in the "replacement" case one would increase the *cost* of prevention (by a factor of 2 if the probability of retardation was 50%, a factor of 4 if 25%, etc.). In the "nonreplacement" case, the same procedure could be followed, but one feels uncomfortable about putting a zero value on the lives of normal fetuses that are aborted in an effort to reduce the incidence of mental retardation. A similar problem could be broached in the replacement case, but the whole matter becomes impossible, since the nonbirth of one normal person makes possible the birth of another.

2) If the world reaches a point where populations must be limited to a given size, then the "nonreplacement" case loses all applicability.

3) In many cases, the prevention of mental retardation will be only one of several goals of a particular program. Rubella, for example, may cause deafness, blindness, and other conditions, as well as mental retardation. From a benefit-cost standpoint, each of these programs

should be individually evaluated and all of their favorable consequences considered, not just the avoidance of mental retardation.

4) It is not necessary to be able to identify the persons for whom mental retardation is averted by a particular program, only that a certain proportion of persons encompassed by a given program will benefit.

5) Each prevention program must be evaluated on an individual basis to determine the category of prevention approaches into which it falls.

Value of prevention. Table 61 shows the components of the measurable economic benefits of the prevention of mental retardation by IQ and sex. The derivation of these data are summarized as follows:

1) The data for earnings and total productivity gain (replacement case only) are based on the information contained in Tables 49 to 52, adjusted for the percentage employed or the percentage in home-making.

2) Savings in costs of *custodial care* in residential facilities were derived by multiplying the estimated custodial costs of lifetime institutionalization (Table 59) by the proportion of persons estimated to be in institutions within the different levels of retardation (29% for persons with IQs below 40, 23% for persons with IQs between 40 and 50, and 1.9% for persons with IQs between 50 and 69: see Chapter V). It was assumed that custodial costs of lifetime institutionalization for the severely and profoundly retarded were the same as for the moderately retarded.

Although only custodial costs incurred in an institution are counted, parents who retain their child at home also have special expenses for purposes other than normal consumption, especially if the mother is prevented from accepting gainful employment. Thus, a substantial amount of social cost is being overlooked.

3) Savings in developmental costs were approximated by calculating savings in educational costs. For the nonreplacement case, lifetime costs of education were taken from Table 54. In the case of the mildly retarded, the intermediate estimate was used (5 years in each type of class). It was assumed that developmental costs for persons with IQs below 40 were the same as for those with IQs between 40 and 49.[45]

The replacement case requires that we estimate the difference in educational costs between the retarded and the nonretarded. In 1970

---

[45] The high cost of developmental services for persons with IQs below 40 is assumed to offset the fact that most are in formal developmental activities for a relatively short time (if at all).

Table 61. Economic value of preventing mental retardation among persons born in 1952 (1970 prices)

	Replacement case				Nonreplacement case			
	Not discounted		Discounted		Not discounted		Discounted	
	Male	Female	Male	Female	Male	Female	Male	Female
IQ below 40								
Earnings gain	$612,000	$161,000	$132,000	$37,000	0	0	0	0
Total productivity gain	764,000	375,000	165,000	82,000	0	0	0	0
Savings in institutional costs (custodial only)	112,000	115,000	49,000	49,000	$112,000	$115,000	$49,000	$49,000
Savings in developmental costs	15,000	15,000	21,000	21,000	26,000	26,000	38,000	38,000
Savings in maintenance costs	a	a	a	a	108,000	113,000	48,000	49,000
IQ 40 to 49								
Earnings gain	550,000	152,000	119,000	35,000	0	0	0	0
Total productivity gain	686,000	336,000	149,000	73,000	0	0	0	0
Savings in institutional costs (custodial only)	89,000	91,000	39,000	39,000	89,000	91,000	39,000	39,000
Savings in developmental costs	15,000	15,000	21,000	21,000	26,000	26,000	38,000	38,000
Savings in maintenance costs	a	a	a	a	78,000	81,000	41,000	41,000
IQ 50 to 69								
Earnings gain	109,000	60,000	20,000	12,000	0	0	0	0
Total productivity gain	135,000	84,000	25,000	17,000	0	0	0	0
Savings in institutional costs (custodial only)	7,000	8,000	3,000	3,000	7,000	8,000	3,000	3,000
Savings in developmental costs	2,000	2,000	2,000	2,000	13,000	13,000	19,000	19,000
Savings in maintenance costs	a	a	a	a	0	0	0	0

aNot applicable.

total average annual per capita costs of regular academic classes were $1,034. The median number of years of education for adults in the United States is about twelve. Using previously described procedures, lifetime educational costs for an 18-year-old person who completed high school in 1970 are estimated at $16,600 if compounded and $10,600 if not. These data were used to make the estimates contained in Table 61.[46]

4) Savings in maintenance expenditures apply only in the non-replacement case. Publicly provided maintenance expenditures for the retarded were of the order of $1,000 per person in 1970, far below the average productivity of most of the mildly retarded. Accordingly, we will not record a maintenance savings to society for preventing cases of mild retardation.

We estimated that 55% of moderately retarded adult males do not work. Median annual earnings of those working were about $1,550 in 1970. However, many workers, especially among those whose earnings were substantially below the median, undoubtedly required additional assistance. We assume that in 1970 moderately retarded male adults (workers and nonworkers) received on the average about $600 from sources other than earnings (public assistance, parents or other relatives, or the value of consumption items received in residential care facilities).

Lifetime savings in maintenance costs were estimated for this group by assuming 100% support from birth to age 18 and 60% support thereafter until age 65. After age 65, we again assume 100% support. The support level is assumed to be $1,000 in 1970 and to vary over time in proportion to productivity change.[47] Lifetime maintenance savings are calculated by applying the usual adjustments for mortality and productivity change and assuming the retarded to be 18 years old in 1970.

We estimated that 81% of moderately retarded females were not working and that the median earnings among those that work was only $816 in 1970. To estimate lifetime maintenance savings for this group, we assume an annual subsidy of 90% between the ages of 18 and 64 and 100% before and after these ages.

Among the profoundly and severely retarded we assume total support throughout their lifetime. The support level is assumed to be

[46] This crude procedure may cause an overstatement of the savings in developmental costs since public school costs are much less than those incurred for college students, so that it is not strictly correct to offset the reduction in costs resulting from high school drop-outs against the costs incurred for college students. The biases involved, however, are small.

[47] Although $1,000 seems low, it is a close approximation to the average income maintenance payment and our estimate of maintenance costs in institutions in 1970.

$1,000 in 1970, and death rates are assumed to be three times normal.

The data in Table 61 are presented in summary form in Table 62. It must be emphasized that these are estimates that are subject to change as better information (or theory) becomes available or as conditions change. In particular, the benefits of preventing moderate retardation may decline if better services enable greater numbers of these individuals to be placed on more productive jobs. On the other hand, an improved quality of maintenance and developmental services may cause an increase in these figures. In addition, these estimates are, as has been emphasized, only partial measures. Although most of the omitted benefits are well known, one that is worth mentioning is that we cannot value the creative and innovative efforts of the scholars and inventors who would be part of the nonretarded groups resulting from the replacement form of prevention.

What conclusions can be drawn? First, the benefits of prevention are large. The prevention of a case of severe retardation (IQ less than 40) among males enables society to make a gross gain (undiscounted) of almost $900,000 over a person's lifetime in the replacement case. This is the value of the resources, saved and created, that would be available to improve the average standard of living. These estimates are in 1970 dollars—continuing inflation and productivity change will increase the per-person value of preventing severe retardation to the million-dollar level in the near future.

Although the social gain of preventing severe retardation among women appears to be considerably less, it must be emphasized that this is a consequence of the lower average earnings of women and that this difference will decrease and perhaps disappear over time, as the earnings of women approach equality with those of men. On a discounted basis, the benefits remained impressive, being over $200,000 in the replacement case of preventing severe retardation among males.

In the nonreplacement case the tangible economic benefits are lower but highly significant. In the case of the severely retarded, the nondiscounted value of prevention is about $250,000 per case and on a discounted basis about $135,000. The value of preventing severe retardation was slightly greater for women than for men, because earnings were not a factor in the calculations, and severely retarded women were assumed to require more subsidized support than severely retarded men.

The value of prevention declines as less severe levels of retardation are considered, although in no case can the value of prevention be regarded as insignificant.

Total output in the United States was about $3.4 billion greater in 1970 than it would have been had the prevalence of persons with IQs

Table 62. Summary of the economic value of preventing mental retardation among persons born in 1952, (1970 prices)

| | Prevention of brain damage or replacement birth | | | | Prevent birth without replacement | | | |
| | Not discounted | | Discounted | | Not discounted | | Discounted | |
	Male	Female	Male	Female	Male	Female	Male	Female
IQ below 40								
Includes earnings gain but not values of housekeeping and other unpaid work	$739,000	$291,000	$202,000	$107,000	$246,000	$254,000	$135,000	$136,000
Includes total productivity gain	891,000	505,000	235,000	152,000				
IQ 40 to 49								
Includes earnings gain but not values of housekeeping and other unpaid work	654,000	258,000	179,000	95,000	193,000	198,000	118,000	118,000
Includes total productivity gain	790,000	442,000	209,000	133,000				
IQ 50 to 69								
Includes earnings gain but not values of housekeeping and other unpaid work	118,000	70,000	25,000	17,000	20,000	21,000	22,000	22,000
Includes total productivity gain	144,000	94,000	30,000	22,000				

below 50 in the general population been the same as was estimated for the children of lower-class nonwhites. As discussed previously, the lower rates of severe retardation among whites and the more favored nonwhites evidently reflect the combination of various factors which cumulatively prevent significant amounts of brain damage among the children born to these groups. To this must be added $1.4 billion in custodial costs and $600 million in the excess costs of educating the trainable mentally retarded that was saved because of this assumed reduction in the number of severely retarded persons. In short, preventive efforts were responsible for an increment of over $5 billion in the resources available to society to enhance living standards. [48]

If the prevalence of persons with IQs below 50 was the same in the general population as it was among the children of middle- and upper-class whites in 1970 (which implies a reduction of about 45% in their numbers) output would have been roughly $500 million greater, and custodial costs and special education costs would have been over $300 million less.

Because of data limitations and the large number of ways of preventing mental retardation, no overall benefit-cost analysis of preventive efforts will be undertaken. We will, however, examine four of the more important methods of preventing this condition.

Down's syndrome (mongolism). Down's syndrome is an abnormality where the cells in the body contain 47 chromosomes instead of the usual complement of 46. In a few cases, the cells appear to contain the normal 46 chromosomes, but one of the chromosomes contains excess genetic material.

Mosaic mongolism occurs when only part of the cells in the human body contain 47 chromosomes. Mosaic mongols have higher IQs and less physical stigmata than other persons with Down's syndrome. Due to the fact that there is little demographic data on mosaic mongolism, our succeeding discussion will be limited to the prevention of cases of complete mongolism. Apparently, less than 10% of the cases of mongolism are inherited; the remainder are due to an accident in the process of cell division shortly after conception.

Since Down's syndrome usually leads to moderate retardation, the economic value of preventing a case of mongolism is represented by the

---

[48] These figures are crudely derived. It was assumed that 20% of the prevented cases of severe and moderate mental retardation would be in institutions at an average annual custodial cost of $3,450, and that half of trainable school age children would be in special classes at an excess cost of $2,500. Average employment rates and earnings were used to estimate output gains, with an adjustment for what the probable productivity of these persons would have been had they suffered brain damage. Almost all prevention would fall into the replacement category.

IQ 40 to 49 category. However, this may understate the benefits of preventing mongolism, since mongols appear to be even less successful in locating work than other retardates of similar IQ.

Estimates of the incidence of Down's syndrome vary widely, ranging from 1 in 1,000 births to 1 in 400, with 1 in 600 or 700 being the most frequently cited. Reed states that the frequency would be in the neighborhood of 1 in 500 births, if undiagnosed cases of infant mortality were taken into account,[49] and Montagu states that the incidence is 1 in 400.[50] Apparently, about 7,000 babies with Down's syndrome are born each year, of whom perhaps 20% fail to live more than a few years.

More important than the overall incidence is the incidence by age and by certain demographic groups. Roughly 1 in 1,000 babies born to mothers under 35 have Down's syndrome (a ratio that would rise sharply for females below age 15 or 16). This ratio rises to 1 in 300 for mothers aged 35 to 39, 1 in 100 for mothers aged 40 to 44, and 1 in 50 for mothers aged 45 to 49.[51]

Three groups in the population have a higher probability of producing a child with Down's syndrome than indicated by their age alone. People who themselves have Down's syndrome have about a 1 in 2 chance of producing a mongol child. The arguments against permitting these individuals to have children are so powerful on other grounds that this group will not be considered further.[52] Mosaic mongols constitute the second group. Their prevalence in the population is unknown (one authority guesses that the ratio is 1 in 3,000).[53] The probability of their giving birth to a mongol child is also unknown, although it is presumed to be above average and to vary with the degree of mosaicism.

The final group is the small proportion of mongols whose condition is inherited from nonmongoloid parents. In these cases one of the par-

[49] Sheldon C. Reed, *Counseling in Medical Genetics* (Philadelphia: W. B. Saunders Company, 1963), p. 50.

[50] Ashley Montagu, *Human Heredity* (Cleveland: The World Publishing Company, 1963), p. 89.

[51] Reed, *Counseling in Medical Genetics*, p. 51; and Ernest M. Gruenberg, "Epidemiology," in *Mental Retardation, A Review of Research*; Harvey A. Stevens and Rick Heber, eds. (Chicago: The University of Chicago Press, 1964), p. 302.

[52] There still remains the question of whether sterilization or segregation is the best means of ensuring nonreproduction. The former is clearly superior on economic grounds, but there are possible moral issues involved. The probability of a mongol having a mongol child is 1 in 2 if one parent is a non-mongol. If both parents are mongols, the probability rises to 2 out of 3.

[53] L. S. Penrose, "Studies of Mosaicism in Down's Anomaly," in *Mental Retardation, a Symposium*, George A. Jervis, ed. (Springfield, Illinois: Charles C Thomas, 1967), p. 9.

ents, usually the mother, has only 45 chromosomes, although one chromosome contains the genetic material normally divided into two chromosomes. A parent with this abnormality has about a 1 in 3 chance of producing a completely normal child, about a 1 in 3 chance of having a normal child who is a carrier of mongolism, and about a 1 in 3 chance of producing an infant with Down's syndrome. It is possible that a mongol fetus is more subject to spontaneous abortion than normal fetuses, and that therefore the probability of a mongol child being born to a carrier parent is less than 1 in 3.

At present, there are three principle methods of preventing mongolism: (1) Women can be encouraged to complete their families before reaching high-risk ages. Reed states that at least one-third of the cases of mongolism could be prevented if the mother completed her family before she was 40. Montagu notes that half of the cases of Down's syndrome were born to mothers of 35 years of age or more. If family size is unchanged, this case is comparable to the replacement case in Table 62. The only possible difference is that one may wish to impute an interest charge on the resources expended on children at an earlier time than would normally be the case.

2) Persons with a high risk of producing mongol children can be encouraged not to have children. This obviously includes mongols, non-mongoloid carriers of the defect, many mosaic mongols, and women over 40. If family size is reduced, this is equivalent to the nonreplacement case of Table 62. Detection of high-risk women (other than those defined by age) is a difficult matter, since it requires mass screening, except in cases where women have already given birth to an infant with Down's syndrome.

3) High-risk cases can be examined by a process called amniocentesis, in which cast-off, floating fetal cells are obtained by inserting a hypodermic needle through the mother's abdominal wall into the amniotic sac encompassing the fetus. These cells are then examined by means of a recently developed process to determine whether the fetus is a mongoloid (47 chromosomes), a carrier of mongolism (45 chromosomes), or normal. If the fetus is abnormal, the parents may opt for abortion at this early stage. If the woman again becomes pregnant and produces a normal child, then the benefits of prevention are best described by the replacement case.

Swanson reports that the current costs of these tests are about $150 and suggests that mass production could conceivably reduce these costs to $100.[54] If *all* pregnant women over 44 underwent this examination,

[54] T. E. Swanson, "A Systems Analysis Approach to the Prevention of Mongolism," Report to the Research and Advancement Subcommittee, The President's

the cost of detecting a mongoloid fetus would be between $5,000 and $7,500 (50 × $100 or $150). An abortion would increase the total cost of prevention to perhaps $5,500 or $8,000. If we use an intermediate figure of $7,000, and adjust it backward eighteen years to allow for interest charges and productivity change, then the present value (in 1970) of the resources used to prevent a case of mongolism among 45- to 49-year-old women in 1952 would be $15,170.[55] This figure is far below any of the estimates of the discounted value of preventing mental retardation with or without replacement.

The comparable cost figures among women in the 40- to 44-year age range are $13,000 and $28,000, and among women in the 35- to 39-year age group $40,000 and $87,000. On a present-value basis, these costs are significantly below the benefits of preventing mental retardation when the IQ would fall below 50.

Among women below age 35, the cost of preventing a case of mongolism by screening all pregnant women is about $130,000, and when adjusted for interest charges and productivity change, on the assumption that the prevention effort took place eighteen years earlier, the present value of this cost rises to $280,000. Economic values alone do not justify the prevention of mongolism among women below the age of 35 (although I suspect that most expectant mothers would gladly accept the cost of ensuring that their child is not born with Down's syndrome).

When high-risk groups can be identified, the economics of prevention are even more startling. When one of the parents has only 45 chromosomes, the present value of the economic benefits of amniotic examination and the replacement of a mongoloid fetus by a normal fetus range between 50 and 110 times the present value of the cost of this procedure (assuming that it requires three examinations to detect a case of mongolism). In the case of mosaic mongolism, the risk of an abnormal child would almost certainly be greater than the 2% estimated for women age 45 and over, and on a benefit-cost basis would be justified.

These statements are true only *after* a high risk population has been identified. To date, identification of a high risk population does not take place until after a mongoloid child has been born. Since no more than 1 out of 10 mongoloid infants is born to a family where one parent has 45 chromosomes, at least 10, possible 20, and perhaps even

---

Committee on Mental Retardation, July 2, 1968, Appendix. Technically, this estimate should be adjusted to 1970 price levels. However, it is likely that improved methods have offset the effect of price increases.

[55] Of course, amniocentesis was not perfected in 1950, but this adjustment is necessary in order to express these figures in present value form.

more of these parents would have to be screened to detect a single carrier. This would increase the total cost of preventing a second case of mongolism among this high-risk group to about $2,000, or in present value terms, about $4,400. Although the economic desirability of such a program cannot be doubted, it would prevent a relatively small proportion of the cases of mongolism.

The economic pinch arises when one considers screening the entire population to ascertain a high-risk group before the birth of a mongoloid infant. As many as 2,000 persons may have to be examined to detect a single case of a mosaic mongol or a person with 45 chromosomes. In terms of present-value calculations, one cannot justify such an effort until the cost of chromosomal examination declines below the figures cited above. Moreover, since most mongolism is not inherited, this type of screening would still be effective in reducing only about 10% of the cases of mongolism.

One more approach to preventing mongolism would be to screen all pregnant women by amniocentesis (rather than the entire population), assuming that adequate facilities were available and that safety to the mother and the developing fetus was assured. Not only could mongolism be eradicated, but cases of mental retardation from many other causes could be eliminated or reduced since there are a growing number of metabolic diseases that cause mental retardation which can be diagnosed in utero prior to birth from study of the amniotic fluid or cells. These disorders include: Tay-Sachs disease, Hurler's syndrome, galactosemia, Gaucher's and glycogen diseases. If a defective fetus is discovered and the pregnancy terminated about once in every 500 cases, such a screening program would cost about $75,500 for each case of severe defect prevented, or about $166,000 in present value terms.

Phenylketonuria. Phenylketonuria (PKU) is a hereditary disease in which individuals lack an enzyme which is needed to convert phenylalanine, an essential amino acid in protein foods, into a form which can be used by the body. If PKU babies are fed milk, phenylalanine and its byproducts accumulate in the body, preventing normal development of the brain and apparently also causing psychological disturbances.

Estimates of the prevalence of PKU have varied between 1 in 25,000 and 1 in 10,000, with the latter figure becoming increasingly accepted as the results of mass screening for PKU become available.[56]

The extent of intellectual damage caused by PKU varies from almost complete mental deterioration to no apparent deterioration. One

[56] I. Jay Brightman, "Mental Retardation Activities of the Department of Health," *Proceedings of the Mental Retardation Assembly*, February 1–2, 1968, Department of Mental Hygiene, New York, p. 50.

authority speculates that possibly one in two PKU infants will not be mentally damaged. Other authorities argue that "On the basis of the evidence thus far presented it would appear that in most, if not practically all, cases continuously elevated blood phenylalanine levels would lead to mental retardation unless treatment is initiated early.[57]

We will assume that only 1 in 2 PKU infants suffer significant brain damage. This may be an understatement and, in any event, does not take account of the gains of averting the psychological disturbances that appear frequently among PKU adults whose intellect appears unharmed.[58]

We will also assume that most PKU infants who suffer brain damage will fall into the moderately retarded category if not treated, although this is probably conservative. Koch et al. reported on 23 PKU children who did not receive treatment. Their average age at diagnosis was 12 and their average IQ was 43. Three years later their estimated average IQ had fallen 19 points.[59]

Screening for PKU among infants is a relatively simple, efficient, and inexpensive procedure requiring a few drops of blood before the infant leaves the hospital. The cost of the procedure is about 25¢ per infant, so that the total cost of detecting a potential phenylketonuric infant is only $2,500.[60]

Once detected, the diagnosis must be confirmed, and if confirmed, the infants are placed on a special diet and monitored carefully by a physician until their middle or late teens. It has been estimated that the total cost of the PKU program per baby discovered and treated in Massachusetts is $10,000.[61] This is perhaps an overstatement, since the cost of food that a normal child would consume should be deducted from the cost of maintaining a special diet for a PKU child.

If only one out of two of these children benefit, the cost of prevention would rise to $20,000 per case, which, on a present-value basis is one-third to one-fifth the resulting benefits (the present value of these resources would be about $40,000, assuming that most costs were incurred prior to the age of 6).

[57] Richard Koch, Phyllis Acosta, and Karol Fishler, "Observations of Phenylketonuria," in *Phenylketonuria and Allied Metabolic Diseases*, John A. Anderson and Kenneth F. Swaiman, eds., USDHEW, SRS (USGPO, 1967), p. 116.

[58] Samuel P. Bassman, "The Implications of the Drive for Screening," in *Phenylketonuria and Allied Metabolic Diseases*, p. 178.

[59] Koch et al., "Observations of Phenylketonuria," p. 123.

[60] Mathilde Krim, "The Prevention of Mental Retardation: Today and Tomorrow," *PCMR Message* (March 1968): 6.

[61] Benjamin D. White, "Case-Finding of Phenylketonuria as a Public Health Approach," in *Phenylketonuria and Allied Metabolic Diseases*, p. 152.

A prerequisite to success in preventing PKU is early treatment.[62] A delay of even a few months may prove catastrophic. Data presented by Koch et al., points up clearly the negative relationship between age of diagnosis and IQ scores after a period of treatment.[63] Damage may even begin prior to birth which, although treatable, is difficult to detect. A number of authorities assert that brain damage cannot always be completely prevented, but emphasize that early treatment may mean the difference between severe (IQ below 40) and mild retardation.[64] The economic benefits of reducing the extent of brain damage in this way are about the same as those of preventing a case of moderate retardation.

A serious consideration remains. A poorly administered diet may have harmful effects and may itself cause brain damage. Since not all PKU children will suffer brain damage, the propriety of subjecting all children who have PKU to a hazardous diet has been questioned, especially since adequate dietary supervision depends upon parental understanding and cooperation and careful supervision by the prescribing physician, conditions which are not always met. Woolf, however, observes that "The only disadvantages of treating all newborn phenylketonurics with the low-phenylalanine diet are the cost, the relatively unpalatable nature of the diet and the danger of dietary deficiencies. . . . treating up to twice as many patients as may be necessary seems a small price to pay for preventing the mental deterioration otherwise inevitable in at least half of them."[65]

Rubella. When rubella is contracted by a woman in the first trimester of pregnancy, the probability of damage to the developing embryo is high and, in the opinion of some authorities, is almost certain. Rubella contracted in the second trimester of pregnancy also creates a serious hazard for an unborn infant. The probability of damage may be as high as two-thirds.[66]

Rubella babies suffer a variety of congenital defects. Heart disease, hearing loss, eye disease, and mental retardation are among the most

---

[62] James Dobson et al., "Cognitive Development and Dietary Therapy in *Phenylketonuric Children,*" New England Journal of Medicine (May 23, 1968): 1142–44.

[63] Koch et al., "Observations of Phenylketonuria," in *Phenylketonuria and Allied Metabolic Diseases*, pp. 119–23.

[64] Dobson et al., "Cognitive Development," p. 1144.

[65] L. I. Woolfe, "Large-Scale Screening for Metabolic Diseases in the Newborn in Great Britain, " in *Phenylketonuria and Allied Metabolic Diseases*, p. 58.

[66] Janet B. Hardy et al., "Adverse Fetal Outcome Following Maternal Rubella *After* the First Trimester of Pregnancy," *Journal of the American Medical Association* (March 31, 1969): 2414.

serious. Apparently about 40% are developmentally retarded. A considerable number are spontaneously aborted, still-born, or die shortly after birth.[67]

The last epidemic of German measles in the United States occurred in 1964 causing congenital defects in an estimated 30,000 infants and an unknown number of fetal deaths.[68] Peaks of the disease occur every six to fifteen years. During epidemic years, about 1% of all live births are rubella babies.[69] During nonepidemic years, the rate is one-twentieth to one-hundredth of this.[70] Assuming a rubella cycle of ten years, this would mean that 1 in every 700 to 900 infants would be born with congenital damage caused by maternal rubella, and 1 in every 1,700 to 2,300, infants would have developmental retardation as a consequence. We will assume that the relevent rates are 1 in 800 and 1 in 2,000.

The severity of retardation caused by rubella ranges from mild to profound, with a high incidence of multiple handicaps. Apparently, it is premature to make a judgment on the "typical" level of retardation caused by maternal rubella.

Until recently, gamma globulin was frequently given to expectant women who were exposed to rubella. The efficacy of this treatment has been sharply questioned. In addition, an increasing number of states permit abortions for women who contract rubella during pregnancy.

The major recent preventive thrust has been the widespread innoculation of children with a rubella vaccine. In principle, this protects pregnant women by reducing the chance of exposure to a child ill with rubella, and should also protect these children when they attain child-bearing age.

It is estimated by the National Communicable Disease Center that the cost of the vaccine for each injection is about $1.25, if purchased in large quantities. If obtained in a physician's office, the cost would be $6 to $8 (of which $2 to $3 would be the physician's cost of buying a single dose of the vaccine). If every child were given a rubella injection, then, with about 3.5 million births per year, and using the lower-cost

[67] Louis Z. Cooper, "German Measles," *Scientific American*, vol. 215, no. 1 (July 1966): 30.

[68] Louis Z. Cooper, "Rubella: A Preventable Cause of Birth Defects," *Birth Defects: Original Article Series*, vol. 10 no. 7. pp. 22–35. *Intrauterine Infections*, Daniel Bergsman, ed. (The National Foundation, December 1968), p. 23.

[69] Cooper, "Rubella: A Preventable Cause," p. 23.

[70] John L. Sever, "Perinatal Infections Affecting the Developing Fetus and Newborn," *The Prevention of Mental Retardation through Control of Infectious Diseases*, USDHEW, NIH, Public Health Service Publication No. 1692 (USGPO), p. 49. Also, Louis Z. Cooper, Report to the First PCMR Staff Development Conference.

figure, the total cost of the vaccine used by the program would be about $4.4 million per year (after the initial backlog was disposed of), or about $1,000 to protect the 1 infant in 800 who would be born with a congenital defect because of rubella, and $2,500 to protect the 1 infant in 2,000 who would be retarded because of rubella. If all injections were given in a physician's office, the average cost of preventing birth defects due to maternal rubella would be considerably higher, perhaps $6,500 per case, and $16,000 for each case of retardation prevented. In present-value terms, these four costs range between $2,000 and $35,000. Inspection of Table 62 shows that the present value of the benefits of preventing moderate or severe retardation is many times these costs. When a case of mild retardation is prevented, the highest estimated cost of so doing is a little less than our calculation of the present value of benefits.

The cost of preventing maternal rubella should be evaluated against all benefits and not just the benefits of preventing mental retardation. If the value of preventing all birth defects due to maternal rubella were calculated, it is likely that the ratio of benefits to cost would be about twice what we have measured.

This assumes a safe, effective vaccine. Apparently there is still a question as to whether existing vaccines confer long-term immunity to the disease, or whether the immunized individual might not inadvertently transmit the disease to another person.

Measles. Most children recover from regular measles without serious after-effects. Once in about every 1,000 cases, however, post-infectious encephalitis occurs. Between 10% and 20% of these persons die and 33% to 50% develop a long-lasting central nervous system defect.[71] About 1 in every 3,000 children who contract measles will become retarded as a result. The degree of retardation ranges from mild to severe.

An effective vaccine for measles has been developed. Purchased in large quantities, the cost is comparable to that of rubella vaccine. On this basis, the cost of preventing a case of post-infectious encephalitis due to measles is between $1,200 and $8,000, depending on the method of providing the injections. The cost of preventing mental retardation is between $3,600 and $24,000. In present-value terms, these costs range between $2,500 and $52,000. As in the case of maternal rubella, the benefits of preventing moderate or severe retardation are far greater than the costs, but the benefits of preventing a case of mild

[71] Charles Kennedy and T. F. McNair Scott, "The Management of Acute Febrile Encephalapathies," in *The Prevention of Mental Retardation through Control of Infectious Diseases*, p. 319.

retardation are less than the most costly method of preventing mental retardation from this cause. The overall benefits would be much higher if we added in the value of preventing premature death, the savings in lengthy hospital stays, and the value of eliminating the discomfort and worry that attend this disease. Since almost every unprotected child will become infected with measles, it is certain that universal use of a measles vaccine is justified on a benefit-cost basis.

Final comment. Since mental retardation has many causes, prevention must be comprised of many programs, each preventing a relatively small number of cases of retardation, but cumulatively making significant inroads on the problem.

We have briefly reviewed four prevention methods. In each case it was concluded that these programs were either clearly or probably economically justified. Full implementation of these four programs would reduce the incidence of severe retardation by 10% to 20%. Although prevention of brain damage is sometimes criticized on the grounds that it can have only a negligible impact on the total problem of mental retardation, this overlooks the very important fact that prevention will have a significant impact on the prevalence of moderate and severe retardation.

There are many other methods of preventing mental retardation. The incidence of lead poisoning was recently estimated to cause an annual toll of 1,900 cases of permanent brain damage among children.[72] Each year, over 345,000 children are left with permanent impairment, and occasionally mental retardation, due to accidents of all kinds.[73] Lead poisoning and accidents are preventable.

A premarital blood test for syphilis is mandatory in almost every state. For pennies more, an RH factor test and a rubella antibody test could be added. If women who did not have rubella as children were inoculated, and if modern techniques for tranfusing RH infants were available, mental retardation due to these agents could be virtually eradicated.

Genetic counseling can identify high-risk parents. This will assist in preventing damage by alerting parents and physicians to possible medical needs among newborn infants and, in some cases, may influence adults to voluntarily refrain from having children. The PKU case is

[72] Garson A. Lutz et al., *Final Report on Technical, Intelligence and Project Information System for the Environmental Health Service, Volume III. Lead Model Case Study* to USDHEW, Environmental Health Service, by Battelle Memorial Institute, Columbus, Ohio, June 29, 1970, p. 35.

[73] National Association for Retarded Children, *Fact Sheet on Prevention of Mental Retardation*, October 1968, p. 4.

worth considering. If a PKU adult (with two recessive PKU genes) marries an adult with two normal genes, *all* of their children will carry the PKU gene in recessive form, although none will have this condition. If PKU adults marry persons with one PKU gene (1 chance in 80) 50% of their children will have PKU. If two adults with one PKU gene each marry, 25% of their children will have PKU.

Efforts to reduce poverty may, by altering the life styles of many poor people, contribute greatly to the prevention of mental retardation (and, in turn, assist in combatting poverty). Malnutrition among parents and children will be eradicated. Prenatal and postnatal care and delivery procedures will be greatly improved. Better pediatric care will reduce the probability that routine childhood diseases will have serious consequences and will cause mental retardation.

CULTURAL DEPRIVATION

Although we concluded that a more stimulating environment would have enabled over half of the retarded to achieve IQ scores above the arbitrary cutoff point of 70, we have not ventured into a comparison of the benefits and costs of environmental enrichment. The following points, however, should be noted.

First, mental retardation due to environmental shortcomings cannot be effectively dealt with except as a part of the overall attack on cultural deprivation. If successful, the benefits will transverse the entire intellectual spectrum. Not only will IQs that would have declined to the 50's and 60's be maintained in the 70's and 80's, but IQs in the 120's and 130's will be prevented from falling to the 100's and 110's.

Second, preventing mental retardation by improving the environment is quite different from preventing mental retardation by preventing brain damage. In the first case, the IQs of the persons for whom retardation is prevented will still be below average. In the second case, the distribution of IQs among persons for whom brain damage is prevented will approximate that of the normal population. However, since environmental enrichment will benefit an entire population, the distribution of IQs among this entire population may approach that of the general population.

Third, the benefits of reducing cultural deprivation are large. If, in 1970, nonwhite men and women had the same unemployment rates and earning levels as whites, aggregate output would have increased by $21 billion. This loss reflects the influence of many factors and it is not possible to estimate, even crudely, the part of this loss that can be attributed solely to lowered IQ due to cultural conditions.

SUMMARY

1. Despite the crucial importance of comparisons of benefits and costs for decisionmaking, benefit-cost analyses of expenditures on the mentally retarded have many limitations which must be fully appreciated if these analyses are to be useful. These limitations are both conceptual and empirical. Among the more important of these limitations are the difficulty of identifying all the costs that should be compared with the lifetime earnings of the retarded (or relating a portion of lifetime earnings to a particular cost) and the problem of determining an appropriate discount rate.

2. The lifetime earnings of retarded workers are high. A mildly retarded male who entered the work force at age 18 in 1970 could expect lifetime earnings of over $600 thousand dollars. This estimate assumed a 2.5% growth rate of productivity and is expressed in terms of 1970 prices. The present value of these earnings when discounted at 7% was $131,000. Among women and the moderately retarded these values were, of course, considerably lower.

3. Each dollar expended on the vocational rehabilitation of 18-year-old mildly retarded adult males generates an estimated increase in future earnings of $14 in present-value terms. The ratios declined among older retardates, women, and the more severely retarded, but in all cases were equal to or greater than the critical value of "1," and in most cases, far above this value.

4. The lifetime educational costs of the mildly retarded were far below their estimated lifetime productivity, stated in present-value terms, even if they attended special education classes for the entire time they were in school. These comparisons were much less favorable for the moderately retarded, although it is probable that the data underestimated their earning potential.

5. The custodial costs (those exclusive of normal consumption and developmental expenditures) of lifetime institutionalization of the retarded are almost $400,000 (1970 dollars). Prevention of institutionalization may be a significant part of the benefits of extending additional community services to the retarded.

6. A substantial share of the benefits of developmental expenditures on the retarded are received by taxpayers, in the form of reduced provision of public maintenance and increased tax payments, probably about one-half of their earnings.

7. The benefits of prevention are large. For each case of severe retardation among males that is averted, the undiscounted total gain to society is almost $900,000 (1970 dollars). For an 18-year-old adult in 1970, this would have a present value of over $200,000.

8. Prevention is important. If all groups in society had the same percentage of persons with IQs below 50 as upper- and middle-class white children, the prevalence of this level of retardation would decrease by almost 80%. In '1970 this would have meant an increase of about $800 million in the resources available to improve living standards.

9. Since the causes of retardation are diverse, prevention must be comprised of many programs. The four programs considered in this chapter appeared justified on the basis of economic returns alone.

Improving
Services

EVALUATION

The meaning of optimality. Many people would define an optimal program in the field of mental retardation as one that: (1) would enable the retarded to achieve the highest possible degree of self-support and personal and social adequacy, and (2) would prevent mental retardation whenever possible.

The hard fact is that these programs require resources. And even as affluent a country as the United States lacks the resources necessary to satisfy all of its citizens' needs and wants. In fact, a large proportion of the population is inadequately educated, in poor health, and subsisting at poverty levels. Existing and future resources must, therefore, be allocated to meet a variety of needs, many of which are urgent, none of which are likely to be completely satisfied, and of which mental retardation is only one.

A more realistic definition of an optimal program tempers humanitarianism with the reality of limited resources. An optimal program would be one that always used the most efficient method of attaining a specified goal and that expanded programs only when the increase in marginal benefits exceeded the increase in marginal costs (and would contract programs if the opposite were true). Unfortunately, funds may not be sufficient to support all programs that are believed to be worthwhile. In this case, projects with the highest benefit-cost ratios should be selected.

Optimality, therefore, may have two meanings. It can refer to all programs that can be economically justified—"social optimality"—or it can refer to the most efficient use of available resources—"resources optimality." Social optimality represents our long-run goal and resource optimality represents our immediate goal.

Limited resources is the usual justification for economic evaluation of social programs. Even if resources were unlimited, however, an evaluation of the alternative uses of resources would still be necessary as long as one type of expenditure precluded another. For example, the retarded cannot live or work in more than one place at a time, and decisions must be made as to which of the many possible alternatives would best promote their welfare.

Program evaluation. Program evaluation has two interrelated purposes. One is to ascertain whether a program should be expanded (or created) or contracted (or eliminated). The other is to determine whether there are modifications to a program which will make it more efficient or whether there are alternative programs which are more efficient in achieving program goals. Sometimes these are referred to as the "how much" and the "how to" problems.

Frequent attempts are made to distinguish between the terms, benefit-cost analysis and cost-effectiveness analysis. One distinction is that benefit-cost analysis refers to determining whether a program shall be expanded (the "how much" problem), and cost-effectiveness analysis refers to the comparison of alternative ways of providing services or achieving goals (the "how to" problem). This distinction is weak, however, because the more efficiently a program is operated, the greater the amount of services it can justifiably render. Thus, no real separation between the "how much" and "how to" problems is possible. Moreover, when benefits and costs can be expressed in monetary terms, the techniques of benefit-cost and cost-effectiveness analyses are identical and no meaningful distinction is possible. In dealing with the mentally retarded, however, we frequently are unable to express many benefits in monetary terms. Another definition of cost-effectiveness analysis is that it refers to evaluations where some of the data, usually on the benefit side, is not expressed in monetary terms. In these cases, both the "how much" and the "how to" questions must be decided on the basis of these evaluations.

When comparing alternative programs, evaluative studies must reach one of the following four conclusions (if they reach any conclusions at all): (1) that one program will achieve the same level of benefits as another, but at a lower cost; (2) that one program will have a higher level of benefits than another, although both have identical costs;

(3) that one program has both lower costs and higher benefits than another; and (4) that *both* the costs and benefits of one program are higher than another.

When one of the first three types of conclusions is reached, it can be positively stated that one program is better than (or worse than) another, even though benefits may not all be expressible in additive (monetary) terms. For the first conclusion only costs need be measured, and these are usually accessible to quantification. For the second, only benefits need to be measured. This can be done by any one of several generally acceptable, available indices, e.g., better health, change in IQs etc. The third conclusion is, of course, a combination of the first two and the same remarks are germane.

Determining the best methods of providing services through such "better than" and "worse than" techniques (the third approach to benefit-cost analysis in the previous chapter) is enormously useful in many cases. The weaknesses of this approach are: (1) it can be used only when special conditions are met—either constant costs, constant benefits, or a lowering of costs and an increase in benefits; and (2) when used, it demonstrates the superiority of one method of providing services only over a small range of alternatives rather than the full range of alternatives that policymakers must consider.

Ultimately, program development will depend largely upon an assessment of alternative situations where both benefits and costs increase (the second approach to benefit-cost analysis in the previous chapter), and if some benefits cannot be expressed in monetary terms, subjective judgments will have to be made by policymakers. The goal of evaluative analyses is to improve the basis on which these decisions are made by measuring the magnitude of the changes and calculating their costs.

Models, systems analysis, operations analysis, PPBS. A model is a set of interrelated hypotheses about a problem or process. It may be expressed in mathematical, geometric, or verbal terms. To be complete, the model should identify all of the relevant variables and demonstrate how they interact with one another. To be useful, a model should eliminate all of the irrelevant or relatively unimportant variables, so that it does not become so cumbersome and unwieldy as to defy interpretation and empirical quantification. Obviously, these goals conflict, and their resolution depends upon the judgment of the analyst in each particular case.

Systems analysis and operations analysis (the two terms may be used interchangeably) can be defined as the process of constructing models and, if possible, of placing quantitative values on the inputs and outputs of the system. Model-building and its extension, systems analysis, are crucial and integral steps in benefit-cost and cost-effectiveness analyses. Because of the complex cause-and-effect relationships inherent in most social problems, a systems analysis is necessary if we are to be certain that we identify (1) all of the costs and benefits of a particular project; and (2) all of the alternative ways of achieving specific goals. A systems analysis also helps to pinpoint bottlenecks and unnecessary activities within the system.

Although many systems analyses present far more complicated models than some benefit-cost or cost-effectiveness analysts are accustomed to using, it is probable that in these days of computerized operations, massive data banks, and ever more refined analysis, the use of these complex models will become the rule rather than the exception.

In 1965 President Johnson ordered all departments and most agencies of the U.S. government to begin to formulate their spending plans in terms of planning-programming-budgeting systems (PPBS). PPBS is best described as applied benefit-cost and cost-effectiveness analysis. It addresses itself to the immediate planning needs of government agencies. It proceeds by identifying all of the various means of attaining the objectives of an agency and evaluating their relative costs, benefits, and time required to attain these benefits. Data limitations require that PPBS analyses utilize data and make assumptions that are highly questionable. However, decisions must be made, and time restraints preclude waiting for the results of more refined analyses. To offset this limitation of PPBS analyses, there is usually a careful description of the major unknowns or uncertainties which could result in errors in the evaluation, and the spending plans are periodically reevaluated and modified when this is deemed appropriate.

Despite the enormous impetus that has been given to applying PPBS methods to social programs in the last few years, many people still view such activities skeptically. In part, this is because many past efforts of this nature have produced little of tangible value, and may, on occasion, have even been harmful. And, in part, it is because they still fail to see that the primary purpose of these exercises is to improve programs, not reduce budgets. In fact, most PPBS analyses of social programs conclude with a recommendation for expansion of programs.

Past failures of PPBS are regrettable, but readily understandable in view of the difficulties that had to be overcome. The PPBS approach was imposed upon many government agencies before being itself properly PPBS'ed. Persons familiar with PPBS lacked sufficient understanding of the programs they were called upon to evaluate. Professional staff of most agencies, although familiar with the programs, lacked sufficient familiarity with PPBS to properly utilize the technique.

Professionals concerned with PPBS have been handicapped by a lack of basic data and ambiguity about program goals. Some despaired that even if program goals were clearly specified, much of the data necessary to measure progress toward these goals was not amenable to empirical quantification. Superimposed upon these limitations were frequent demands that program decisions be made quickly and with supporting analyses through the use of PPBS. It is not surprising that many PPBS analyses were, and still are, superficial, misleading, self-serving, and now lying unopened and unmourned in forgotten corners.

The problems associated with PPBS in the past have not been due to PPBS itself, but to its misuse. A PPBS system suitable for evaluating social programs is still not adequately developed. However, if properly developed, and if used with a full appreciation of its limitations, PPBS is an enormous aid. It is, in fact, an essential element in the development of programs in mental retardation and other human service programs.

Additional comments. (1) Final resolution of the question of what constitutes an optimal program requires a long interim period during which many programs must be evaluated and jugmental errors rectified.

2) The problem of a control group is far less serious when comparing one program with another than when a program is being compared with the alternative of no program. Since people are not being denied services, we need only assure that there is random distribution of persons among alternative programs.

3) High benefit-cost ratios do not prove that a program is efficient, since it is possible that if the people served by this program were served by a different program, these ratios would be even higher. Similarly, low benefit-cost ratios do not prove that a program is inefficient, since they may represent the maximum development of some people's potential.

4) Benefit-cost or cost-effectiveness analysis becomes extremely complicated, since we are seeking to determine whether services to a particular group should be expanded, while simultaneously ascertaining which would be the most efficient way of providing this service. In addition, these analyses should be separately carried out for different demographic groups (e.g., by level of IQ, type of handicapping condition, etc.).

5) The ultimate test of mental retardation programs is the improvement of the social and vocational adjustment of the retarded as adults. Children's programs must, for the most part, therefore, be evaluated by variables that are assumed to improve eventual social and

vocational adjustment. Academic progress is one such variable. It is of equal and perhaps greater importance to measure such things as peer relationships, work habits, and attitudes toward work.

GENERAL CHARACTERISTICS OF AN OPTIMAL PROGRAM

We should distinguish between the general and the specific characteristics of an optimal program in mental retardation. General characteristics refer to program guides that will be as necessary in the future as they are today. Specific program characteristics refer to such things as the number of various types of facilities needed, the optimal size of residential institutions, etc.

Specific program characteristics will vary over time as knowledge increases and growing affluence makes society more able, and perhaps more willing, to increase the resources set aside for the benefit of the retarded. Clearly one general characteristic of an optimal program is that its specific characteristics are being continuously evaluated and modified as circumstances warrant.

At least six other general characteristics of an optimal program can be identified. One is that it must be based on a deep social concern with the *quality* of the lives of the retarded. Low productivity should not condemn them to poverty. Institutionalization should not mean deprivation of all but the essentials of life.

The normalization principle is one way of defining operational standards for the quality of the lives of the retarded. This principle, developed and long applied in the Scandinavian countries, was defined by Nirje as follows: ". . . the normalization principle means making available to the mentally retarded patterns and conditions of everyday life which are as close as possible to the norms and patterns of the mainstream of society."[1] It requires that the latent capabilities of the retarded be developed so that their personal habits, social relationships, and productive endeavors can be as nearly normal as possible. It also requires that society tolerate behavior which diverges from the norm, when such behavior is essentially harmless. It eschews, whenever possible, a paternalistic attitude. Implicitly the normalization principle places a high value on the nonmarket benefits of programs for the retarded, but needs to be modified to take account of the costs of achieving these benefits.

[1] Bengt Nirje, "The Normalization Principle and Its Human Management Implications," in *Changing Patterns in Residential Services for the Mentally Retarded*, Robert B. Kugel and Wolf Wolfensberger, eds. (Washington: President's Committee on Mental Retardation, 1969), p. 181.

Since this second general principle of an optimal program is a value judgment, its inclusion cannot be defended on scientific grounds. I have included it for two reasons: (1) Researchers have an obligation to make explicit the social philosophy underlying their work; (2) such preconceived philosophies are common. Much, for example, has been written on strategies of eliminating poverty with no justification other than that poverty ought to be eliminated.

The third general characteristic of an optimal program is that it must be efficient. Efficiency does not require that the resources expended on the retarded should be minimized. Such a practice is itself wasteful if restricting expenditures causes a greater loss of benefits. Efficiency is attained by selecting the treatment method that will bring the mentally retarded to a *given* level of social functioning at the lowest cost. This comparison, and *not* one of actual costs, is the relevant one from an economic standpoint.

The remaining general characteristics of an optimal program are familiar to health professionals. The program must be comprehensive, coordinated, continuous and accessible. A comprehensive program is one in which treatment and a full range of preventive and other services are available. A coordinated program provides for the activities of different groups dealing with the retarded to be combined to work toward a common goal. A continuous program is one in which appropriate services are available as needed to each retarded person throughout his lifetime. And an accessible program means that persons requiring services are able to obtain them regardless of geographic location, arbitrary eligibility requirements, or lack of funds.

In terms of assisting the retarded to achieve a *given* level of social functioning (the efficiency criterion), a program with these four characteristics *cannot* lead to higher costs and in many cases will lead to lower costs than a program lacking one or more of these characteristics. To see that it cannot lead to higher costs we must observe that a program with these characteristics (hereafter called a balanced program) will have all of the services that a less balanced program would have and that there should be no difference in the costs of specific services (vocational training, counseling, residential care, etc.). A balanced program, therefore, can always provide the retarded with the same services that they would receive in an unbalanced program at no greater cost. If, therefore, the services chosen for the retarded in a balanced program differ in type or quality from those in an unbalanced program, it must be because costs are expected to be lower or benefits are expected to be greater. If this were not the case, there would be no purpose in providing services different from those which would have been provided in an unbalanced program.

There are five possible outcomes if the retarded are treated in a balanced rather than an unbalanced program. They can be helped to the same level of social functioning as they would have achieved in an unbalanced program at equal or less cost, or they can be helped to a superior level of social functioning at costs that are less than, equal to, or higher than would have been incurred in an unbalanced program. The broad range of services offered in a balanced program precludes the necessity of choosing treatment that would be more expensive though no more effective.

It is those cases where the costs of treatment increase that are apt to cause concern. However, costs of treatment should never be evaluated independently of the benefits of treatment. In a balanced program costs will be higher than in an unbalanced program only if superior results are expected. If we assume that any additional costs are justified by additional benefits (the more expensive services should not be provided if they are not), then the relevant economic comparison is between the relative cost of attaining the higher benefit level in a balanced and in an unbalanced program. But since a balanced program can always offer the same services as an unbalanced program, costs in the former need never be higher than those of the latter for achieving a given benefit level.

The important question is how many cases would there be where the costs of helping the retarded to achieve a given level of social functioning would be less in a balanced system than in an unbalanced one. The following reasons suggest that the number would be significant:

1) Because services are comprehensive, coordinated, continuous, and accessible to all, a balanced program will make more effective use of its resources than one which lacks one or more of these characteristics. In an unbalanced program, the mentally retarded will sometimes have to be provided with types of care that are not the most suitable for their needs. It necessarily follows that more resources will be required to restore these persons to a given level of social competence than if more effective types of care were available. In some cases, because of the delay of treatment, inferior treatment settings, and limited ability to provide services, it will be impossible for unbalanced programs to match the effectiveness of balanced ones.

2) Increased accessibility to care should influence some of the retarded and their parents to seek assistance earlier than they otherwise would. In general, earlier care improves the prognosis for the mentally retarded.

3) Large-scale coordinated planning for comprehensive treatment of the retarded will make it possible to achieve a better balance in the development of services and will afford greater latitude for innovation in ways of preventing and detecting retardation and in methods of caring for the retarded.

Several objections might be made to the above analysis. The assumption that a balanced program can always offer the same services as an unbalanced program will not be valid if the latter contains services that are considered undesirable. Thus, if large institutions for the retarded are phased out in the future, the possibility of identical services will not always exist. Moreover, if there are economies of scale in large institutions then the costs of residential care will not be identical between the two programs and, in this case, would be higher in a balanced than in an unbalanced program. However, these possibilities do not invalidate our analysis; in fact, they support it. If a service is not available, it must be because it has been judged inferior in terms of cost and benefits to another service, even though the latter may involve higher cost. Since the nonexistent service is economically inferior to the service which replaces it, it necessarily follows that it would be less costly to achieve a given level of social competence through the superior service.

Basically, an optimal program in the field of mental retardation would consist of a wide range of services designed to meet a broad variety of needs in the areas of both prevention and treatment. The services actually provided to individuals will depend upon their particular needs at a point in time. The heart of the matter is that a choice of services must be available. In no other way can the enormous diversity of needs of the retarded be adequately met.

The remainder of this chapter will consider selected areas in services to the retarded. Most of the discussion will focus on needs of adult retardates. Despite the increased attention that has been given to the retarded in recent years, the problems of adult retardates are among the most neglected in our society.

EMPLOYMENT OF THE RETARDED

Employment needs. In Chapter V we estimated that in 1970 an additional 136,000 male and 204,000 female retardates, age 20 to 64, living in the community, would be employed if they had the same employment rates as the general population. In addition, another 124,000 male and 770,000 female retardates in this age range were not working because of normal unemployment and nonparticipation in the labor force. If we assume that the proportion of full-time homemakers among mildly retarded women is the same as for the general population, and take account of the estimated 9,000 homemakers among women with IQs of between 40 and 50, this would account for about 682,000 of the nonworking women. Given this latter assumption, there are about 260,000 noninstitutionalized retarded men and 291,000 noninstitutionalized retarded women, age 20 to 64, who are economically idle, i.e., who are neither employed for wages nor keeping house full-time.

To estimate the total number of economically idle retardates, we must also consider the number in residential care. This would increase these totals to 340,000 retarded men and 350,000 retarded women.[2]

Although almost half of these retardates, even if not retarded, would not be in the labor force because of school attendance, early retirement, discouragement, or disability, this is a largely irrelevant consideration from a policy standpoint. Policy must be formulated on the basis of conditions that actually exist, not on hypothetical calculations of what conditions would be if the impossible could be accomplished, i.e., if retardation could be wished out of existence. Few retardates attend school after age 20, and voluntary early retirement is unlikely to be an important consideration. Discouragement and disability, the other causes of labor force nonparticipation, are the very conditions that we are seeking to ameliorate.

We conclude, therefore, that almost all of these 690,000 economically idle or institutionalized retardates would accept work if work were available that was within their capabilities. Unfortunately, not all of these persons are capable of gainful work. It can be reasonably assumed that almost all persons with IQs below 25 are unemployable, even in strongly sheltered situations.

Although we earlier assumed that all persons with IQs between 25 and 39 were economically idle, this is not true in all cases. Saenger, for example, retested 27 severely retarded employed persons and reported that 9 received IQ scores below 40. Loos and Tizard reported on 6 retarded youths with IQs between 24 and 37 who, after careful training, became regularly employed in a sheltered workshop with minimal supervision.[3] Although employment for persons in this IQ range is only

---

[2] Since a large proportion of adult retardates in institutional care are employed on institution work, it is not altogether accurate to label all of these persons as economically idle.

[3] F. M. Loos and J. Tizard, "The Employment of Adult Imbeciles in a Hospital Workshop," *American Journal of Mental Deficiency* (January 955): 395–403.

feasible under strongly sheltered conditions, one suspects that if sufficient sheltered work were made available, a majority would be capable
of some gainful activity.

Gainful work is almost always feasible for persons with IQs above 40,
unless precluded by physical or emotional handicaps. The vocational
failure of a substantial number of retardates is largely attributable to a
lack of supportive services. There are a number of bits of evidence for
this belief.

1) Saenger reported that only one out of five persons who sought
employment among severely retarded persons in his sample received
assistance from established employment services or organizations for
the retarded.

2) In a study of 258 retarded persons whose cases were closed as
unfeasible by vocational rehabilitation agencies in 1958 and 1959,
Rockower found that only 14% were actually considered incapable of
work (a few were institutionalized). The rest required long-term personal adjustment or workshop training which was not available (58%)
or encountered parental opposition to the rehabilitation plan because
of low wages or occupational prospects (28%).[4]

3) In 1968 state vocational rehabilitation agencies reported that
three times as many of the moderately retarded were being rehabilitated as not rehabilitated at closure.[5] Many of those closed as not
rehabilitated voluntarily declined services because they found work independently. It is worth noting that of almost 40,000 retarded persons
whose cases were closed by vocational rehabilitation agencies in 1967,
less than 6% were denied further service because of the severity of their
handicaps.[6]

4) In a sample of retarded residents in institutions in three English
counties, Tizard and O'Connor reported that less than 10% of the
feebleminded (mildly retarded), 45% of the imbeciles, (moderately retarded), and 88% of the "idiots" (severely and profoundly retarded)

[4] Leonard W. Rockower, "A Study of Mentally Retarded Applicants for Vocational Rehabilitation in New York City," *Vocational Rehabilitation of the Mentally
Retarded*, USDHEW, Rehabilitation Service Series, No. 123, p. 132.

[5] USDHEW, SRS, RSA, *Major Disabling Condition of Rehabilitated and Not
Rehabilitated Clients of State Vocational Rehabilitation Agencies—Fiscal Year
1968*, Statistical Note No. 17, September 1969.

[6] Computed from data from USDHEW, SRS, RSA, *Rehabilitation Rates and
Types of Closures from the Vocational Rehabilitation Process among Selected
Groups of Clients, Fiscal Year 1967*, Statistical Note No. 2, October 1968; and
*Reasons for Unsuccessful Closures among Selected Groups of Clients, Fiscal Year
1967*, Statistical Note No. 1, September 1968.

were unemployable.[7] Apparently employability was defined as actually working in the hospital or on license outside the hospital at the time of survey and therefore can be assumed to understate actual employability.

5) In Chapter IV we estimated that about half of the adult residents in public institutions were ward helpers, almost one-fifth were employed on other work projects, and almost one-sixth were candidates for these positions.[8] Clearly the great majority of the adult residents of public institutions are capable of gainful work. Moreover, it is probable that these retardates face more severe employment impediments than unemployed retardates not in institutions.

6) Cowan and Goldman compared 20 retarded persons who received services from a vocational rehabilitation agency with 20 retarded persons who were known to a private agency but had not received vocational training or job placement. The subjects were closely matched for age and IQ. Most were mildly retarded. About three years had transpired since they had contacted their respective agencies.

At evaluation, 60% of the rehabilitation group was employed as compared to 20% of the control group. The successful nonrehabilitants had a mean grade level of 6.75, the successful rehabilitants a mean grade level of 4.92, unsuccessful nonrehabilitants a mean grade level of 4.75, and unsuccessful rehabilitants a mean grade level of 3.0. There were no statistically significant differences in the average IQs of the four groups.[9]

The sample size was too small for the authors to attach statistical significance to these differences. However, these differences suggest that prior education and the availability of rehabilitation services are crucial and interacting factors in the vocational success of the retarded.

7) Home conditions have an important effect on the vocational success of the retarded. In the Ferguson study, an experienced social worker rated the homes of the parents or guardians of the retardates. Of those retardates from homes assessed as "good" (N=75), 14% were in skilled or nonmanual jobs and 8% were unemployed. But of those

[7] N. O'Connor and J. Tizard, *The Social Problem of Mental Deficiency* (New York: Pergamon Press, 1956), p. 42.

[8] Dan Payne, Ronald C. Johnson, and Robert B. Abelson, *A Comprehensive Description of Institutionalized Retardates in the Western United States* (Boulder, Colorado: Western Interstate Commission for Higher Education, 1969), pp. 110, 134–35.

[9] Lawrence Cowan and Morton Goldman, "The Selection of the Mentally Deficient for Vocational Training and the Effect of this Training on Vocational Success," *Journal of Consulting Psychology* (February 1959): 78–84.

from homes rated as "bad" (N=17), only one was in skilled work and 35% were unemployed.

8) Behavior, rather than ability to work, is often the factor that determines the employability of the retarded. As expressed by Grate:

For most of the retarded, the necessity of learning good work habits is primary. Learning good job skills is secondary. Of 53 project clients who entered a training program at Goodwill, 34 were recommended for work adjustment training as opposed to vocational training. In each of these cases the primary reason for work adjustment training was the opportunity needed by the client to learn how to work and what constituted good work habits. By and large, the project population could give evidence of very little previous work experience. In any case significant stress had to be placed on items such as personal hygiene and appearance, punctuality and absenteeism, appropriate response to supervision and peers, and the relationship between effort and monetary reward.

It is probable that at least 400,000 of the 690,000 currently idle or institutionalized retardates could be employed if appropriate services were available. This speculative estimate was derived by assuming that most of the 200,000 adults of working age with IQs below 40 would not work and that about one-fifth of those with IQs above this level would be too severely physically or emotionally disabled to work. Our estimate of employment needs would be greater if we considered employment needs among teenage retardates, or took account of the desirability of upgrading the employment of some currently employed retardates, or were more optimistic about the employment potential of persons with IQs between 25 and 40.

A precise estimate of the number of potential workers among this group of economically inactive retardates is not necessary. It is only important to establish that the number is substantial.

Theory of employment. Two conditions are essential if everyone capable of work is to be: (1) employed (or unemployed for only short periods); and (2) placed on jobs which make the best use of their abilities. One is that the aggregate demand for goods and services be sufficiently high to generate enough jobs for the available labor force, and the other is that there be an effective method for channeling unemployed and underemployed workers to suitable jobs.

Since 1946 the responsibility for maintaining full employment has been assumed by the federal government with varying levels of success, while the major function of state employment services is to implement the second condition. Even when these two conditions are filled, some workers will be unemployed or employed on jobs where their earnings are below what they are potentially capable of achieving, because of a lack of training or other supportive services and lack of availability of suitable jobs.

Efforts to overcome these problems take three forms: (1) Workers can be trained for occupations in which the demand for workers exceeds the supply, increasing the number of persons employed in these occupations.

2) Workers can be trained for those occupations for which their abilities are best suited. If no change is occurring in the number of persons employed in these occupations then some persons who would have been hired will be forced to find jobs elsewhere. The justification for the use of this approach is that the persons who seek jobs elsewhere are better able to adjust to other occupations than persons whose skills are so limited that they must be trained for particular occupations. This will not impose a substantial hardship on the displaced group, since in a dynamic labor market where new workers are constantly replacing those who have retired, died, or moved to another occupation, it merely means that some persons who would have found employment in one occupation will accept presumably comparable jobs elsewhere.

3) Finally, disabled or disadvantaged workers unable to function satisfactorily in competitive jobs may have to be employed under sheltered conditions, which may be in sheltered workshops or regular employment channels.

In general, the first approach is considered superior to the second and the second to the third. The second approach is preferable, however, if the worker's limitations are such that he cannot be trained for jobs in which there are existing vacancies or if his abilities are such that his productivity would be substantially greater if trained for other occupations. The third approach is preferable if the person is unable to perform any job in the competitive sector of the labor market, or if his productivity in sheltered employment would be higher than could be achieved elsewhere (as will sometimes be the case).

Jobs for the retarded. Because of their limited capabilities, the second and third approaches to finding jobs for the unemployed are most appropriate for those retardates who are currently idle or institutionalized. In fact, a very substantial number will have to be employed under sheltered conditions—perhaps over half of those who could be employed.

Sheltered employment is probably best described as employment under conditions that differ in some way from what they would be if a nondisabled worker did the same task. The worker may not be expected to work as fast, as consistently, or for as many hours as usual. Extra supervision may be required or unusual behavioral patterns tolerated. The tasks performed may be simplified. Workers may be hired with the understanding that they will not receive normal promotions into more difficult jobs. Jobs that are created specifically for the disabled (e.g., some salvage operations) should also be considered as a form of sheltered employment.

Where can 400,000 or more jobs for retarded workers, almost all of which must be of an unskilled nature and many of which must be under sheltered conditions, be found? There are four possibilities:

1) For reasons to be discussed, the majority of these jobs, whether of a competitive or sheltered nature, should be sought through *regular* employment channels in private industry or government.

2) Some jobs will be located in sheltered workshops. We should emphasize the distinction between sheltered workshops and sheltered work. Sheltered workshops are organizations that are specifically organized to provide sheltered work for the disabled and to prepare them for gainful employment. Sheltered work refers to jobs that are modified to meet the special needs of handicapped workers and which may be provided through sheltered workshops or regular employment channels.

3) Work may be brought to the home of the homebound retarded.

4) The government can attempt to influence the composition of demand for labor in such a way as to increase the demand for retarded workers.

In general, one can dismiss homebound programs as being of negligible importance. Although some nonretarded homebound individuals achieve considerable economic success doing such tasks as typing, telephone soliciting, bookkeeping, etc., most such jobs are beyond the capability of homebound retardates.

The government is justified in influencing the composition of the demand for labor to create jobs for the retarded if the types of jobs generated by normal market processes are beyond their skills. For example, a general expansion of aggregate demand may primarily increase the availability of semi-skilled and skilled jobs rather than unskilled jobs. The demand for retarded workers may be increased by hiring the retarded directly, or by expanding government expenditures on goods and services that will create a need for unskilled workers. For example, the government could maintain cleaner parks and roads, creating jobs within the capabilities of the retarded.

Taxpayers, although they may prefer other goods to cleaner streets and parks, are still better off than they would be if the retarded were not hired for this purpose. The choice is not between alternative types of goods or services, but between idleness and some form of productive activity. The taxpayer pays in either case—in the form of public assistance in the first case and wages for services in the second.

The possibility of restructuring aggregate demand to create jobs for the retarded merits consideration but not immediate action. It does, after all, force consumers into consumption patterns that they would not select of their own accord. Before undertaking such a step it must be established that the retarded cannot produce with reasonable efficiency the types of goods that consumers prefer. It will be argued that the vast majority can, either in sheltered workshops or through regular employment channels.

Sheltered workshops. The earnings of clients in sheltered workshops are low, especially if they are retarded. In a survey of 8,556 clients (all diagnostic categories) in 123 workshops in New York, New Jersey, and Pennsylvania in 1966, Button reported that median weekly earnings were $16.54. One-third earned less than $10.00 per week.[10] The U.S. Department of Labor reported that average hourly earnings for clients in all workshops in the United States were $.72 in February 1967 and that 42% of the clients made less than $.50 per hour.[11] Button reported that clients worked an average of 33 hours per week which would, if applicable nationally, mean that average weekly earnings in workshops were $23.76 and that 42% of the clients earned less than $16 per week. These data include the earnings of clients in work activity centers.

The earnings of retarded clients were even more dismal. Average hourly earnings in workshops serving the retarded exclusively were only $.35, which amounted to $11.55 weekly if retardates worked 33 hours per week. Button reported that average hourly earnings in workshops decreased as the percentage of retarded clients increased $(r=-.63)$.

One reason for these low earnings is that many workshop clients are being prepared for jobs in regular employment channels. Productivity may, in fact, be sacrificed in order to expedite the rehabilitation process. In principle, workshops should be evaluated on the basis of the earnings of clients who have completed training. Button reported that average hourly earnings in workshops increased as the average length of stay of clients increased $(r=.41)$. However, this would not change our conclusion that earnings in workshops are dismally low.

[10] William H. Button, *Wage Levels in Sheltered Employment* (Ithaca, New York: Region II Rehabilitation Research Institute, New York State School of Industrial and Labor Relations, Cornell University, 1969).

[11] U.S. Department of Labor, Wage and Hour and Public Contracts Divisions, *Sheltered Workshop Report of the Secretary of Labor*, September 1967. These figures were calculated from wage data contained in applications submitted by sheltered workshops and activity centers for exemptions from the minimum wage.

Another reason for the low productivity of workshop clients is that they tend to be among the more severely disabled. Button concluded "that the proportion of clients served by sheltered workshops is drawn from that segment of the State agency caseload with greater vocational and educational deficits than those confronted by the average rehabilitant, more severe impairments, and greater economic deprivation." In a California survey it was estimated that a majority of clients in workshops for the retarded were severely retarded.[12]

Retarded clients in sheltered workshops are apparently even more severely disabled than other workshop clients. In 1967 almost 80% of the clients in workshops serving only the retarded were given work activity exemption in contrast to less than one-fourth of the clients of all other workshops.[13] A work activity exemption is granted when a client's physical or mental handicap is so severe as to make his productive capacity inconsequential.[14]

Still another reason for the low earnings of workshop clients is that most workshops are themselves inherently inefficient producing units. There are three conditions that are generally necessary if a workshop is to be economically efficient (i.e., able to pay meaningful wages to long-term clients). It must have a source of profitable work. The work must be continuous. And there must be a variety of types of work. The last requirement merits elaboration. Sheltered workshop clients are usually severely limited in the number of job tasks they can perform. In addition there is great diversity in the types of job tasks for which workshop clients are best suited. The greater the diversity of job tasks available, therefore, the greater the likelihood that workshop clients can be placed on tasks that make the best use of their residual abilities.

The work performed in sheltered workshops is of three types: (1) prime manufacturing (e.g., candles, brooms and mops, light bulbs); (2) subcontract work from industry (excluding salvage and reclamation); and (3) salvage and reclamation (from public donations or subcontracts from industry). Button estimated that subcontract operations accounted for 28% of aggregate workshop income (which apparently

[12] Nathan Nelson, *Workshops for the Mentally Retarded in California* (Sacramento: State Department of Education, Vocational Rehabilitation Service, February 1962), p. 16.

[13] *Sheltered Workshop Report*, p. 41.

[14] In practice these exemptions are granted when workers are unable to earn at least half of the federal minimum wage. In fact, only a little over 5% of the retarded were able to earn or exceed half the federal minimum wage, in contrast to almost 60% of all other clients. All clients in work activity centers were reported as exempted workers.

included salvage and reclamation projects from industry), prime manufacturing 32%, and salvage and reclamation 33%. Salvage and reclamation operations and prime manufacturing tend to be concentrated in a few large workshops. In consequence, subcontract operations are the most important source of work for most workshops.[15]

Prime manufacturing has the advantage that the flow of work is not subject to contract cancellation or variability. Its disadvantages are that it requires extensive marketing arrangements, a greater need for fixed and working capital, and often a wide range of skills among workers. In addition, the workshop may compete with private industry where it will be substantially disadvantaged, since it will usually face superior technical knowledge and more modern and extensive capital equipment. In consequence, output is usually limited to a few labor-intensive commodities with relatively low profit potential.

The supply of salvage and reclamation work from industry is almost boundless. The problem is that the income flow generated by such work is usually low. Dolnick presented data which showed that the average hourly income flow from industrial salvage and reclamation projects ranged between one-half and one-fourth of other subcontract operations.[16]

Subcontracting operations (other than industrial salvage and reclamation) appear to be work well-suited to workshops. Usually, little investment in raw materials is required. Since the work would have to be done with or without the workshop's services, the contractor is usually willing to pay the going price.

Private industry abounds in opportunities for subcontract operations. The work flow through business establishments is rarely even throughout the year and many businessmen prefer to subcontract irregular increases in work loads rather than go through the painful process of hiring and discharging workers.

Unfortunately, the following structural characteristics of most sheltered workshops greatly impede their efforts to become economically efficient producing units:

1) Many workshops are poorly managed from a business standpoint. Because of a lack of qualified production managers, production is often organized in an inefficient manner. Opportunities for profitable

---

[15] These percentages do not add up to 100% because of income from other sources.

[16] Michael M. Dolnick, *Contract Procurement Practices of Sheltered Workshops* (Chicago: National Society for Crippled Children and Adults, Inc., 1963), p. 10. The procedure was to divide median income per contract by median hours worked per contract in each category of subcontracts.

subcontracting frequently go unrecognized because of a lack of capable contract procurement personnel. In a survey of 35 well established workshops, for example, it was found that only 15 employed contract procurement personnel, 7 of whom were part-time.[17]

2) Most workshops are small. The average workshop had 43 clients in 1967. Workshops serving retardates only were even smaller, averaging 33 clients.[18] Small workshops are unable to accept large subcontracts and may need to turn down offers of work if employed on other projects.

3) Most workshops specialize in particular disabilities, particularly workshops that serve the retarded. In 1967 about 80% of the retarded were in single-disability workshops (compared to 36% of all the other workshop clients). The limited range of abilities in single-disability workshops limits the variety of contracts they can accept. In multiple-disability workshops the capabilities of one client compensate for the limitations of another, enabling the workshop to accept many more types of subcontracts.[19]

4) Finally, many workshops lack sufficient funds to purchase needed machinery. The result may be to create jobs, since human power must substitute for machine power, but the resulting inefficiency is one factor behind the low earnings of workshop clients.

The consequence of these workshop features are that industry is likely to regard the services of most workshops as inconsequential and unreliable (industry often needs work done immediately and can't wait for a workshop to complete other work). The flow of work to workshops is often irregular and the diversity of workshop jobs is inevitably limited. In consequence, workshops are usually inefficient in their production methods, and a large part of workshop work is in low productivity salvage operations.

These four characteristics of workshops are interrelated, since it is the small workshops which are least likely to be adequately capitalized, most likely to be single-disability, and least likely to have business-

[17] Ibid., p. 49. The fact that most workshops are concerned with rehabilitation as well as production does not justify an unbusiness-like approach to business operations. Management should seek to maximize productivity, subject to the constraint that some rehabilitation needs will have priority over production (e.g., the most efficient workers will not always be used if other workers need experience in particular jobs.

[18] Sheltered Workshop Report, p. 41.

[19] Retardates in single disability workshops are apparently more severely retarded than those in multiple-disability workshops, which would explain part of the low earnings of the former group. See Nelson, Workshops for the Mentally Retarded in California, p. 16.

oriented management. The 1967 survey of sheltered workshops did not find a relationship between the average hourly earnings of all clients (including trainees and exceptions) and workshop size for workshops with client populations below 75, as we would hypothesize on the basis of the preceding comments. It is probable that this does not represent a stabilizing of productivity among very small workshops, but rather, an increasing amount of wage subsidization from outside sources. Among larger facilities, average earnings increased sharply with facility size. Average hourly earnings in workshops with over 200 clients were 35% higher than in workshops with 75 to 99 clients.

When the earnings of regular clients, trainees, and exceptions from the minimum wage (the three client statuses in workshops) were considered separately, there was no relationship between facility size and earnings. This should occasion no surprise, since client status is itself largely determined by the client's earnings. A crucial difference between large and small workshops was that the percentage of exceptions among clients was much greater in the latter. Only 14% of the employees of workshops with over 200 clients were excepted from the federal minimum wage laws, as compared to 45% in workshops with 75 to 99 clients. Although part of this difference may be ascribable to more severe disabilities among clients in small workshops, it is probable that most of this difference is due to the greater efficiency of large workshops.[20]

Using data on 73 workshops in 5 states, Vladimir Stoikov evaluated the importance of size on workshop productivity. Rough adjustments were made for demographic differences among clients in different workshops, the efficiency of workshop management, and differences in the number of clients being rehabilitated. He concluded that all workshops with under 150 clients in average daily attendance were operating at a highly inefficient level. This encompassed 86% of all workshops serving 50% of all workshop clients.[21]

A number of important observations have been drawn. Most workshop clients earn low wages. Small workshops pay considerably lower wages than large workshops, an observation that is obscured because of the large number of exceptions among clients in small workshops (due to low productivity). There are many reasons why small workshops

---

[20] The Department of Labor reported average hourly earnings by workshop size and their client status, but did not report earnings for all clients in a workshop. As a result, the most important observation to be derived from this data was overlooked, i.e., the relationship between workshop size and client earnings.

[21] Vladimir Stoikov, "Economics of Scale in Sheltered Workshop Operations," *Rehabilitation, Sheltered Workshops and the Disadvantaged* (Ithaca, New York: Cornell University, 1970), p. 66.

Table 63. Earnings of sheltered workshop clients by status and size of facility, 1967[a]

	Number of clients in workshop								
	1–9	10–19	20–29	30–39	40–49	50–74	75–99	100–199	200+
Total number of clients	431	1,861	2,960	3,391	2,696	5,680	3 649	8,129	6,663
Status of clients:									
Regular	43%	33%	22%	32%	29%	27%	38%	48%	66%
Trainee	15	15	16	19	18	20	17	17	20
Exception	42	52	63	49	53	53	45	36	14
Average hourly earnings:									
Regular	$1.03	$1.12	$1.07	$1.17	$1.13	$1.09	$1.18	$1.23	$1.19
Trainees	0.64	0.53	0.47	0.47	0.49	0.50	0.49	0.44	0.48
Exceptions	0.31	0.34	0.34	0.33	0.34	0.35	0.38	0.43	0.50
All	0.67	0.62	0.52	0.62	0.60	0.58	0.70	0.81	0.95

[a]Source: This table was consolidated from information contained in Tables A–2, A–18, and A–30 of Sheltered Workshop Report. The average hourly earnings for all clients had to be calculated from data presented for each of the three separate categories of clients. These data include clients in work activity centers.

may be more economically inefficient than large ones. It is possible that part of the low earnings of clients in small workshops may be due to exceptionally severe disabilities among these clients. It is probable, however, that most of the reasons for the differences in productivity between large and small workshops are due to the greater inefficiency of the latter.

Regular employment channels. In most cases, retarded adults will earn far more if employed through regular employment channels rather than sheltered workshops. This is, in part, due to the inherent inefficiency of sheltered workshops and in part to the amazing diversity of types of jobs available in regular employment channels. Few retardates are so vocationally limited that jobs within their capabilities cannot be found in regular employment channels.

The term "vocationally limited" should be used cautiously. No individual is so versatile as to be able to move into any available job. In that sense, everybody has some degree of vocational limitation. The difference between the vocational limitations of the retarded and the non-retarded is that the retarded have a smaller range of jobs that they can accomplish.

If carefully placed, however, most retardates work satisfactorily. The key to this process is placement. "Placement of the mentally retarded is not a job that can be done by well-wishers, do-gooders, nor through the use of snappy slogans. It is a job requiring professional skills and knowledge, and must be done on an individualized basis . . . individualized in terms of knowing the capabilities of the mental retardate, and individualized in terms of knowing employers' requirements intimately by visiting the place of employment and knowing not only the job skill requirements, but the kind of people and the working climate in which the mental retardate is to work."[22]

Most of the 400,000 additional jobs needed for the retarded should be sought through regular employment channels. The following examples illustrate the abundant opportunities that exist.

A couple of years ago, it would never have occurred to me to deliberately select a mentally retarded person to fill a vacancy in my plant. That was before—quite accidentally—I stumbled upon this reservoir of skills.

It happened in the pre-Christmas rush, when a shipment of defective motors was returned for repair. I needed some men to unpack and break down the motors and then re-pack the parts. And I needed them fast.

---

[22] Janet I. Pinner, "New York State Employment Service's Experience in Placing the Mentally Retarded," in *Outlook for the Adult Retarded, Proceedings of the 35th Spring Conference of the Woods Schools*, Langhorne, Pennsylvania, p. 46.

I put in a call to the nearby State Training School for the Retarded. They sent me two men—retarded youths who had never worked before. Working together, the two did the job in less than four hours—half the time previously required for a similar job.

I now have about 34 retarded men and women among my 600 employees. Their flying fingers, devotion to the job, and even dispositions more than compensate for their lack of intellect. Some of them are doing work which normal employees wouldn't want to do—and they're taking pride in doing it well. You couldn't ask for better workers.[23]

Some years ago Remco Industries, one of the nation's largest toy-makers, hired sixty retarded workers on a trial basis. Forty qualified for permanent employment. A company official observed that their efficiency was a little below average and the cost of their training was a little above average, but believed that this was offset by the lower turnover rates and superior attendance, punctuality, quality consciousness, and dependability of retarded workers as compared to other workers. The same official remarked, "We could use more of this type of personnel than we are getting."[24]

The W. T. Grant Company, a chain of 1,100 variety stores, reported that 103 retarded workers were employed in early 1968. Only 3 had been given a poor performance rating. One reason why more had not been hired was that only 10% of their stores had ever been contacted by professional agencies.[25]

In 1964 a program to place mentally retarded adults in federal jobs was initiated. This was not an attempt to provide sheltered employment, but to locate routine, repetitive—but necessary—jobs that retardates could perform well. Two and one-half years later over 1,500 retarded adults had been appointed to federal jobs. Only 9% had to have their employment terminated.[26] By January 1972 the total number hired under this program had risen to over 7,000 of whom 3,800 were still employed by the federal government. Undoubtedly many moved on to nonfederal jobs.

As a final example, 1,500 job openings for the retarded in 5 major companies (4 in the food industry) were located by a project jointly

[23] William Sleith, "What a Mentally Retarded Worker Can Do," *Supervisory Management* (January 1966): 24–28.

[24] James C. G. Conniff, "Business 'Si! Charity—No!," *Columbia Magazine* (November 1961).

[25] The President's Committee on Employment of the Handicapped Special Report, "Why We Hire the Retarded—An Employer Speaks" (January 1968).

[26] John W. Macy, Jr., *Federal Employment of the Mentally Retarded*, The President's Committee on Mental Retardation, August 1966.

sponsored by the National Association for Retarded Children (NARC) and the United States Department of Labor. Persons placed on these jobs were paid not less than $50 per week, of which the company was reimbursed $27.50 for 10 weeks to pay for training and administration. All placements were referred by vocational rehabilitation agencies. Only about 500 job openings were filled during a two-year period. Most of the retarded were employed as kitchen helpers, porters, busboys, pantrymen, or dishwashers. About 80% were retained as full-time permanent employees.[27]

Successful job placement of the retarded is made possible by the fact that many jobs do not require a high level of intellectual ability. Dinger's observations about jobs held by students who had attended classes for the educable retarded are relevant:

Thirty-three percent of the jobs held by these subjects required no reading skills, and, in all but a very few cases, the remaining jobs required reading ability of a very simple nature. Reading of printed tags, signs, inventory sheets, and labels on boxes were the most frequent types of required reading.

Only 31% of the group are required to perform any writing function other than to sign their check or complete an application form. Much of the required writing consists of filling in data or tally marks on inventory sheets or other printed forms in repetitive situations.

Ten percent of the group have no arithmetic function to perform and an additional 47% use no arithmetic process higher than counting. Only 5% to 6% of the total group use any mathematical process higher than third or fourth grade level.[28]

Two questions arise. One is, will there be enough unskilled and semi-skilled jobs for retarded workers? The answer is probably affirmative. To begin with, there appears to be a shortage of retardates available for work, not a shortage of suitable jobs. Repeatedly, employers of the retarded remark that more such workers could be utilized if available.

In addition, modern industrial processes are remarkably flexible and resilient. There are usually a variety of ways of producing goods which utilize varying amounts of skilled and unskilled labor. The purpose of production is profit. Profits cannot be gained if production is forgone. We may expect, therefore, that employers will organize production in

[27] National Association for Retarded Children, *Final Report of National MDTA-OJT Project Promotional Contract with the United States Department of Labor, Bureau of Apprenticeship and Training, to Promote Job Opportunities for the Mentally Retarded*, no date.

[28] Jack C. Dinger, "Post-School Adjustment of Former Educable Retarded Pupils," *Exceptional Children* (March 1961): 357.

order to make the best use of the skills of the available work force, if they are made aware of its capabilities and limitations.

This brings us to the next question. If indeed there are large numbers of noninstitutionalized retardates needing jobs, and if low-skill jobs within their capabilities are available, what is preventing these retardates from being hired on these jobs? In view of the observations that NARC filled only one-third of the 1,500 jobs located specifically for the retarded, and that unemployment is concentrated among youth, minority groups, and the uneducated, one might question both of the premises of the question. These concentrations of unemployment are probably explained by poor work habits and discrimination rather than lack of jobs or inability to work.

Prolonged idleness among retardates is explained by the difficulty that many have in locating available jobs. The retarded may not know how to look for work, may be unable to fill out job application forms, and may encounter restrictive and unnecessary conditions of employment and employer discrimination. They may abandon the effort to locate work, especially after frustrating and sometimes humiliating efforts. They are usually unaware of, or suspicious of, services available from state vocational rehabilitation agencies or employment services.

Although state vocational rehabilitation agencies and employment services have begun to place a stronger emphasis on finding jobs for mental retardates, these programs have the overwhelming defect that rehabilitation and employment service counselors passively wait until retardates find their way to their offices before initiating any positive action to assist the retarded. Most adult retardates are unaware of these services and apparently do not come in contact with agencies or groups that could guide them toward help. In consequence, most retardates referred for vocational rehabilitation are referred directly from the public school system, the one organization that has established strong links with vocational rehabilitation agencies. The great majority of retardates who are rehabilitated are under age 20. Tens of thousands of adult retardates apparently languish in the community, unaware of existing services. It is not surprising that vocational rehabilitation agencies were unable to refer enough retardates to fill the jobs located for them in the NARC project.

Another reason for idleness among adult retardates is that years of neglect have left them untrained and unprepared to accept the responsibilities of regular employment. Extensive work adjustment training is required.

Finally, the fact must be faced that many retardates are unable to *fully* qualify for normal employment. Employment must be under sheltered conditions. The critical question is not whether sheltered work is needed, but where it should be provided—in sheltered workshops or in regular employment channels.

Normally employers have specific jobs for which they hire workers. In consequence, rehabilitation agencies usually prepare the disabled to meet specific job requirements—i.e., they try to enable the disabled to do the same work as the nondisabled. This approach is successful for most of the handicapped, including most retardates. But inevitably a reservoir of the more severely handicapped remain who cannot be trained for existing jobs. In these cases jobs must be engineered to fall within the capabilities of the specific workers—(i.e., the work must be sheltered).

Locating sheltered work in regular employment channels has enormous advantages over locating it in sheltered workshops. Since it is part of the regular production process, the work will be continuous and will not vary greatly in content. Moreover, the diversity of jobs is enormous, and even the more severely retarded can usually be placed in productive roles.

Sheltered workshops, even the bigger and better ones, are almost certain to have fluctuations in work. They will be continuously retooling for the different types of work generated by successive contracts and at a point in time will have a limited number of types of jobs available. Clients will occasionally be idle, will frequently have to be retrained for new tasks, and at the same time, may be ill-fitted for the types of work currently available. Productivity will almost always be less than could be attained by placing the same workers in regular employment channels.

There are several obstacles to creating sheltered work in regular employment channels. One is that most managers will have to adopt new attitudes toward the employment of the severely disabled. In addition, some severely disabled workers will have to be paid less than the established wage for a particular job because of below average productivity; occasionally, the wage will be below the federal minimum wage standards. This may create difficulties with unions and coworkers. Further, some employers are reluctant to hire high-risk workers for the understandable reason that they wish to avoid the unpleasant prospect of having to fire them if they prove unsatisfactory.

Finally, it requires time and resources to re-engineer jobs, provide extra supervision, bring materials to the work bench, etc. Similarly, although the federal Fair Labor Standards Act permits employers to pay less than the minimum wage if they establish that the workers are sufficiently handicapped, this also requires considerable time and expense. Many employers are understandably reluctant to incur these additional expenses for the sake of marginal employees.

Policy implications. The policy implications of the preceding remarks are summarized as follows:

1) Most of the additional 400,000 jobs needed for retardates should be sought in regular employment channels.

2) Sheltered workshops have a crucial rehabilitation role and are the employer of last resort for disabled persons with unacceptable behavior problems and the very seriously disabled.

3) Whenever possible, workshops should be encouraged to take steps to improve their productive efficiency by consolidating into larger multidisability workshops and by adopting a business-like approach to production. Areas with a number of workshops should centralize contract procurements so that larger subcontracts can be accepted (and subdivided) and in order to take advantage of the enormous economies of scale for this activity.

4) The two agencies most concerned with the employment of the retarded are the state employment services and vocational rehabilitation agencies. In order to effectively serve the more severely disabled, the traditional approaches of these agencies must be modified: (a) A means of locating retarded persons in the community in need of vocational services must be developed—probably by extensive publicity oriented toward professional groups likely to come in contact with the retarded; (b) Instead of placing clients in jobs and closing the case after a short follow-up, a means of long-term, and in some instances life-long, monitoring of the vocational (and social) adjustment of the severely disabled must be developed—presumably involving interagency cooperation and employer and family involvement, as well as planned periodic contacts.

5) Employers should be encouraged to assess the possibility of hiring the severely disabled for existing jobs, and also the possibilities of modifying these jobs if necessary, to bring them within the capabilities of the severely disabled. Possible salvage operations should also be explored. Expert assistance should be available to employers for this task from either the employment service or vocational rehabilitation agencies. In fact, a professional group of workers whose sole concern is with the development of sheltered work should be developed to work with rehabilitation counselors. Listings of the types of disabled persons for whom jobs are needed should be compiled. Such lists should also contain examples of the types of jobs these persons have been placed in, as a guide to employers and rehabilitation counselors.

6) At least part of the additional burden of employing the disabled should be removed from employers. The unpleasant task of discharging

handicapped workers may be performed by rehabilitation counselors. The rehabilitation counselor and not the employer could assume the responsibility for justifying wages below the statutory minimum.

Comments on unemployment and technical progress. The advisability of preparing additional persons for gainful employment when 4%, 5%, or even 6% of the labor force is unemployed has often been questioned. If jobs for unemployed retardates were found, would this cause the unemployment of others?

This question cannot be answered without a more detailed explanation of the causes of unemployment. One such cause is a deficiency of aggregate demand. This occurs when total spending for goods and services (aggregate demand)[29] is less than the value of what the economy produces (aggregate supply). Inventories accumulate and businessmen restrict production and thereby reduce employment.

Fortunately, the federal government has the power to increase the level of aggregate demand to any desired level through such means as increasing government spending, reducing taxes, and increasing the supply of loanable funds. Short-run problems may arise, since it takes time for these policies to be effective, and the effectiveness of different policies has not been accurately ascertained, but we can expect that a deficiency of aggregate demand will not be a major cause of unemployment over an extended period of time.

Public manpower policy should always be based on the assumption that aggregate demand will be maintained sufficiently high so that jobs will be available for qualified persons. To assume otherwise would mean the existence of an unnecessary and intolerable situation and would, in effect, penalize persons who could be prepared for gainful employment.

In a dynamic, changing economy there will always be some workers who are temporarily unemployed. There are many reasons for this. Some workers will have lost their previous jobs because of a change in production methods, or a shift in the composition of aggregate demand which reduced the demand for the goods or services they produced, or the failure of their employers to compete successfully with other firms producing similar goods. Other workers will be reentering the job market after a spell of illness. Still other workers will be in the process of changing jobs because of dissatisfaction with their previous jobs or a desire to live in a different area. A small amount of unemployment from these causes is unavoidable. Such "normal" unemployment will in no way impede the efforts to employ additional workers.

---

[29] Total spending is the sum of spending on consumption, investment, public services, and the excess of exports over imports.

A third type of unemployment, usually termed "structural" or "hard core" results when unemployed persons are unable or unwilling to work on available jobs, or lack knowledge of how to obtain jobs within their capabilities. The problem is not deficiency of jobs, but rather one of preparing people for existing jobs through training and other rehabilitative services. In sum, the existence of a pool of unemployed workers should not discourage efforts to employ all potentially employable persons.

Another frequently expressed concern is that technological changes and automation will eliminate many of the relatively unskilled jobs on which the retarded are employed, creating unsolvable structural unemployment. This fear also appears groundless, at least for the foreseeable future. Technological change has two effects. It leads to new and improved products and to more efficient methods of production. More efficient methods of production are achieved by making labor more specialized and substituting machinery for labor.

The effect of the specialization of labor and an increasing diversity in production goods has been to increase the number and types of jobs available to the mentally retarded. Specialization of labor, which in earlier years was typified by the adoption of assembly-line methods, breaks down a complicated production operation into specific and usually uncomplicated tasks. This enables workers to become highly proficient in a limited area and, in addition, enables employers to utilize relatively unskilled labor. This makes it possible for the mentally retarded to participate in such complicated productive tasks as the assembly of automobiles, as jobs may become so specialized as to consist of no more than tightening a few screws.

A wide diversity of products increases the number of assembly-line operations, widening the variety of specialized and uncomplicated jobs. Even the retarded with physical and psychological impairments find jobs. For example, retarded persons with limited mobility may do such tasks as stuffing envelopes or assembling small electrical appliances. Retarded persons with impaired use of the upper extremities may become messengers. When an economy becomes as specialized and as diverse as the American economy is, the vast majority of the retarded, including the physically and psychologically handicapped, can be placed on jobs in which their residual abilities can be utilized.

Automation, the replacement of men with machinery, has the opposite effect. In part, such substitution is made possible by the very specialization of labor which originally simplified jobs. As individual jobs are reduced to simpler movements, it becomes technologically feasible to substitute a machine to perform these movements, especially as the development of sophisticated electronic devices progresses. This creates a need for highly skilled workers capable of operating and maintaining mechanical equipment.

Automation is occurring at all levels. It is taking over jobs that are designated blue-collar and white-collar, unskilled, semiskilled, and skilled. But it is the least skilled jobs that are most amenable to automation. In agriculture, mechanical pickers are replacing hand pickers. Automatic dishwashers are used in most restaurants. Large-scale ditch digging and dirt removal is mechanically performed. Even domestic work usually requires an understanding of the operations of an increasingly complicated array of household appliances.

The net effect of technological change on the availability of jobs for the retarded cannot be ascertained. It is worth noting that even if the supply of unskilled jobs should decline, the demand for these jobs should also decline, due to a general improvement in the education and training of the work force. There is no evidence from follow-up studies to suggest that employment opportunities for the retarded have decreased as a result of technological progress. And so far as the future is concerned, Russell Nixon reviewed forecasts of future skill requirements for the work force and concluded that "regardless of these gaps and limits in our research and data, existing evidence is overwhelming that technological change is not changing worker requirements in such a way as significantly to reduce the opportunities for successful vocational rehabilitation of the mentally retarded. These changes in our technology may actually increase such job opportunities."[30]

This is not to suggest that technological change will not create problems for those directly affected. In particular, the retarded may have difficulty locating new jobs. This is one reason why adequate employment programs are necessary.

SHELTERED LIVING

Sheltered living may range from complete and total care in an institution to periodic visits by a social worker. In between these extremes are a number of possibilities, offering varying degrees of protection and supervision, including group homes or boarding houses. One fact is clear. The choices available at present are extremely limited. If a retardate cannot live independently, or with relatives, then usually he must be committed to full-time institutional care. The lack of alternatives to

---

[30] Russell A. Nixon, "The Impact of Automation and Technological Change on the Employability of the Mentally Retarded," *Rehabilitation and Health* (August 1969): 7.

full-time institutional care constitutes a glaring gap in the services provided to the retarded.

Size of institution. No aspect of the care offered to retardates has been so roundly deplored as the large size of most residential institutions. It is asserted that bureaucratic procedures become more important than residents and that the care is usually custodial rather than rehabilitative, especially for adults. Conditions in most institutions are described as dehumanizing. Proponents of large institutions (and there are few) reply that large facilities are less expensive to operate and make possible a wide diversity of skilled personnel and treatment programs.

In spite of the criticism that has been directed toward "largeness" in institutions it should be emphasized that the underlying issue is not size, per se, but the low quality of care that exists in most institutions. Size itself would not preclude a high quality of care if funding were adequate. However, there are other grounds on which large institutions can be criticized. A decision on the optimal size of residential facilities depends upon the answers to three questions: Do economies of scale exist in residential care? If so, are there compensating advantages to small facilities that would make up for the loss of economies of scale? And if there are compensating advantages, under what conditions will they be realized?

Data on public institutions in 1968 that were described in Chapter IV were utilized to investigate the importance of economies of scale. It was found that per patient cost declined rapidly as institution size increased ($r=-.69$). When restricted to institutions with 500 or more persons in average daily residence, the relationship was less pronounced ($r=-.31$).[31]

Multiple-regression analyses were employed to identify different factors that contribute to these correlations. The dependent variable was average per patient cost. Institution size was, of course, one of the independent variables. Two variables, the resident-to-staff ratio and the ratio of full-time professional staff to total staff were used as proxy variables for differences in quality of care among institutions. The percentages of the resident populations that were under 20 years of age, that had IQs below 35, and that had IQs between 35 and 50 were

[31] There were 107 institutions with 500 or more residents. There were 150 institutions of all sizes but 11 were dropped from the calculations because of inadequate data. Among these were the 8 smallest institutions. The smallest institution included in the calculations had 69 residents. In Chapter IV, the calculations were presented only for institutions with over 500 persons in average daily attendance.

variables used as indicators of differential treatment needs among resident populations.

Two other independent variables were average staff earnings in 1965 by state (which was used to adjust for wage differentials among states) and whether the facility was located in a Standard Metropolitan Statistical Area (SMSA). These regressions were calculated in log linear form. Two regressions were run. One for all institutions and one for those with 500 or more persons in average daily residence. The R^2's for the two equations were 0.85 and 0.88.

These regressions indicate that substantial economies of scale exist. Among facilities with 500 or more residents, a 100% rise in the resident population is associated with a decline in per capita costs of slightly less than 8%. Based on this regression equation, in 1968 a facility with 4,000 residents should incur average costs that are about $560 ($3,650 to $3,100) less than a facility with 500 residents, if salaries, staffing patterns, and the demographic characteristics of the residents were similar.[32]

When the regression was calculated for all institutions, the coefficient for facility size more than doubled. A 100% increase in the resident population was associated with an 18% decline in average cost per patient. Between a 4,000-bed facility and a 100-bed facility, a difference of about $2,500 per resident per year would be expected.[33]

These apparent economies of scale should be viewed skeptically. There may be important differences in the quality of care provided in large and small facilities which may not have been adequately accounted for in these regressions. Small facilities do not crowd 25 to 100 persons into a single large sleeping area. Light, heat, air conditioning, and plant maintenance costs will surely rise when residents are housed in rooms of 2 to 4 persons. Cost differences due to these factors should be least partly attributable to differences in quality of care, although our regressions would consider these differences as due to economies of scale.[34]

[32] When the regression was run using the absolute values of the variables the estimated cost difference between facilities of these two sizes was $760, again holding all other variables constant.

[33] When run in linear form, the estimated difference between these two facility sizes was $2,300.

[34] Michael Grossman observed that the average daily population was divided into total costs to estimate the dependent variable and was an independent variable as well. If this variable is subject to measurement error, its regression coefficient will be biased downward. Thus part of the coefficient indicating economies of scale could be spurious.

On the other hand, we may have underestimated economies of scale. We assumed that differences in the resident-to-staff ratio reflected differences in the quality of care. These differences could also, however, reflect a more efficient use of manpower by large institutions, which should be attributed to economies of scale. Since the resident-to-staff ratio declines markedly as institution size increases ($r=-.42$ in the regression run for facilities with over 500 residents), this is an important consideration.

We can conclude that there are some economies of scale in institutions, which may be somewhat greater or less than estimated through the multiple-regression equations. Based on visual inspection of a scatter diagram, it was also concluded that economies of scale decline rapidly after institution size reaches 500 residents and are of minor importance for institutions of over 1,000 residents. This is the conclusion one would expect in a labor-intensive industry.

Advantages of small facilities. Despite the loss of economies of scale, small facilities, if properly developed, may be less costly to operate and will produce more benefits than the present large residential institutions. Small facilities may cost less for several reasons: (1) Because small facilities can be located in communities, it should be possible for them to obtain many services at a cost lower than would be incurred if the services were provided in a large institution—a surprising possibility in view of the loss of economies of scale. A large residential facility is frequently a self-contained unit that provides its own schools, medical facilities, power, water, waste disposal, roads, etc. With the possible exception of schools, there are significant economies of scale in the provision of these services. Even the largest institutions, however, operate on a small scale compared to the populations given these services in communities. Facilities located in the community, therefore, will usually be able to purchase these services at a cost lower than that for which they could produce them. Since there is likely to be a flat rate for these services, an important source of economies of scale would be eliminated. In short, one reason for the existence of economies of scale is the inefficient way in which typical institutions maintain themselves.

In the regression equations it was predicted that facilities located in SMSAs would have slightly higher costs (about $300) than those not in SMSAs, which is contrary to what was expected, since these facilities are most likely to have access to city services. The probable explanation is that wage scales are higher for institutions located in SMSAs than for institutions located outside of SMSAs. Our adjustment for differences in salaries between facilities was based on statewide data and could not take account of these intrastate differences. Thus, our hypothesis that small facilities obtain many services at lower cost than large facilities may still be valid. Our data is insufficiently refined to test this hypothesis.

2) Since small facilities can be specialized, only those services needed by retardates in each facility need to be provided. In large institutions the retarded are compelled to accept the full range of custodial services. In addition, because of specialization, the cost of constructing or acquiring small facilities should be considerably less, on a per-resident basis, than for a larger brick and mortar building, because cheaper methods of construction can be used. The buildings will not need to be made to last forever. Hallways can be narrower. Fire regulations may be less stringent. In some cases, these costs can be brought down to the level of residential housing. The interest savings would be enormous. Conceivably, a reduction in capital cost could also be realized.[35]

The benefits of placing persons in small rather than large facilities are as follows:

1) Geographic dispersion of smaller facilities will enable institutionalized retardates to be nearer home, helping to maintain family contacts,[36] and will also make possible greater integration into the community (they can attend public schools, use local recreational facilities, etc). This may expedite the earlier release of retardates. In addition, access to community services may make possible a wider range of services from a greater variety of professional personnel than could be obtained in a large residential institution located in a remote area.

2) Small community-based facilities will enable many residents to locate employment through regular employment channels or sheltered workshops. We have already observed that many retardates are institutionalized because they need supervision in their day-to-day living, not because they can't work. It is manifestly impossible to find adequate employment opportunities for retardates when they are concentrated in large institutions, especially if located in remote areas or if public transportation is not convenient. Of course, many work within the institu-

---

[35] For example, if the cost of a resident bed was lowered from $15,000 to $5,000, then assuming an interest rate of 7% the interest saving would be $700. If depreciation was at a rate of 2% in the first case and 5% in the second there would be a further saving of $50.

[36] However, at least one investigator was unable to detect a meaningful relationship between the distance of a facility from an institutionalized retardate's home and the number of visits to the retardate by his family. M. Michael Klaber, "A Study of Institutions," *Conference on Residential Care, Proceedings of a Working Conference*, June 13–14, 1968, University of Hartford, West Hartford, Connecticut, p. 76.

tion, but the limited number of available jobs and the lack of any strong orientation toward productive activity means that their abilities will usually be misused. Only if they are able to avail themselves of the opportunities offered by regular employment channels can this problem be corrected.

The economic arguments in favor of small, community-based, sheltered living arrangements for the retarded are strong. Potentially, the social benefits are substantial, ranging to as high as $8,000 per person if we consider both productivity and savings in the cost of institutional care.

Criteria of optimal program. An optimal program of sheltered living for the retarded would have the following characteristics:[37]

1) Because of the tremendous diversity in the needs and capabilities of the retarded, there must be a wide range of types of sheltered living arrangements. At one extreme would be nursing homes and institutions. At the other extreme, the retarded may live in regular apartments with supportive services—e.g., financial management or periodic visits by a social worker or other "benefactor" to ensure that the retarded person has not encountered unforeseen difficulties. In between are group homes which may be little more than sleeping quarters, or which may provide a complete range of hotel services, including food preparation, or which may go even further and maintain strict supervision over the day-to-day activities of the retarded. Retardates may also be placed with sympathetic landlords in boarding houses or hotels.

2) All of the anticipated advantages of small institutions depend upon location as well as size. Scattering numerous small residential facilities in remote areas would achieve nothing but the loss of economies of scale.

Location has two aspects. One is dispersion. The other is that facilities be community-based. The community is necessary if the retarded are to have access to community life, services, and jobs. Dispersion is necessary in order to avoid overtaxing community resources.

A few professionals argue that all retardates should be placed in facilities in their home communities. Although this emphasizes the maintenance of family ties, not all communities would be able to provide the services or jobs needed by the retarded. Or perhaps more accurately, the cost of services would be excessive and available jobs unsatisfactory.

[37] See Gunnar Dybwad, "Action Implications, USA-Today," in *Changing Patterns in Residential Services for the Mentally Retarded*, Robert B. Kugel and Wolf Wolfensberger, eds. (Washington: USGPO, 1969), pp. 387–89, for a discussion of the first four of these requirements (although there are variations in orientation and terminology).

3) Community-based facilities must be integrated with other services, such as vocational rehabilitation, public assistance, etc.

4) Placement in a particular style of sheltered living should never be regarded as permanent, since changing needs on the part of the retarded will enable some to move into less sheltered situations and may require others to move into more sheltered situations.

Implicit in the third and fourth requirements are the concepts of comprehensive, coordinated, and continuous services.

5) Finally, community acceptance of the retarded is necessary.

Demand for limited sheltered living. There were about 140,000 retarded adults in various types of residential institutions in the United States in 1970. Of these, about 35,000 had IQs below 25, about 28,000 had IQs between 25 and 39, and an estimated 77,000 had IQs of 40 or more. Clearly, those with IQs below 25 and many of those with IQs between 25 and 39 require full-time, closely supervised residential care. It is doubtful if any substantial advantage could be derived from placing them in small community-based group homes. Some residents with IQs over 40 would also fall into this category, because of severe physical incapacities or behavioral problems. Nevertheless, it is probable that over half of the adult residents with IQs over 40, and at least one-fourth of those with IQs between 25 and 39 could be advantageously placed in less sheltered situations—about 45,000 persons.

There is a tremendous potential demand for community-based sheltered living accomodations among noninstitutionalized adult retardates. In a study of 48 ex-patients from Pacific State Hospital, Edgerton found that almost all had located "benefactors," i.e., normal people who helped them cope with everyday problems. The extent of assistance varied widely, ranging from the complete provision of food, shelter, and clothing, to occasional counseling and guidance. Thirteen benefactors were spouses or lovers, twelve were employers, ten were landladies or neighbors, four were social workers, and ten were relatives. Edgerton concluded that "the ex-patient succeeds in his efforts to sustain a life in the community only as well as he succeeds in locating and holding a benefactor."[38] A benefactor, in effect, provides the retardate with the necessary shelter in his day-to-day living. Unfortunately, locating a suitable benefactor is largely a matter of chance, with no assurance that the relationship will be adequate or enduring.

There is no way of ascertaining how many noninstitutionalized adult retardates will want or would benefit from a limited sheltered living situation other than that provided by relatives or friends. In 1970 there

---

[38] Robert B. Edgerton, *The Cloak of Competence* (Berkeley: University of California Press, 1967), pp. 202–3.

were about 180,000 adults with IQs between 25 and 50 and over 2.5 million with IQs between 50 and 70 living in the community. Many live independently. Others require full-time, closely supervised care, which is provided by parents in most cases. Of the remainder, some would choose to continue under the protection of friends or relatives.

As an indication of potential demand, assume that 25% of those with IQs between 25 and 40, 50% of the 40 to 49 IQ group, and 5% of the 50 to 69 IQ group, or about 195,000 persons not now in institutions, would seek this type of accommodation if available. And this estimate may well be low. Parents and other relatives would often welcome the opportunity for the retardate to reside in a protected situation which offered as normal a life as he was capable of, and where family relationships could be maintained. Placement in such a home need not imbue the parent with a sense of guilt and loss. The retarded person would have a new-found independence.

Such sheltered living arrangements need not be costly to the government, since most residents could defray part or all of the cost of their maintenance out of their earnings. We have estimated that about 240,000 retarded adults, in or out of institutions, would benefit from being placed in a sheltered living arrangement less restrictive than full-time residential care. The number of retarded children who could benefit from such living arrangements may equal or exceed the estimate for the number of retarded adults.

POVERTY AMONG THE RETARDED

Institutionalized retardates. In these days of concern about the poor in America, it is strange that little attention has been directed toward the conditions existing in residential facilities for the mentally retarded and mentally ill, despite the vigorous efforts of professionals in these fields. Together such facilities house over 500,000 persons. Living conditions range from pleasant to deplorable. The latter adjective is usually the more appropriate. The cruelty of life in some institutions can be described, but must be seen to be fully understood.

One ward, in a large state institution that I visited, was occupied by young girls. Most were in their late teens, mildly retarded, without visible physical handicaps, and quite attractive. Half of the ward was used for sleeping quarters. Two passages for walking were the only free space. The beds, so close together as to touch, lined the walls and formed three rows down the center of the room. To get to a bed in the middle row, a resident had to climb over a bed in an outside row. The ward housed about 100 residents, 50 to 75 fewer than had been in the ward several years previously. The ward was immaculate. Every bed was made, the tile floor polished, the footlockers closed. No pictures, no toys, no books, no slippers disrupted the unbroken display of uniformity. The only flaw was an odor of urine. A visitor might be impressed, but a resident might find life infinitely drab.

The other half of the ward was used as a day room. The residents spent many hours here—only a small part of the day was devoted to outside activities. In one corner was a television set. The walls were lined with chairs. There were a few tables on which were games. The day room, like the sleeping quarters, was immaculate. For the most part, the children sat passively in the chairs lining the walls. One was impressed by a regimen that imposed such cleanliness and quiet among 100 healthy, adolescent girls.

As we walked around the ward, some of the children crowded around us asking for "daddy," or "mommy." Many wanted to shake hands or be picked up. Some just tried to touch us. Almost all sought a kind or comforting word. Two attendants cared for these 100 children.

As we left the building, a group of adult retarded males marched by on their way to outdoor activities. Their apparel was shocking. On their feet they wore tennis shoes, sandals, work shoes, dress shoes, and some that were not identifiable. Every possible defect that shoes could have was observed—holes in the sides and soles, broken down backs, shoe-laces untied (if, indeed, there were shoelaces), worn down or missing heels, etc. Few wore socks. The diversity in their clothing was in marked contrast to the uniformity of the physical components of the ward we had just left. T-shirts, with and without air ports, shorts, overalls, although sometimes held up by only one strap, were typical. In general, it was a disreputable looking group, although all were sufficiently well-behaved to march in quiet order.

Visits to other wards replicated the same clean, disciplined, monotonous, dreary scenes. The most vivid recollection is of a ward for adult severely retarded males. Their clothes and shoes, with a few exceptions, were as rag-tag as those previously described. The exceptions were persons sans shoes, sans shirt, sans trousers, sans everything. The tile floor shone. In the middle was a drain. Periodically the floor was hosed down to cleanse it of human urine and defecation.[39]

This is not the worst or the best institution in the United States. It is directed by extremely capable, dedicated individuals who have managed to greatly improve conditions over the last few years. There is, however,

[39] For a more elaborate description of conditions in another state institution, see Craig MacAndrew and Robert Edgerton, "The Everyday Life of Institutionalized Idiots," *Human Organization* (Winter 1964): 312–18. Also, Geraldo Rivera, *Willowbrook, A Report on How It Is and Why It Doesn't Have To Be That Way* (New York: Vintage Books, 1972).

only so much that can be accomplished with a limited budget and antiquated buildings.

For the most part, living standards in residential institutions are intolerable. The problem will be partly solved when community living arrangements for the retarded are developed. But for the immediate future the major solution must be an increased social concern for the quality of life of the institutionalized mentally retarded and mentally ill. Overcrowded conditions must be eliminated. Ward-type accommodations should be phased out. Residents should be given opportunities to express their individuality. Their lives must consist of more than aimless wandering around in a day room.

Noninstitutionalized retardates. Earlier we estimated that there were almost 550,000 noninstitutionalized adult retardates who are economically idle (not working and, in the case of women, not married). In addition, the earnings of many employed retardates are insufficient to maintain an adequate standard of living. The day-to-day survival of most of these persons depends upon the willingness of others to provide support. Most of them are supported either by parents or other close relatives or by income-maintenance payments (public assistance or "childhood" disability benefits from one of the trust funds). Earlier we estimated that about 360,000 adult retardates received publicly funded income maintenance payments in 1970, a few of whom are in institutions. Apparently about half of retardates who are economically idle or whose productivity is very low are totally dependent upon relatives.

Publicly provided income maintenance payments support life, but at current levels (about $1,000 per person in 1970) would not suffice to prevent poverty. The only protection these retardates have against poverty is the willingness and ability of their parents or other relatives to provide supplemental support. The number actually living in poverty cannot be determined.

One solution to this problem is to provide the services that will enable many of these retardates to be employed in jobs that will provide an adequate income. There will always remain, however, some retardates who are unable to work or whose earnings are inadequate to support a minimally acceptable standard of living. Poverty can only be averted by the intercession of parents or public income maintenance. This raises three problems:

1) What is the minimally acceptable standard of living that society will guarantee to the economically dependent? Present levels of income maintenance payments are clearly too low. But should they be increased by 50%, 100%, or more?

2) How can a minimum standard of living be guaranteed without impairing work incentives? This becomes an especially difficult problem

in the case of persons whose potential earnings are below the income-maintenance payments they would receive if not working. If their income-maintenance payments are reduced by the same amount as their earnings, there is little or no incentive to locate work or to increase their earnings if working. Even when earnings exceed income-maintenance payments, low-productivity workers may not always feel that the difference justifies a full-time work effort.

One solution to the problem is to deny income-maintenance payments to individuals who, in the judgement of the vocational counselor or social worker assigned to the case, could work but refuse to do so. Before adversely judging such a system, consider the alternatives. One is to accept abuses of the system. This will either increase costs or reduce the average level of income support. The other alternative is to keep income maintenance payments low, so that individuals would lack a financial incentive to avoid work. Either alternative punishes those truly in need of public support.

Another solution that should probably be combined with the power to deny income maintenance payments is to permit low-productivity workers to retain some part of their earnings. For every $2.00 of earnings, for example, income-maintenance payments may be reduced by only $1.00.

Current income-maintenance programs provide too little incentive for marginal workers. In some states, any income earned by recipients of APTD must be reported and the amount deducted from the monthly allotment. In other states, only a small amount of earnings is permitted. Recipients of Social Security benefits or Aid to the Blind, are permitted a somewhat higher level of earnings before a reduction in benefits takes place; in both cases, however, the amounts involved are less than $100 per month.

3) At present, nonworking adult retardates who live with their parents are not normally eligible for either public assistance or Social Security payments.[40] The equity of this arrangement will be discussed below. It suffices to point out that a solution to the problem of poverty among the retarded also requires a judgment as to whether this situation should continue.

FINANCING AND PROVIDING SERVICES

The private sector. "Consumer sovereignty," "competition," and the necessity for producing firms to avoid losses are forces which auto-

---

[40]Payments will be made for these individuals if the head of household is retired, disabled, or deceased.

matically guide most resources used in the private sector to their most productive uses.

"Consumer sovereignty" is the right of any individual to consume, within the limits of his income, whatever goods and services he chooses. This dictates to the private sector what they must produce. Recalcitrance by private producers cannot last because it leads to business failure. We assume that most consumers are rational, i.e., that they select those goods and services which make the greatest contribution to their welfare.

Competition will cause firms to seek advantages over their competitors by setting slightly lower prices. Unless there is collusion, prices will fall to the average cost of the most efficient producers. Firms that cannot match this price will be forced to terminate their operations.

The system is technologically dynamic. In the competitive struggle, firms seek ways of further reducing costs, or ways of improving and differentiating their products (or of giving the illusion of so doing). Firms that cannot maintain the pace are eliminated.

In sum, due to the pressures of consumer sovereignty, competition, and the necessity of profits, the private sector of the economy has automatic mechanisms that favor the survival of those firms and the activities of those individuals that produce the most desired goods and services at the lowest possible price and that promote continued technological improvement.

These three forces also stimulate and guide new investments. It is the expectation of future profits that encourages businessmen to invest in plant equipment, research, and people. Many firms train employees, usually by on-the-job training, especially if the skills acquired are of primary benefit to the firm providing the training.[41] Similarly, the high earnings of persons in professions where there is a shortage of personnel induces people to obtain this training in colleges, vocational schools, apprenticeship programs, etc.

Obviously, this description of the "moving" forces in the private sector is highly schematic. People respond to many motivations other than a simple desire to maximize economic welfare. And, certainly, these "moving" forces do not operate as perfectly or as rapidly as economic theory sometimes suggests. In particular, the assumption of vigorous competition would be challenged in many cases.

Nevertheless, the entire rationale for maintaining a large autonomous private sector is that these three forces will combine to make this sector

[41] Gary Becker, "Investment in Human Capital—A Theoretical Analysis," *Journal of Political Economy*, supplement (October 1962): 13.

more responsive to consumer preference and more dynamic than any alternative economic system. In cases where it does not work well, we must either strengthen the operation of these moving forces or consider government intervention.

Reasons for public intervention. Fortunately, the bulk of evidence indicates that the capitalistic system works very well in technologically advanced and affluent societies and apparently is superior to any alternative mode of production. Nevertheless, there are times when the government must influence the allocation of resources if we are to achieve the goals of society.

1) Some persons, because of age, mental or physical defects, or other impediments to employment are unable to command an income that provides them with a minimally acceptable standard of living. In addition, families may lack funds to purchase needed medical care and education for their handicapped members.

2) Investments in the education and health of people often have external benefits. A prospective student would not take account of his increased tax payments in determining whether or not to initiate training—only net pay. Public sharing of the costs of training is necessary if marginal social benefits are to be equated to marginal social costs.

3) A third reason why public intervention is needed is that the private sector does not always respond in the most appropriate manner to the economic forces which are supposed to guide it, especially when it comes to investing in people. Most people do not have the resources for extended training and rehabilitation. Most lending institutions are unwilling to make loans to develop such an intangible asset as human capital, and most people are unwilling to incur large debts for the uncertain prospect of increased future earnings. In addition, some people lack knowledge; others are discouraged. Still others require services, such as sheltered living, which the private sector has not made available.

4) The private sector normally responds only to monetary benefits, while the public sector considers all of the tangible and intangible benefits that contribute to general welfare. The mentally retarded are among those most likely to need public intervention if their minimal consumption and medical needs are to be met and if their limited productive skills are to be properly utilized.

Issues in public intervention. Public intervention to ensure that needed services are provided to the retarded brings up a number of interrelated issues as to how services should be financed and produced. Public intervention can take three forms. Services can be publicly produced and tax-supported, privately produced and tax-supported, or publicly produced and privately supported. The last alternative raises the question of the appropriate division of financial responsibility between the government and the families of the retarded—a topic that will be discussed below.

Publicly produced services (e.g., public institutions, public special education classes) do not face competition. Nor are they faced with the necessity of avoiding losses, since the benefits they produce are enjoyed by others. In consequence, there are no automatic mechanisms that impel the public sector to an optimal use of resources. Lacking profit motivation, managers of public programs often take refuge in bureaucratic procedures which stress avoidance of mistakes rather than innovation. The correct procedure, rather than the greatest output, becomes of paramount importance. Methods of operations rarely change, and when change does come, it is usually a product of the demands and entreaties of organized pressure groups.

This does not mean that an optimal use of resources in the public sector is impossible, but it will not be an easily achieved goal. Benefit-cost calculations, which must substitute for the discipline of competition, have many empirical and conceptual limitations that have been noted previously.

Public intervention can be equally well achieved by government purchase of services from private producers. For example, residential services may be purchased from private facilities by states when their public facilities are overcrowded or nonexistent. From a cost standpoint, there is no disadvantage to so doing. To provide comparable care, private and public facilities must utilize equivalent manpower, building, equipment, and supplies. Public facilities may appear somewhat less costly, since they are exempted from excise taxes on equipment and supplies and often fail to properly cost out the use of buildings, but this is an artificial difference.

This reasoning is plausible in the case of nonprofit facilities but what of profit-making private facilities? It is strange that profit, which has impelled a part of the world's population to spectacular heights, should be viewed with such disdain when made by providing services to people. In any event, economists reason that if excessive profits are being made, new firms will enter the industry, competition will force prices down, and that this process will continue until profits are sufficiently low so as to just pay a fair return for the use of land and capital and a fair wage to management. These are costs that public and private nonprofit facilities must also incur. In sum, the costs of providing services should be roughly equivalent in public or private facilities over time, regardless of whether the private facilities are profit-making or nonprofit.

Are there advantages to having services provided by profit-seeking facilities? Strangely enough, yes. Private facilities, lured by the hope of profit, will seek new and better ways to provide services, hoping to gain business by providing a better service or the same service at lower cost.[42] The system is dynamic and expansive.

In recent years, a number of professionals in the field of mental retardation, cognizant of the inadequacies of present programs serving the retarded and despairing at the unwillingness of state governments to improve services, have proposed that such services be publicly funded, but that parents and other persons involved in the decision to obtain services be able to purchase them from public or private providers. The primary concern would be to obtain the best care possible with the available money. Undoubtedly, a number of private facilities would spring up offering a wide diversity of types of care.

This approach to obtaining and financing services is not a concept unique to mental retardation. It has been proposed for the field of education generally. Most publicly financed medical services are provided under this principle (e.g., Medicare, Medicaid).

The argument for this approach is stronger for services to the retarded than for education generally. Education services are usually well developed, and, for the most part, fairly standard over much of a child's elementary and junior high school years. Inferior school systems need to be improved, but this may not be best achieved by permitting students to flee the system.

In contrast, many of the services needed for the mentally retarded are virtually nonexistent. Moreover, many diverse types of care are needed by the retarded, especially the severely retarded. A program must often be developed on an individual basis rather than on a group basis, and the individual will need to be able to utilize a number of various services. Permitting the purchase of these services from any available source is obviously more satisfactory than restricting the retarded to those services available from a few public programs.

Financing services. Services to the retarded may be financed publicly or privately through voluntary contributions or patient fees.

It can be categorically stated that essential services to the retarded should not be dependent upon voluntary efforts. Experience has demonstrated that contributions of money are usually inadequate, and a volunteer staff is often deficient in essential skills.

Nevertheless, there is much to be said in favor of encouraging voluntary services, especially of time. Volunteers are usually quite young or

---

[42] Presumably, guidelines and standards would be enforced to assure that a facility does not seek a competitive advantage by reducing the quality of services.

in the 50-and-over age group. They frequently work on a one-to-one basis with the retarded and bring an important personal relationship to their lives. On occasion, these efforts achieve remarkable results.

Donations of time are relatively costless to society. Volunteers usually work part-time, during hours when they would not otherwise be engaged in gainful work. Donations of money, in contrast, usually require that resources be bid away from other gainful activities.

Logically, one would be less enthusiastic about voluntary contributions of money if such contributions merely represented an alternative to public funding of services and imposed a burden on a small segment of society that should be borne by society as a whole. Realistically, however, donations make possible the provision of many services that would not be publicly funded. A great deal of research is privately funded, as are the public information activities of many private organizations that work on behalf of the retarded. New and innovative ways of providing services are often stimulated by private funds.

In general, parents are responsible for the physical necessities of life and medical care for their children, while the cost of education is publicly borne, provided parents are willing to send their children to public schools. Such a division of financial responsibility is also satisfactory for retarded children in most cases.

In some cases, however, caring for the retarded, especially the more severely retarded with physical or psychiatric handicaps, will impose horrifying financial and personal burdens. Extra bedroom space may be needed. Costs of medical care and physical therapy may be unusually high. Local public schools may not have classrooms appropriate to the needs of the retarded. Parents must then seek educational services from private facilities, usually bearing the full cost burden. And the daily, unending, monotonous routine of continued surveillance, feeding, bathing, and sometimes medication, coupled with chronic sorrow, will eventually grind down the most devoted mother.

Although it can be argued that parents have a moral obligation to provide all needed services to their children, the facts are that inability to do so causes many retarded children to be denied services, and when services are provided, it is often at enormous sacrifice to the family. In the interests of the needs of retarded children and their families, it is more appealing to argue that *unusual* financial burdens caused by a handicapped child should be spread out among the population. This can be justified on the grounds that no potential parent is exempt from the possibility of having such a child. Payment should be made to the families of handicapped children from public funds to enable them to obtain educational services, if locally unavailable or inappropriate, to compensate them for unusual medical and therapy expenses, and to provide needed respite.

Families who place a retarded child in an institution should not, on the other hand, be excused from what would normally be expended on a child's support. This would not cover the full costs of institutional care. Educational, unusual medical, and other non-normal costs should be publicly financed, as was suggested for the retarded child who is kept at home.

It is, however, extremely difficult to determine the marginal cost of a child to a family. The amount varies by family size, income, and personal taste. An estimate of the average marginal cost is of little value, since some families would be unable to pay such a sum and others could only do so with substantial hardship.

One solution would be to require families with institutionalized children to pay a percentage of the average annual operating costs of institutions, with the stipulation that no family would be required to pay more than a given percentage of their net taxable income under the federal income tax (gross income less deductions) for the year.[43]

What of retarded adults? Normally, parents expect to be relieved of the expense of caring for their children as they approach adulthood. If retarded and dependent, however, the burden may last as long as the children live at home with their parents. A more equitable solution would be to make noninstitutionalized retarded adults living with parents eligible for income maintenance, presumably through the "childhood disability" provisions of one of the trust funds, supplemented, if necessary, by public assistance (if, for example, a person is not eligible for "childhood disability" because his parents were not covered by one of the trust funds).

Obviously, parents should not be responsible for either the unusual or the normal expenses of institutionalized offspring beyond adulthood—certainly not past the age of 21. Most states already have such a provision in their laws governing commitment.[44]

[43] Suppose the percentage of operating costs that a family was required to pay was 25%. If operating costs averaged $4,000 per year, a family's liability would be fixed at $1,000. If the maximum payment were limited to 5% of taxable income, only families with taxable income of $20,000 or more per year would actually pay this amount. Average operating costs could be based on individual facility costs or an average for a state, for purposes of charging fees. The first approach might reflect differences in the quality of care, but the second approach is probably the more applicable if we are interested in reimbursement only for normal costs of child care.

[44] Norman F. Smith, *Charges for Residential Care of the Mentally Retarded in State Institutions in the United States, A Comparison of Present Charge Systems with the Policy Set Forth by NARC* (New York: National Association for Retarded

In sum, reasonable judgments would indicate that parents of retarded children should be responsible for the normal cost of their maintenance as children whether institutionalized or not, while extraordinary costs should be assumed publicly. The full costs of the care of dependent retarded adults should be publicly assumed.

One may recognize in these judgments an extension of the normalization principle. The retarded, *and their families*, should be enabled to lead lives as near normal as possible.

FINAL REMARKS

Many topics have been covered in this study, most prefaced with a lament about the inadequacy of the data. Scholarly researchers may be tempted to dismiss part of the analysis as too intuitive to be of scientific value. Humanists won't care. Both have a point.

Mental retardation is a problem of large dimension and horrifying consequences. Efforts to mitigate these consequences cannot await the results of rigorous research. Wrong decisions may involve waste. But doing nothing will cause even greater waste.

A full-scale program to deal with mental retardation is, however, an expensive undertaking that must be compared with other worthwhile uses of resources. Thus, we are confronted with a problem that involves a large use of resources and one that cannot await a scientific determination of the optimal use of these resources. However poor the data may be, we must make the best use of it. The mentally retarded are human beings, with as much capacity for love, hate, hope, fear, contentment, frustration, and anger as any of us. Most of the retarded can live reasonably useful and happy lives if provision is made for their special needs.

If services for the retarded are not improved, future generations will consider our neglect cruel, incomprehensible, and outrageous. Descriptions of public institutions will fill them with the same horror we feel at the barbarities of the Spanish inquisition and Aztec human sacrifice.

Implementation of a comprehensive program of services for the retarded may appear expensive. The increase could be of the order of $3 to $4 billion more than is currently being spent. A more exact increased cost figure is not possible until the effectiveness of the programs can be evaluated. In the long run, such a program is less expensive than initially appears. Many expenditures are one-time costs required to resolve

---

Children, 1966), p. 8. A few states define financial liability in terms of a set number of years which creates obvious inequities in the case of persons institutionalized as adults.

a backlog of cases. This is especially true in rehabilitation of adult retardates and the development of sheltered living arrangements. Many of these expenditures will be income generating. If 400,000 retardates were currently successfully placed at minimum wage levels, output would increase by almost $1.6 billion per year, which is more than their rehabilitation is likely to cost.

Some expenditures will reduce other costs. Childhood development efforts will reduce adult dependency. Group homes are less expensive than state residential facilities.

Part of the increase in cost will be lifted from the families of the retarded and redistributed among society in general, with no increase in social cost. Income maintenance payments and payments for extraordinary cost of care fall into this category. Part of the increase in cost will be used to improve the quality of life of the dependent retarded, and are therefore transfer payments rather than social costs.

Comprehensive prevention programs, which will reduce the incidence of severe retardation, will have striking effects and eventually reduce the need for other types of services.

In most cases mental retardation programs will increase GNP by more than they cost. As for the remainder, a society with a trillion dollar GNP can afford to be concerned about the quality of life of all of its citizens.

In this chapter, we have covered only a few of the many needs of the retarded. In particular, there are critical problems in transportation, recreation, and education for the severely retarded and the multiply-handicapped retarded that have not been covered.

SUMMARY

1. An optimal program for the retarded would be undergoing continuous reassessment and change. It would be humanitarian in philosophy, efficient in the use of resources, comprehensive, coordinated, and accessible.

2. An estimated 690,000 adult retardates are economically idle, of whom about 400,000 could be gainfully employed if appropriate services were made available. Many of these retardates have physical or emotional handicaps and are in the middle range of intellectual deficiency.

3. Most sheltered workshops pay inordinately low wages to employees. In large part this is due to inefficient operation, because of the small size, single-disability status, and lack of a business-like approach in most workshops.

4. Although workshop efficiency could be improved, workshops could not match the efficiency and job diversity available through regular employment channels. Most jobs for idle retardates should therefore be sought from normal places of business. In some cases, sheltered employment situations could be developed for the severely disabled in regular employment channels.

5. Small community-based facilities offering various degrees of sheltered living to retardates would be less costly than large institutions in many cases. Possibly 240,000 adult retardates would benefit from sheltered living accommodations of this nature.

6. Living conditions in most public institutions are intolerable.

7. A strong case can be made for financing the "excess" costs of services to the retarded out of public funds. This includes most childhood developmental expenditures and maintenance costs among adults.

Index

Library of Congress Cataloging in Publication Data

Conley, Ronald W
 The economics of mental retardation.

 Includes bibliographical references.
  1. Mentally handicapped. I. Title.
[DNLM: 1. Costs and cost analysis. 2. Mental
retardation. WM 300 C752e 1972]
HV3004.C65 1973 362.3 72-12345
ISBN 0-8018-1410-3